METHODS IN MOLECULAR BIOLOGY

Series Editor
John M. Walker
School of Life and Medical Sciences
University of Hertfordshire
Hatfield, Hertfordshire, AL10 9AB, UK

For further volumes:
http://www.springer.com/series/7651

Handbook of ELISPOT

Methods and Protocols

Third Edition

Edited by

Alexander E. Kalyuzhny

Bio-Techne, Inc., Minneapolis, MN, USA

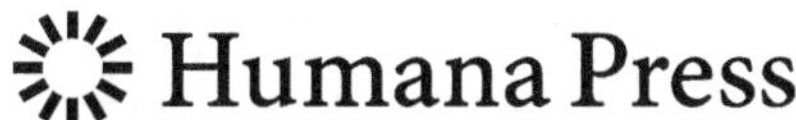

Humana Press

Editor
Alexander E. Kalyuzhny
Bio-Techne, Inc.
Minneapolis, MN, USA

ISSN 1064-3745   ISSN 1940-6029   (electronic)
Methods in Molecular Biology
ISBN 978-1-4939-8566-1   ISBN 978-1-4939-8567-8   (eBook)
https://doi.org/10.1007/978-1-4939-8567-8

Library of Congress Control Number: 2018946639

Preface

Despite technological advancements and the availability of ultrasensitive analytical methods, ELISpot assay, which is technically quite simple, is firmly holding its ground for studying the cytokine-secreting activity of immune system cells. Furthermore, this assay is gaining a reputation as a robust and reliable research and diagnostic tool. To refresh readers' memories, it is worth mentioning that the first edition of the *Handbook of ELISpot* was released in 2005. Due to a strong interest from the scientific community, it was followed by a second edition published in 2012. We were excited to learn that our second edition also received strong positive feedback, which prompted us to continue with a third edition. It appears that ELISpot remains to be a very dynamic technique that can be easily modified to meet challenging experimental needs. However, the simplicity of ELISpot may be deceptive as it requires a clear understanding of its bioassay and immunoassay components and how they blend together. In addition to learning basic ELISpot technique, researchers should understand the principles of analyzing ELISpot images and spot quantification, how to digest the biological information from the images with arrays of spots, and how to perform statistical analysis.

The third edition of the *Handbook of ELISpot* expands upon our first and second editions, and we are adhering to the same principles as before: the book should help researchers learn new protocols and become proficient in using this technique. Due to a strong interest in multiplex ELISpot, our current volume includes numerous chapters on ELISpot's sibling, known as FluoroSpot, disclosing vast details on how to set, run, and analyze multiplex data. To address the challenges in studying and diagnosing infectious diseases, we included chapters on using ELISpot for tuberculosis, influenza, Dengue virus, and feline immunodeficiency virus analysis. Other chapters are focused on ELISpot for vaccine research, essential controls, image analysis of spots, assay evaluation, ELISpot automation, and challenges in analyzing antibody-secreting cells and designing the assay. As with the first and second editions, the goal of compiling this volume was to make an additional technical reference and a troubleshooting guide both for researchers who are new to the field and for experienced ELISpot users. All the chapters were written by experts who were excited to have an opportunity to share their experience and skills with colleagues worldwide.

I wish to express my sincere thanks to our contributing authors for committing their time and effort to work on their chapters and submitting them in a timely manner. As the book's editor, I was privileged to connect with many exceptional and passionate scholars from whom I learned a lot about advances in ELISpot technology.

We hope this book will serve as a stepping stone for novices as well as food for thought for ELISpot experts.

Minneapolis, MN, USA   *Alexander E. Kalyuzhny*

Contents

Contributors

NIKLAS AHLBORG • *Mabtech, Nacka Strand, Sweden; Department of Immunology, Stockholm University, Stockholm, Sweden*

PAULINA ANDRADE • *Division of Infectious Diseases and Vaccinology, School of Public Health, University of California, Berkeley, CA, USA; University of San Francisco de Quito, Quito, Ecuador*

ALEK M. ARANYOS • *Department of Infectious Diseases and Immunology, College of Veterinary Medicine, University of Florida, Gainesville, FL, USA*

RICHARD CASPELL • *Cellular Technology Ltd., Shaker Heights, OH, USA*

YI-YING CHEN • *Graduate Institute of Pharmacology, College of Medicine, National Taiwan University, Taipei, Taiwan*

JOSEFINA COLOMA • *Division of Infectious Diseases and Vaccinology, School of Public Health, University of California, Berkeley, Berkeley, CA, USA*

A. GERMANN • *Fraunhofer Institute for Biomedical Engineering, Sulzbach, Germany*

JODI HAGEN • *Bio-Techne, Minneapolis, MN, USA*

JODI HANSON • *Cellular Technology Ltd., Shaker Heights, OH, USA*

IANA H. HARALAMBIEVA • *Mayo Clinic Vaccine Research Group, Mayo Clinic, Rochester, MN, USA*

EVA HARRIS • *Division of Infectious Diseases and Vaccinology, School of Public Health, University of California, Berkeley, CA, USA*

HAW HWAI • *Department of Medicine, College of Medicine, National Taiwan University, Taipei, Taiwan*

PETER JAHNMATZ • *Department of Medicine, Karolinska Institutet, Stockholm, Sweden; Mabtech, Nacka Strand, Sweden*

SYLVIA JANETZKI • *ZellNet Consulting, Inc., Fort Lee, NJ, USA*

CHANDIMA JEEWANDARA • *Centre for Dengue Research, Faculty of Medical Sciences, University of Sri Jayewardenapura, Nugegoda, Sri Lanka*

ALISON J. JOHNSON • *Department of Microbiology and Immunology, Albert Einstein College of Medicine, Bronx, NY, USA*

ALEXANDER E. KALYUZHNY • *Bio-Techne, Inc., Minneapolis, MN, USA*

ACHALA INDIKA KAMALADASA • *Centre for Dengue Research, Faculty of Medical Sciences, University of Sri Jayewardenapura, Nugegoda, Sri Lanka*

ALEXEY Y. KARULIN • *Cellular Technology Ltd., Shaker Heights, OH, USA*

RICHARD B. KENNEDY • *Mayo Clinic Vaccine Research Group, Mayo Clinic, Rochester, MN, USA*

STEVEN C. KENNEDY • *Department of Microbiology and Immunology, Albert Einstein College of Medicine, Bronx, NY, USA*

PAUL V. LEHMANN • *Cellular Technology Ltd., Shaker Heights, OH, USA*

GATHSAURIE NEELIKA MALAVIGE • *Centre for Dengue Research, Faculty of Medical Sciences, University of Sri Jayewardenapura, Nugegoda, Sri Lanka; MRC Human Immunology Unit, Weatherall Institute of Molecular Medicine, John Radcliffe Hospital, Oxford, UK*

NIKOLAI N. MARTYNOV • *MZ Computers Ltd, Moscow, Russian Federation*

ANDREW MCAVOY • *Department of Infectious Diseases and Immunology, College of Veterinary Medicine, University of Florida, Gainesville, FL, USA*

ZOLTÁN MEGYESI • *Cellular Technology Ltd., Shaker Heights, OH, USA*

J. C. NEUBAUER • *Fraunhofer Institute for Biomedical Engineering, Sulzbach, Germany; Fraunhofer Project Centre for Stem Cell Process Engineering, Wurzburg, Germany*

TONY W. NG • *Department of Microbiology and Immunology, Albert Einstein College of Medicine, Bronx, NY, USA*

GRAHAM S. OGG • *MRC Human Immunology Unit, Weatherall Institute of Molecular Medicine, John Radcliffe Hospital, Oxford, UK*

OSAMU OHARA • *Laboratory for Integrative Genomics, RIKEN Center for Integrative Medical Sciences, Tokyo, Japan; Department of Genome Research and Development, Kazusa DNA Research Institute, Chiba, Japan; The Futuristic Medical Care Education and Research Organization, Chiba University, Chiba, Japan*

INNA G. OVSYANNIKOVA • *Mayo Clinic Vaccine Research Group, Mayo Clinic, Rochester, MN, USA*

GREGORY A. POLAND • *Mayo Clinic Vaccine Research Group, Mayo Clinic, Rochester, MN, USA*

STEVEN A. PORCELLI • *Department of Microbiology and Immunology, Albert Einstein College of Medicine, Bronx, NY, USA; Department of Medicine, Albert Einstein College of Medicine, Bronx, NY, USA*

DIANA R. ROEN • *Cellular Technology Ltd., Shaker Heights, OH, USA*

BIKASH SAHAY • *Department of Infectious Diseases and Immunology, College of Veterinary Medicine, University of Florida, Gainesville, FL, USA*

I. SÉBASTIEN • *Fraunhofer Project Centre for Stem Cell Process Engineering, Würzburg, Germany*

YOSHITAKA SHIRASAKI • *PRESTO, Japan Science and Technology Agency, Tokyo, Japan; Department of Biological Science, Graduate School of Science, The University of Tokyo, Tokyo, Japan; Laboratory for Integrative Genomics, RIKEN Center for Integrative Medical Sciences, Tokyo, Japan*

MONIKA SIMMONS • *Naval Medical Research Center, Silver Spring, MD, USA*

PEIFANG SUN • *Henry Jackson Foundation for the Advancement of Military Medicine, Bethesda, MD, USA*

SHIANG-JONG TZENG • *Graduate Institute of Pharmacology, College of Medicine, National Taiwan University, Taipei, Taiwan*

H. VON BRIESEN • *Fraunhofer Institute for Biomedical Engineering, Sulzbach, Germany*

JANET K. YAMAMOTO • *Department of Infectious Diseases and Immunology, College of Veterinary Medicine, University of Florida, Gainesville, FL, USA*

SERGEY S. ZADOROZHNY • *MZ Computers Ltd, Moscow, Russian Federation*

H. ZIMMERMANN • *Fraunhofer Institute for Biomedical Engineering, Sulzbach, Germany; Fraunhofer Project Centre for Stem Cell Process Engineering, Würzburg, Germany; Molecular and Cellular Biotechnology/Nanotechnology, Saarland University, Saarbrucken, Germany; Facultad de Ciencias del Mar, Universidad Catolica del Norte, Coquimbo, Chile*

Chapter 1

Challenges in Developing Protein Secretion Assays at a Single-Cell Level

Yoshitaka Shirasaki and Osamu Ohara

Abstract

In addition to direct physical interactions between/among cells, the secretion of humoral factors from living cells is a critical process for cell-cell communications. A well-known extracellular signaling event is mediated by immune cell cytokines/chemokines. Because cell-cell communication is crucial in immune cell sociology, protein secretion assays first attracted a broad range of immunology interests. Now that we have entered an era of systems biology, cell-cell interactions mediated by secreted molecules should be revisited to understand the dynamics and homeostasis of the cell society as a whole. Of more importance, recent advances in detection and microfluidics technologies enable us to monitor protein secretion in real time rather than as a snapshot from the past, which gives us an opportunity to more deeply understand the logic of mammalian cell sociology. This chapter reviews the recent progress in and future direction of protein secretion assays, particularly from a mammalian cell sociology viewpoint.

Key words Cell sociology, Protein secretion, Real-time monitoring, Single cell, Snapshot, Systems biology

1 Introduction

It is well known that cell-cell communication plays a crucial role in cellular dynamics and homeostasis. In particular, long-range interactions among cells are key for homeostasis of the whole cell society, and short-range interactions evoked by direct physical contact between cells are indispensable routes for the local cell system. Although long-range interactions can also be mediated physically (e.g., through electric signals and/or cellular nanotubes), humoral factors secreted from cells are the most prominent players for long-range cell-cell interactions in this sense. This chapter focuses on protein secretion as a representative humoral factor.

The concentration of secreted proteins is conventionally measured by enzyme-linked immunosorbent assay (ELISA) as a sum of humoral factors secreted from many cells into culture media. Such a measurement cannot clarify how many cells are contributing to

Alexander E. Kalyuzhny (ed.), *Handbook of ELISPOT: Methods and Protocols*, Methods in Molecular Biology, vol. 1808, https://doi.org/10.1007/978-1-4939-8567-8_1, © Springer Science+Business Media, LLC, part of Springer Nature 2018

secretion of the humoral factors of interest, which is frequently crucial to figure out the activation state of the cell society. To address this problem, Czerkinsky et al. [1] introduced the Enzyme-Linked ImmunoSpot (ELISPOT) assay in 1983. The ELISPOT assay was the first method that enabled us to monitor protein secretion at the single-cell level. Once this breakthrough was introduced, this field's technological progress gained momentum and is continuously improving. In fact, recent advances in detection and microfluidics technologies have enabled us to further improve the ELISPOT method; even real-time monitoring of protein secretion at the single-cell level has become possible with extremely high sensitivity [2].

In this chapter, we review currently available technologies for single-cell protein secretion assays. We then introduce some discussion points for considering future challenges associated with protein secretion assays at the single-cell level.

2 Comparison of Technologies for Protein Secretion Assays

Tables 1 and 2 present comprehensive lists of currently available technologies for single-cell protein secretion assays found in the published literature. Although protein secretion from a single cell is easily monitored if the secretory protein of interest is tagged for detection by recombinant DNA technology, the lists provided in Tables 1 and 2 focus on secretion assays of endogenous proteins without any recombinant tag.

The reported single-cell protein secretion assay methods can be classified into two categories: intermittent (Table 1) and continuous (Table 2). Although we can follow the time course of protein secretion from single cells using the intermittent measurement method, the time resolution of continuous measurements is much higher than that of intermittent measurements, where we obtain snapshots of single-cell protein secretion over time successively but discontinuously. Each technology presented in Tables 1 and 2 can measure protein secretion at a single-cell resolution, but the sensitivity, throughput, and target multiplicity of protein detection vary widely. While considering how cost effective and labor intensive each option is, researchers can now select a method that best fits their needs.

Because the original aim of the ELISPOT assay was to detect cells that secrete the protein of interest in a mixture of cells, the intermittent method is well suited and powerful enough for immunology. The assays in this field have been greatly improved in terms of throughput and sensitivity, as shown in Table 1 [3–21]. In this sense, the protein secretion assay as a snapshot is well matured for the identification of cells that secrete the protein of interest. However, there is still room to enhance quantitative assay performance in terms of secretion rate and biological properties (e.g., affinity of the secreted antibody). This will be briefly described in the next section.

Table 1
Intermittent protein secretion assays in the published literature

Report	Detection method	Assay format	Throughput[a]
Irish et al., 2004 [3]	Fluorescence signal (intracellular staining)	Flow cytometry	High
Manz et al., 1995 [4]	Fluorescence signal on cell surface	Flow cytometry	High
Turcanu and Williams, 2001 [5]	Fluorescence signal in agarose gel	Flow cytometry	High
Akbari and Pirbodaghi, 2014 [6]	Fluorescence signal in alginate gel	Flow cytometry	Medium
Mazutis et al., 2013 [7]	Fluorescence signal on beads	Flow cytometry (droplet)	High
Henn et al., 2009 [8]	ELISPOT[b]	Open space	Medium
Das et al., 2017 [9]	Fluorescence signal	Open space	Low
Jin et al., 2009 [10]	Fluorescence signal	Open-chamber array	High
Yoshimoto et al., 2013 [11]	Fluorescence signal on cell surface	Open-chamber array	High
Ma et al., 2011 [12] Shi et al., 2012 [13] Kravchenko-Balasha et al., 2016 [14]	Fluorescence signal	Closed chamber/ valve	Medium
Lu et al., 2015 [15] Xue et al., 2015 [16]	Fluorescence signal	Closed chamber/ stamp	Medium
George et al., 2016 [17]	Fluorescence signal	Closed chamber/ stamp	Medium
Love et al., 2006 [18] Lohr et al., 2014 [19] Han et al., 2012 [20]	Fluorescence signal	Closed chamber/ stamp	High
Chiu et al., 2016 [21]	Fluorescence signal	Arrayed cells in open space	Medium

[a]High: >10,000 cells/assay; Medium: 1000 cells/assay to 10,000 cells/assay; Low: <1000 cells/assay
[b]ELISPOT: Enzyme-Linked ImmunoSpot

It is interesting to note that real-time protein secretion monitoring systems became available relatively recently (Table 2) [2, 22–28]. In general, real-world biological experiments cannot be performed under "ergodic" conditions in which the population average of cell states in a cell society is not equal to the time-average of a single cell's state. Despite this fact, in the past, there was no way to monitor protein secretion from single cells with a high time resolution. The emergence of real-time monitoring of protein

Table 2
Continuous protein secretion assays in the published literature

Report	Detection method	Assay format	Throughput[a]	Compatibility with live-cell imaging
Shirasaki et al., 2014 [2] Liu et al., 2014 [22]	Fluorescence signal	Open-chamber array	High	Yes
Junkin et al., 2016 [23]	Fluorescence signal on beads	Microfluidic circuit	Low	Yes
Son et al., 2016 [24]	Fluorescence signal on beads	Closed chamber	High	Yes
Raphael et al., 2013 [25] Raghu et al., 2015 [26]	Surface plasmon resonance	Open space	Low	Yes
Liu et al., 2015 [27]	Electrochemical signal	Flow cell	Low	Yes
Matharu et al., 2015 [28]	Electrochemical signal	Closed chamber	Low	Yes

[a]When the acceptable number of cells per assay is larger or smaller than 40, the throughput is shown as "High" or "Low," respectively

secretion from single cells could drastically change our understanding of cell signaling processes from a systems biology viewpoint.

3 Ongoing Challenges of Protein Secretion Assays

Although the single-cell protein secretion assay is one of the technologies used in single-cell analysis, the most prominent advances in single-cell analysis are in single-cell omics based on next-generation DNA sequencing (NGS). Many methods are already available for single-cell transcriptome analysis by NGS, and various bioinformatics pipelines specific for single-cell RNA sequence data have been reported [29]. It is worth noting that it is possible to count the protein molecule numbers in parallel with RNA profiling by NGS [30]. In other words, it is an obvious trend in systems biology to think at the single-cell level. Together with these lines of molecular information of intracellular space, protein secretion measurements at the single-cell level are attracting more interest than ever before.

As for characterization of a large number of single cells, microfluidics technology has tremendous power. For example, Eyer et al. [31] recently reported a method, termed "DropMap," which enables us to analyze the secretion rate and affinity of immunoglobulin G from more than 5×10^5 enriched B cells. Because this method offers us quantitative information about secretion processes and characteristics of secreted proteins, it opens new frontiers for characterizing many single cells by protein secretion.

The single-cell protein secretion assay has been a powerful tool for characterizing single cells without damaging them. Although this provides highly important information regarding cell relationships, the challenge remains to delineate the dynamics of a cell society at the single-cell level. For example, if we would like to determine how the cell society transitions from a resting to an activated state by an external signal, information about temporal changes of protein secretion from single cells combined with monitoring intracellular signaling processes is crucial because the secreted proteins are expected to provide the cell society with cooperativity against a response to the external signal. Some methods listed in Table 2 were developed with this in mind, and plenty of efforts have been made to achieve real-time monitoring of the secretion of multiple proteins together with intracellular signaling and retrieval of single cells for intracellular omics analysis.

4 Future Challenges

The ELISPOT assay was originally developed to detect a particular cell that secretes a protein of interest in a cell group, and many modifications have been made to improve its sensitivity, quantitative accuracy, and throughput (Table 1). Consequently, the range of applications for a single-cell protein secretion assay is broadening from use in basic research to clinical research. One goal of the assay in this direction is to characterize the state of each cell as a snapshot, and we are certainly approaching this goal.

However, we should remember that this type of protein secretion assay has a clear limitation from a cell sociology viewpoint: because secreted proteins are almost irreversibly captured by antibodies or other affinity reagents for detection in the assay, they can no longer behave as an external signaling molecule. In other words, the higher the quantitative power of the assay, the more detrimental the effect of the measurement on the behavior of the cell society. This means we might miss the system's dynamics when we prioritize the accuracy of the quantitative performance of a protein secretion assay from single cells. If the next challenges of the single-cell protein secretion assay are to open a new avenue for acquiring a comprehensive understanding of the cooperation of single cells in a group, we must seriously consider how to obviate this "observer effect" of the protein secretion assay.

Another important challenge from a biological viewpoint is to determine how to monitor the secretion of proteins in/from a solid organ or tissue. While single-cell transcriptional profiling is challenging to use when analyzing secretion in a multicellular organism [32] and/or a solid tumor [33], the spatiotemporal dynamics of protein secretion in solid tissue/organ at the single-cell level has currently not been greatly explored. Although protein secretion is usually monitored ex vivo, understanding the dynamics of protein secretion in situ is highly intriguing from a biological viewpoint. For this purpose, we probably need a new assay principle to detect protein secretion from single cells. Tissue- or organ-on-a-chip technology may serve as a realistic platform to address this need [34].

The well-matured protein secretion assay for the characterization of individual cells will soon be used not only in research laboratories but in clinical settings as well. However, the application of a single-cell protein secretion assay to help understand the mechanism of cell society homeostasis is still in its infancy. We believe such an application will attract more interest as single-cell biology becomes more popular because the exploration of long-range communications among cells is highly intriguing in that field.

References

1. Czerkinsky C, Nilsson L, Nygren H, Ouchterlony O, Tarkowski A (1983) A solid-phase enzyme-linked immunospot (ELISPOT) assay for enumeration of specific antibody-secreting cells. J Immunol Methods 65(1–2):109–121

2. Shirasaki Y, Yamagishi M, Suzuki N et al (2014) Real-time single-cell imaging of protein secretion. Sci Rep 4:4736

3. Irish JM, Hovland R, Krutzik PO et al (2004) Single cell profiling of potentiated phospho-protein networks in cancer cells. Cell 118:217–228

4. Manz R, Assenmacher M, Pflugert E et al (1995) Analysis and sorting of live cells according to secreted molecules, relocated to a cell-surface affinity matrix. Immunology 92:1921–1925

5. Turcanu V, Williams NA (2001) Cell identification and isolation on the basis of cytokine secretion: a novel tool for investigating immune responses. Nat Med 7:373–376

6. Akbari S, Pirbodaghi T (2014) A droplet-based heterogeneous immunoassay for screening single cells secreting antigen-specific antibodies. Lab Chip 14:3275

7. Mazutis L, Gilbert J, Ung WL et al (2013) Single-cell analysis and sorting using droplet-based microfluidics. Nat Protoc 8:870–891

8. Henn AAD, Rebhahn J, Brown MA et al (2009) Modulation of single-cell IgG secretion frequency and rates in human memory B cells by CpG DNA, CD40L, IL-21, and cell division. J Immunol 183:3177–3187

9. Das A, Rouault-Pierre K, Kamdar S et al (2017) Adaptive from innate: human IFN-γ⁺ CD4⁺ T cells can arise directly from CXCL8-producing recent thymic emigrants in babies and adults. J Immunol 199(5):1696–1705

10. Jin A, Ozawa T, Tajiri K et al (2009) A rapid and efficient single-cell manipulation method for screening antigen-specific antibody–secreting cells from human peripheral blood. Nat Med 15:1088–1092

11. Yoshimoto N, Kida A, Jie X et al (2013) An automated system for high-throughput single cell-based breeding. Sci Rep 3:1191

12. Ma C, Fan R, Ahmad H et al (2011) A clinical microchip for evaluation of single immune cells reveals high functional heterogeneity in phenotypically similar T cells. Nat Med 17(6):738–743

13. Shi Q, Qin L, Wei W et al (2012) Single-cell proteomic chip for profiling intracellular signaling pathways in single tumor cells. Proc Natl Acad Sci U S A 109:419–424

14. Kravchenko-Balasha N, Shin YS, Sutherland A et al (2016) Intercellular signaling through

secreted proteins induces free-energy gradient-directed cell movement. Proc Natl Acad Sci U S A 113:5520–5525

15. Lu Y, Xue Q, Eisele MR et al (2015) Highly multiplexed profiling of single-cell effector functions reveals deep functional heterogeneity in response to pathogenic ligands. Proc Natl Acad Sci U S A 112:E607–E615

16. Xue Q, Lu Y, Eisele MR et al (2015) Analysis of single-cell cytokine secretion reveals a role for paracrine signaling in coordinating macrophage responses to TLR4 stimulation. Sci Signal 8:ra59

17. George J, Wang J (2016) Assay of genome-wide transcriptome and secreted proteins on the same single immune cells by microfluidics and RNA sequencing. Anal Chem 88:10309–10315

18. Love JC, Ronan JL, Grotenbreg GM et al (2006) A microengraving method for rapid selection of single cells producing antigen-specific antibodies. Nat Biotechnol 24:703–707

19. Lohr JG, Adalsteinsson VA, Cibulskis K et al (2014) Whole-exome sequencing of circulating tumor cells provides a window into metastatic prostate cancer. Nat Biotechnol 32:479–484

20. Han Q, Bagheri N, Bradshaw EM et al (2012) Polyfunctional responses by human T cells result from sequential release of cytokines. Proc Natl Acad Sci U S A 109:1607–1612

21. Chiu YJ, Cai W, Shih YRV et al (2016) A single-cell assay for time lapse studies of exosome secretion and cell behaviors. Small 12:3658–3666

22. Liu T, Yamaguchi Y, Shirasaki Y et al (2014) Single-cell imaging of caspase-1 dynamics reveals an all-or-none inflammasome signaling response. Cell Rep 8(4):974–982

23. Junkin M, Kaestli AJ, Cheng Z et al (2016) High-content quantification of single-cell immune dynamics. Cell Rep 15:411–422

24. Son KJ, Rahimian A, Shin D-S et al (2016) Microfluidic compartments with sensing microbeads for dynamic monitoring of cytokine and exosome release from single cells. Analyst 141:679–688

25. Raphael MP, Christodoulides JA, Delehanty JB et al (2013) Quantitative imaging of protein secretions from single cells in real time. Biophys J 105:602–608

26. Raghu D, Christodoulides JA, Delehanty JB et al (2015) A label-free technique for the spatio-temporal imaging of single cell secretions. J Vis Exp 1:1–11

27. Liu Y, Liu Y, Matharu Z et al (2015) Detecting multiple cell-secreted cytokines from the same aptamer-functionalized electrode. Biosens Bioelectron 64:43–50

28. Matharu Z, Patel D, Gao Y et al (2014) Detecting transforming growth factor - β release from liver cells using an aptasensor integrated with micro fluidics. Anal Chem 86:8865–8872

29. Neu KE, Tang Q, Wilson PC et al (2017) Single-cell genomics: approaches and utility in immunology. Trends Immunol 38:140–149

30. Peterson VM, Zhang KX, Kumar N et al (2017) Multiplexed quantification of proteins and transcripts in single cells. Nat Biotechnol 35:936–939

31. Eyer K, Doineau RC, Castrillon CE et al (2017) Single-cell deep phenotyping of IgG-secreting cells for high-resolution immune monitoring. Nat Biotechnol 35:977–982

32. Cao J, Packer JS, Ramani V et al (2017) Comprehensive single-cell transcriptional profiling of a multicellular organism. Science 357:661–667

33. Li H et al (2017) Reference component analysis of single-cell transcriptomes elucidates cellular heterogeneity in human colorectal tumors. Nat Genet 49:708–718

34. Zhang B, Radisic M (2017) Organ-on-a-chip devices advance to market. Lab Chip 17:2395–2420

Chapter 2

Mastering the Computational Challenges
of Elispot Plate Evaluation

Sylvia Janetzki

Abstract

Much has been written about Elispot and how to optimally run the assay for a wide variety of applications. But only a limited number of articles exist addressing the analysis step, the plate evaluation. Comparing that fact with the vast amount of analysis advise available for other single cell immune assay, for example, intracellular cytokine staining, the overall impression may be that Elispot evaluation is just simple enough to not require extensive elaboration and guidance. At first thought this appears reasonable because how difficult can it be counting colored spots on a white background. In addition, automated Elispot readers were already introduced more than 20 years ago (Herr et al., J Immunol Methods 203, 141–152, 1997), easing the strenuous load of manual counting and providing means to decrease the subjectivity in Elispot analysis. Just shortly thereafter however, the first report was published about the subjectivity and operator-dependency of plate evaluation even when using automated reader systems (Janetzki et al., J Immunol Methods 291, 175–183, 2004). Later, the plate evaluation was identified as a main factor causing variability in Elispot results, triggering the inclusion of recommendations on handling of artifacts and the audits of plate reading results in the Initial Elispot Harmonization guidelines (Janetzki et al., Cancer Immunol Immunother 57, 303–315, 2008; Britten et al., Cancer Immunol Immunother 57, 289–302, 2008). In follow-up, a large international study with 75 laboratories was conducted to address the current approaches taken to evaluate Elispot plates and to establish consensus guidelines for plate evaluation (Janetzki et al., Nat Protoc 10, 1098–1115, 2015). This article addresses the special challenges of plate evaluation, gives explanations for unusual observation, and provides overall recommendations on how to work through the labyrinth of available algorithms and reader settings to obtain reliable Elispot data.

Key words Elispot, Elispot evaluation, Elispot reader, Elispot images, Elispot software, Elispot analysis

---

1 Introduction

Elispot has been around for more than 35 years [1] and is one of the most commonly used assays for the functional assessment of single immune cells. This fact is driven by the assay's simplicity, but most of all its sensitivity, allowing the detection of cells in very low frequency. Supporting its continuous and increasing usage has been the development of materials and reagents with increasing

Alexander E. Kalyuzhny (ed.), *Handbook of ELISPOT: Methods and Protocols*, Methods in Molecular Biology, vol. 1808, https://doi.org/10.1007/978-1-4939-8567-8_2, © Springer Science+Business Media, LLC, part of Springer Nature 2018

reliability, like improved Elispot plates [2, 3] and antibody kits. Activities of large networks from the fields of infectious diseases, cancer, and autoimmunity have provided guidance and guidelines for sample handling and assay performance [4–10]. Notably, the impressive international collaboration and efforts of the European Cancer Immunotherapy Consortium (CIP/CIMT) and the North American Cancer Immunotherapy Consortium (CIC/CRI) have established large proficiency panel programs with over hundred laboratories from all walks of immunological background that allowed to identify critical protocol steps that influence the assay outcome, on which basis the Harmonization guidelines for Elispot have been established and made available to the immune monitoring field [4, 5, 11] (Fig. 1). It was shown that the integration of these guidelines into a laboratory's SOP improves the overall Elispot performance [7, 11]. Further, the available guidance and relative ease to not only standardize, but qualify/validate the assay in accordance to the ICH guidelines [12–14] has made it a highly valuable tool in early clinical trials with immunological endpoints [15–19]. Based on these positive developments, Elispot has also become one of the go to assays in the arena of neo-antigen discovery and personalized vaccine development [18, 20]. The assay has also entered the diagnostic field, for example, in tuberculosis [21]. In addition, efforts are on their way to have the assay being established as a diagnostic indicator for organ rejection in kidney transplantation [22].

With all that being said, two of the three steps of the assay remain a challenge, which pertain to the preparation of the sample (Step 1) and spot counting (Step 3) (Fig. 2).

<table>
<tr><td colspan="3">Initial Elispot Harmonization Guidelines to Optimize Assay Performance</td></tr>
<tr><td>A</td><td colspan="2">Establish laboratory SOP for Elispot testing procedures, including:</td></tr>
<tr><td></td><td>A1</td><td>Counting method for apoptotic cells for determining adequate cell dilution for plating</td></tr>
<tr><td></td><td>A2</td><td>Overnight rest of cells prior to plating and incubation</td></tr>
<tr><td>B</td><td colspan="2">Use only pre-tested and optimized serum allowing for low background : high signal ratio</td></tr>
<tr><td>C</td><td colspan="2">Establish SOP for plate reading, including:</td></tr>
<tr><td></td><td>C1</td><td>Human auditing during reading process</td></tr>
<tr><td></td><td>C2</td><td>Adequate adjustments for technical artifacts</td></tr>
<tr><td>D</td><td colspan="2">Only allow trained personnel, which is certified per laboratory SOP, to conduct assays</td></tr>
</table>

Fig. 1 Initial Elispot Harmonization guidelines, as published in [4]

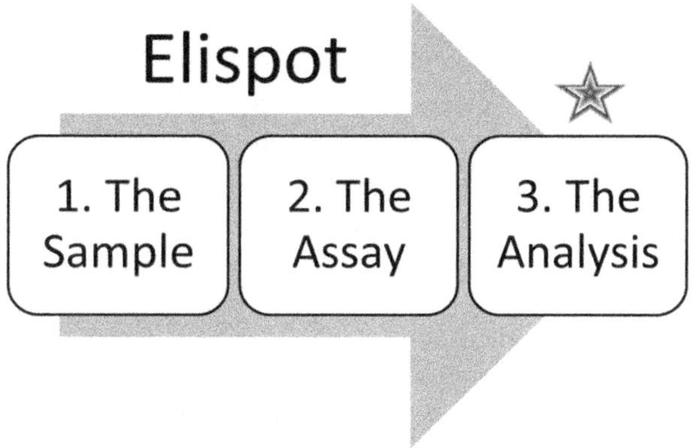

Fig. 2 Steps of an Elispot experiment. The first step pertains to the preparation of the sample (guidance available in [6, 25]), which may include cell isolation (e.g., PBMC from whole blood), freezing, thawing, resting, counting and viability assessment, and perhaps isolation of subpopulations or expansion of cells. The second step, the assay (guidance available in [25, 31]), typically includes the coating and blocking of the Elispot plate, the plating of the sample and stimulants, incubation, and removal of cells and spot development. The third step, labeled by a star above the box, includes the enumeration of spots (guidance available in [24, 32]), and the analysis of raw spot numbers for obtaining measures for response definition (guidance available in [33, 34]). This article focuses on the first part of step 3, the spot enumeration

The enumeration of spots (part of the Analysis Step 3) is the focus of this article.

Shortly after the introduction of automated Elispot readers, the first report was published about the subjectivity and operator-dependency of plate evaluation even when using automated reader systems [23]. Later, the plate evaluation was identified as a main protocol step causing variability in Elispot results, triggering the inclusion of recommendations on handling of artifacts and the audits of plate reading results in the Initial Elispot Harmonization guidelines [4, 5]. In follow-up, a large international study with 75 laboratories was conducted to address the current approaches taken to evaluate Elispot plates and to establish consensus guidelines for plate evaluation [24]. These efforts demonstrated the enormous and shocking variability caused by plate evaluation. In the above study, only Elispot well images were made available to the participants, excluding any variability that could be introduced due to the individual reader and camera setup. And to no surprise, there was no difference identified based on the reader system the participants used to analyze the provided Elispot images. Rather, the results were dependent on laboratories' flexibility and know-how about

1. Adapting previously established reading algorithms and parameters to the new well images provided

2. Adapting algorithms and parameters to the special circumstances present in various sets of well images provided (each set contained triplicates of at least the negative control = cells alone and the antigen-stimulated wells)

3. Adapting algorithms and parameters to the special circumstances present in a subset of wells within image sets provided

With other words, how well did labs handle situations that were different to what they were accustomed to as being "normal," e.g., crowded wells, high background reactivity, presence of artifacts? The most common overall strategies to handle unexpected and challenging observations reported by the participants were:

(a) Reject the sample and readout and attempt retesting of the entire sample

(b) Reject the sample and readout without attempting retesting

(c) Adapt algorithm and reader settings as necessary, and document observation and changes in reading attempts made.

In a laborious effort, the large panel of participants (a list of the more than 100 scientists who participated is provided in [24]) came to an agreement on how to best handle the evaluation approach of Elispot plates to ensure reliable Elispot results. A step-by-step flow chart was created and published, with detailed explanations for each choice of adjustments of reading approaches that are triggered by the plate appearance [24]. It is strongly recommended to consider incorporating those outlined steps, recommendations, and explanations in the plate evaluation SOP of a laboratory.

What follows is a closer look at the influence of adapting algorithms and reading parameters for plate evaluation. The chapter will discuss how to approach challenging conditions and unusual observations, including the explanation of what causes those challenges (*see* **Note 1**).

2   Materials

1. Elispot plate, fully developed and dried (*see* **Notes 2** and **3**).

2. Automated Elispot reader (*see* **Notes 4** and **5**).

3. Suitable Elispot software (*see* **Note 6**).

3   Methods

3.1   Elispot Reader Setup

3.1.1   Camera

Current reader systems are equipped with a digital camera exposing multiple megapixels of resolution. For highly accurate color acquisition, RGB cameras are typically being used which acquire three different color signals (R = Red, G = Green, B = Blue) on three separate sensors. There are multiple settings of a camera that can and have to be adapted to obtain an image that reflects a true presentation of the well's condition. That appears to be a given, but in reality it often is overlooked, as demonstrated in Fig. 3. Artificially enhanced images and spots often give raise to overestimated spot counts. One of the most important features to discriminate true spots from background signals, the spot intensity (also called contrast; see below under Subsection "Spot Parameters") is rendered to a less useful state in artificially enhanced images. This is important to realize since the spot intensity is a correlate of the amount of cytokine that was secreted by a cell. The intensity parameter can hence be an excellent tool to discriminate background signals and true spots.

Two camera settings are of crucial importance. These are the exposure time, and the alignment of the RGB signals for true color presentation. How these two factors work together is demonstrated in Fig. 4. An attempt should be made to obtain images that are an accurate reflection of the Elispot plate wells (*see* **Note 7**).

An important camera feature that needs to be continuously used is the autofocus. This feature allows the camera to focus on the center of each new well. It is important since wells in a 96-well plate are often located not entirely on the same plane. More peripheral wells and especially corner wells in a 96-well plate may be on a different plane level. Also, wells from different plates altogether may be in different focus planes. Older format plates with an open frame design may be slightly deformed due to missing support from a stable frame structure, adding to focus issues.

A special challenge is found in older Elispot plates different from the more recently improved HTS plates which contain a straightened membrane (*see* **Note 8**). Since those older format plates were designed for applications different to Elispot, they contain membranes that were allowed to expand and retract; hence, the center and the periphery of a well are significantly different in their plane location. The issue is demonstrated in Fig. 5.

3.1.2   Software features

While Elispot reader software programs may appear very different from reader system to system, overall they contain similar features and apply similar algorithms and settings, mostly hidden behind different terminology. In this section, we look at three different aspects important for the evaluation of Elispot plates:

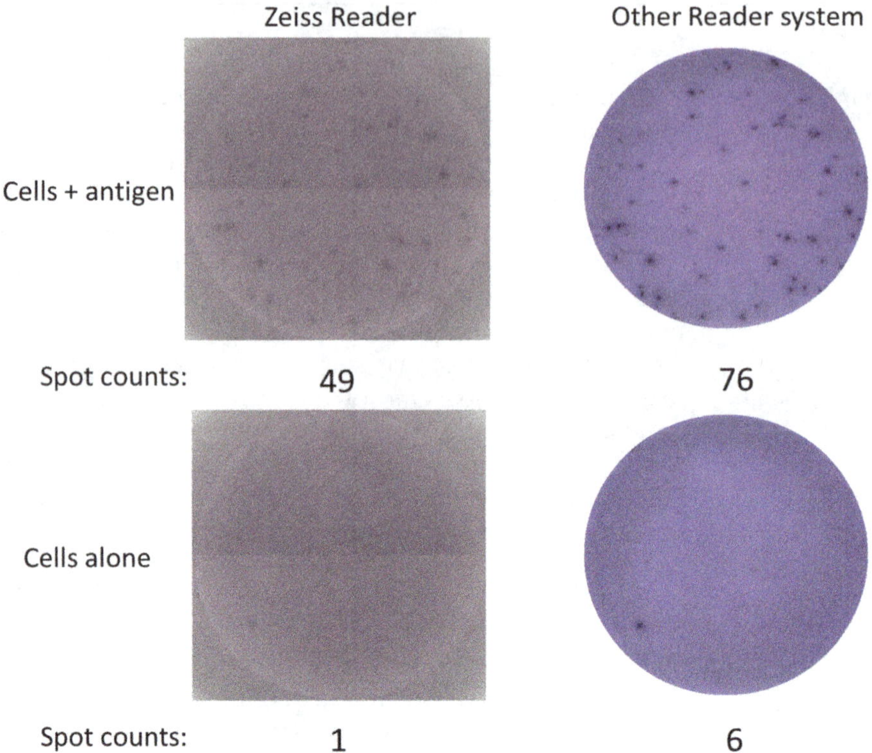

Fig. 3 True and artificially altered well images. Images on the left hand side were taken with a Zeiss reader, with the RGB alignment and exposure settings optimally set as demonstrated in Fig. 4. The real specimen (Elispot plate) exposed high bluish-grey background staining, caused by typical overstaining with BCIP/NBT, and faint spots which were barely recognizable by eye. The upper panel image was taken from a well containing cells stimulated with an antigen. The negative control (cells plus medium only) is shown in the lower panel. The right side images were obtained with a different reader system that performed automated color and intensity adjustments to artificially change the image to highly intense blue staining with nonrealistically strong spots, a process that was not controlled appropriately. Due to the falsely increased presentation of signals (and high sensitivity settings), counted spot numbers in the antigen-stimulated well and the negative control are inaccurately high. While perhaps looking more pleasing to the eye; the images on the right hand side are deceitful and do not reflect the true conditions of that Elispot plate. A part of the well periphery was also cut out and is not represented in the image

1. The area of a well that is actually considered for spot counting

2. The algorithm that defines how signals in a well are separated

3. The parameters that define what a spot is

The Area of Interest (AOI)

The area of interest defines the area of a well that is actually being evaluated. It is typically defined by a ring that can be expanded and retracted to a size that fits the well diameter (which may somewhat differ depending on the kind of plate used) and that allows the exclusion of potential artifacts in the well periphery. In that regard,

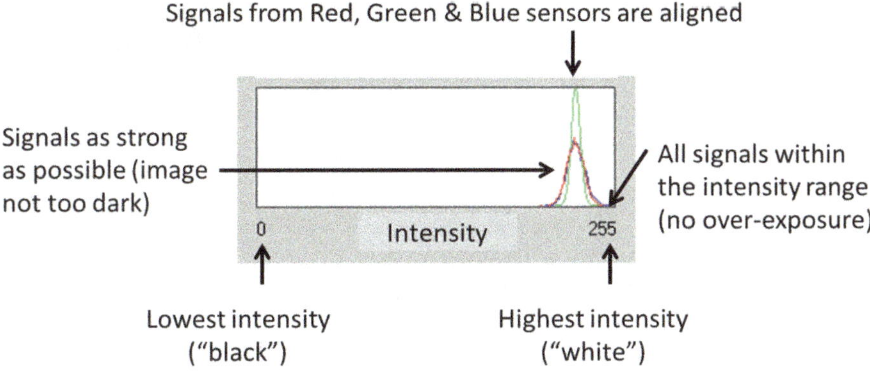

Fig. 4 Optimal camera adaption of exposure and RGB alignment. The intensity of each of the three light channels (RGB) is converted onto a grey scale that per definition has the lowest value set as zero (black, see arrow at left side of diagram) and the highest value at 255 (white, see arrow at right side of diagram). The camera should be adjusted so that all three signals have the same intensity (arrow pointing to the tops of the RGB curves). If this is not the case, the image may appear more red, blue, or green, depending on which signal has the highest intensity. Elispot reader systems have typically a command that allows the automated adjustment of the signal strength and the alignment of the RGB channels (also called Auto-White Balance = AWB). Further, the exposure determines how dark or bright an image will appear. It is important to adjust the exposure settings in a way that none of the signals from the RGB channels are lost in overexposure ("too bright," arrow pointing to the right end bottom of RGB signal curves). Underexposure leads to too dark images

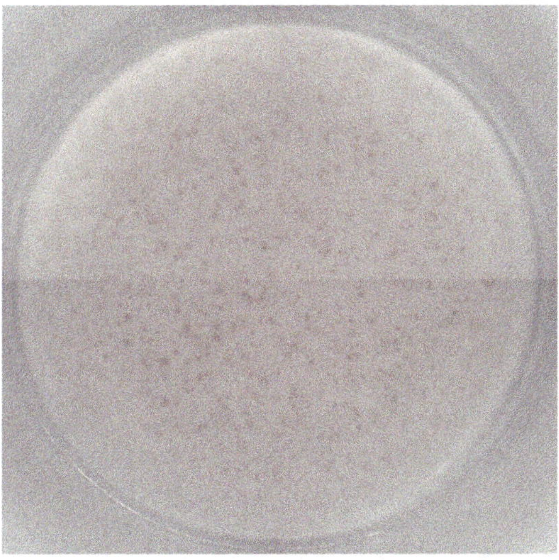

Fig. 5 Concave well membrane. A well image from an old format MAHA well plate with many spots is shown. The image was taken with a KS Elispot reader system (Carl Zeiss, Inc., Thornwood, NY, USA). While spots in the well center are in focus, the well is shaped highly concave with the well periphery being completely out of focus and spots cannot be accurately discriminated and counted

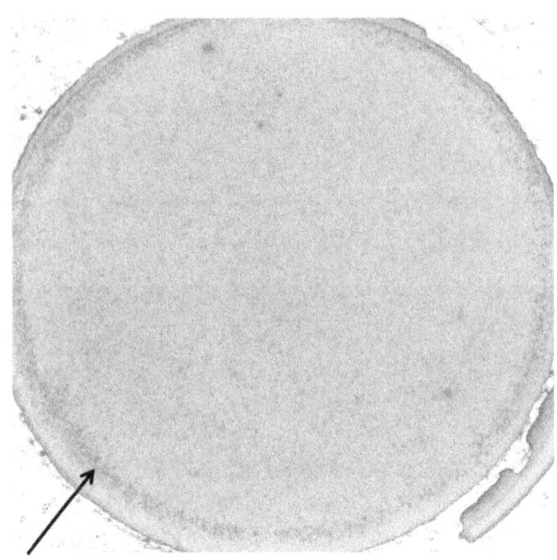

Fig. 6 Elispot well with artifact ring. PBMC were tested for IFNɣ release. A ring of small artifacts is recognizable in the well periphery (arrow), indicative of cell death. A few true spots are also detectable, among a faint cover of artifacts across the membrane. It is advisable to minimize the AOI to exclude the artifact ring in the well periphery. The image was taken with a KS Elispot reader system (Carl Zeiss, Inc., Thornwood, NY, USA)

it is often easier to exclude a small section of the well periphery across all wells in order to exclude artifacts which are, for example, caused by dying cells (Fig. 6), instead of trying to adjust reading parameters for artifact exclusion, what can be extremely challenging.

The Algorithm

The algorithm determines how well signals are distinguished. This is not a trivial task since it determines not only if close by signals or spots are counted as one or as multiple signals, but it also determines the reported size of a spot. Figure 7 demonstrates the change in spot number and spot size with different algorithm settings applied for the same well.

It is important to check the optimal reader settings depending on the spot appearance. If spots are small and well defined, it is good to use algorithm settings that distinguish each signal in the well. If spots are large, it is important to adjust algorithm settings focusing on large spots and prevent the reader recognizing all small staining differences within a spot which would otherwise be counted as multiple spots within a large spot (what can lead to false high spot counts). Large spots are often found in B-cell Elispot, especially when coating was done with the antigen. An example of a well image from a B-cell Elispot is given in Fig. 8.

Another challenge and necessary adaption of the algorithm occurs when wells have so many spots that the spot peripheries touch each other, and it is becoming increasingly difficult to

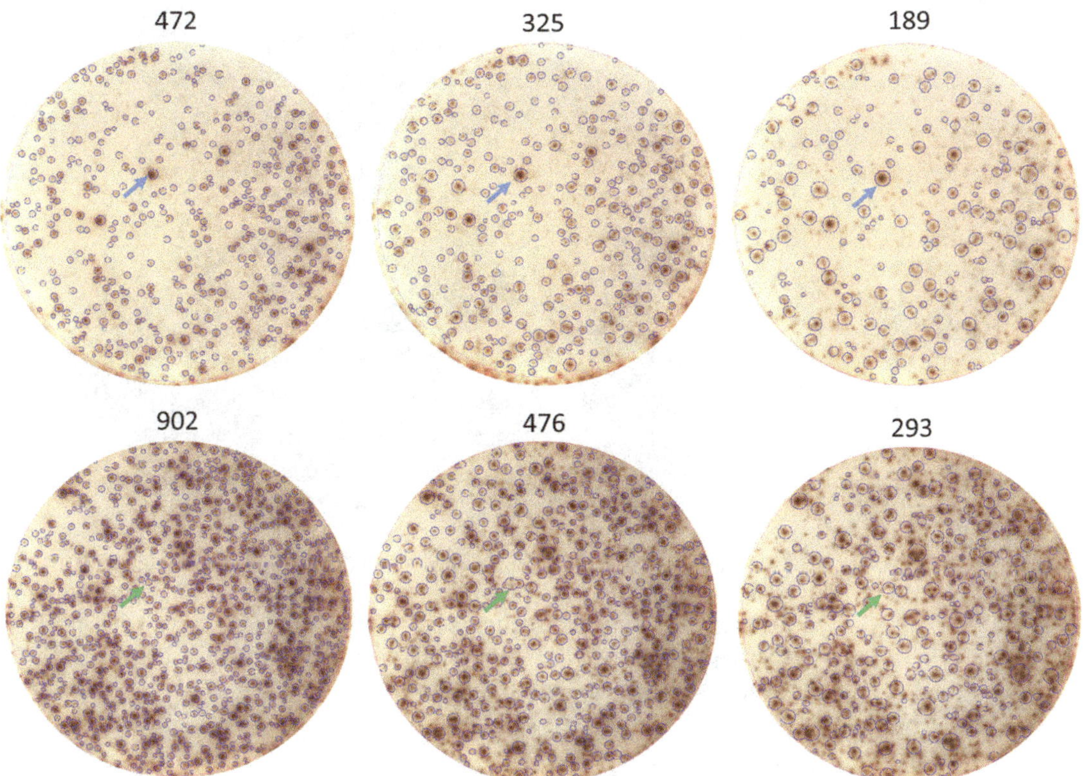

Fig. 7 The influence of the algorithm settings on counted spot number and spot size. The upper and lower panels depict two wells with different spot crowdedness. Images on the left side were evaluated with an algorithm focusing on tiny spots in crowded wells, the center images on large spots, and the right hand images on huge spots. Spot counts are listed on top of each well image. All wells were counted with the same spot parameters in place. Note the decrease in spot numbers counted from left to right and increase in spot size. The blue arrows in the top panel point to one large spot that clearly increases in reported spot size (indicated by the colored ring around the spot). The green arrows in the lower panel point to an area with multiple spots that are well separated in the left image, not separated in the center image, and which contains ignored spots in the right image. The images were taken with an AID iSpot Reader System (Strassberg, Germany)

distinguish single spots. This situation is commonly seen in positive control wells using mitogen for nonspecific stimulation of cells. The scenario is demonstrated in Fig. 9. It is possible that spots form a confluent stained area which cannot be reliably evaluated. Approaches how to handle evaluation results from wells with spot confluence are presented in **Note 9**.

It is possible that only one condition in an experiment requires the adjustment of algorithms (and potentially parameters), for example, the positive control wells. It is recommended to establish a separate set of reader settings for those exceptions, and apply them only to these wells. Applying those "high sensitivity" settings to all wells may lead to false high spot counts in the remaining conditions. Vice versa, applying the reader settings used for the remaining wells to

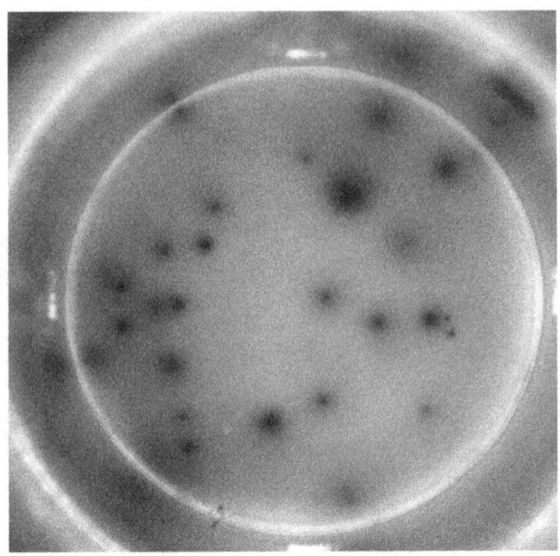

Fig. 8 Example of a B-cell Elispot well testing human B cells for IgG release. The well was coated with the antigen (whole protein) of interest. Spots are very large, requiring algorithm settings focusing on detecting large spots, combing small staining differences within a spot to one spot. The image was taken with an AID iSpot Reader system (Strassberg, Germany)

wells that appear very different (e.g., highly crowded) will lead to too low spot counts (e.g., in the positive control wells).

The distance between signals detected by the software on one hand and the applied algorithm on the other hand determine if both signals will be seen as being caused by one and the same signal (e.g., by inhomogeneity within a spot)—typically when the focus is on larger spots—or by separate signals (higher sensitivity with focus on smaller spots). Clearly, the spot diameter reported with the algorithm focusing on large spots will be larger than the diameter reported with a more sensitive algorithm that may discriminate more than one spot in that same area (also see lower panel in Fig. 7, green arrows). However, changes in the spot size for one and the same signal when different algorithms are applied (as indicated in the upper panel of Fig. 7, blue arrows) are a more complicated matter. Figure 10 explains the underlying mechanism for spot size changes when changing the spot algorithm. This phenomenon has to be kept in mind when using the spot sizes to present experimental results.

Spot Parameters

Spot parameters define an actual spot that is allowed to be counted by the software. Those parameters should distinguish a spot from other, artificial signals. Further, spot parameters have the crucial task to allow the definition of meaningful spots and to exclude spots that are caused by factors that are not meaningful for the study performed and the question asked. Defining spot parameters

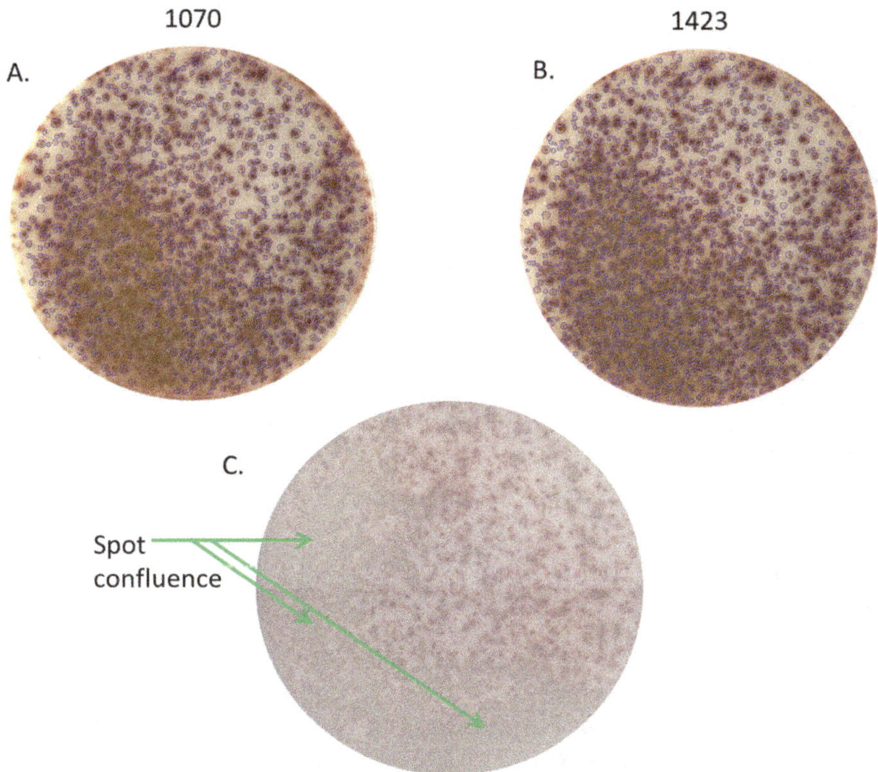

Fig. 9 Spot crowdedness. The upper panel (**a**+**b**) depicts the same well image. The algorithm was adjusted to focus on the detection of all spots. However, since spots are located so close to each other in parts of the well (lower left part of well), the overall background staining is very high in that area and not all spots are picked up (**a**). Further adjustments to the spot intensity (=contrast) had to be made to include spots in that crowded area (**b**). The image was taken with an AID iSpot Reader system (Strassberg, Germany). The lower panel (**c**) demonstrates extreme spot crowdedness. Single spots cannot be distinguished in the crowded area (see arrow). The area is excluded from evaluation (*see* **Note 9**). The image was taken with a Zeiss reader (Carl Zeiss, Inc., Thornwood, NY)

can be straightforward, but may in other cases be extremely challenging. There are two important points to consider:

1. Are the correct spots included, and excluded, from being counted?

2. Do the parameters defined for spot recognition allow a realistic reflection of meaningful biological conditions in a well?

With other words, do my reading results present a transparent picture of the experiment or study without artificially skewing results in favor of anticipated results? Skewing results has been observed [24], for example, when applying different parameter sets for the negative control (lower sensitivity to keep background reactivity levels low) and the experimental wells (higher sensitivity for increase of the signal to noise ratio). In other scenarios, where increased reactivity in negative controls is apparent, parameters

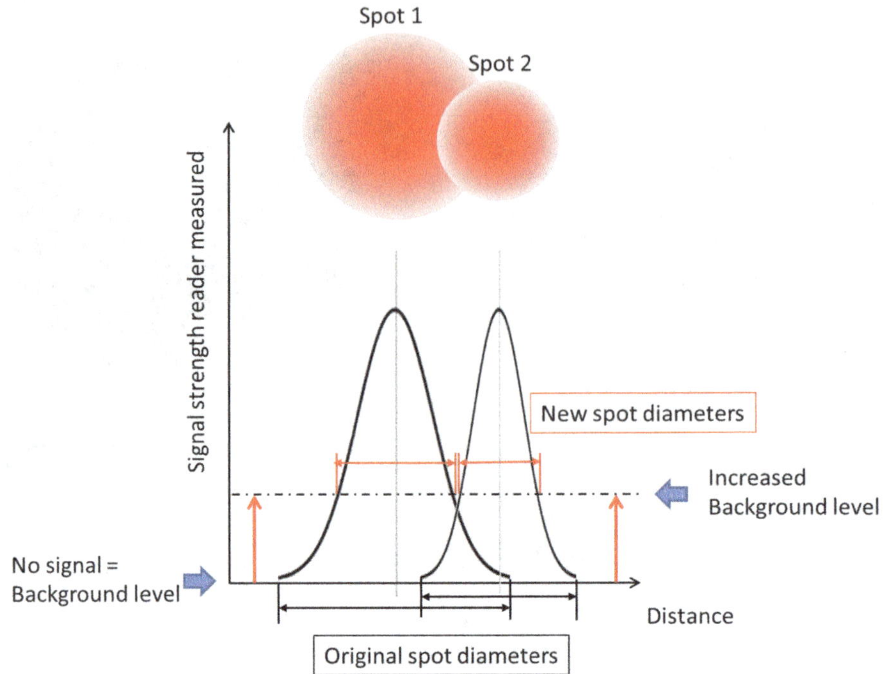

Fig. 10 Algorithm-dependent spot diameter changes. Two partially overlapping spots are illustrated on the top of the graph. The curves indicate the strength of signal for each spot recorded by the software across the spot diameter. The software would discriminate these two spots based on the curves descending fully back to the background level (overall membrane staining), and report the spot size as indicated by the black double arrow lines. The spot size extends across the spot for the lowest peripheral staining the software can distinguish from background staining. Since both spots partially overlap, both curves do not reach the background level undisturbed, hence are not separated. In order to effectively discriminate both spots, the algorithm is set to a higher sensitivity by artificially increasing the background level that would indicate "background staining only" (specified by the red arrows). Now, the staining curves for the two spots are separated at their "new" base again, and the reader can reliably discriminate both spots. However, since the curve is "cut off" at a higher staining intensity, the spot diameter reported is smaller (indicated by the red double arrows)

were adjusted to exclude true, well-defined spots and only count very large spots (which were present in low frequency in experimental wells, but almost absent in the negative control), hence results presented a clean background reactivity (no or close to no spots), and small but significant increase in spot counts for the experimental wells (e.g., 5 spots), while the actual counts for true, well-defined spots, which differed clearly from smaller spots caused by nonspecific stimulation, was indeed insignificant (e.g., 30 spots in the background control, and 35 spots in the experimental well). Prone to such approach are software features that promise the user to scientifically adjust the reading parameters automatically. It is strongly advised to NOT rely on such program features, due to the complexity of and variability in biological responses that can occur and be measured with Elispot.

There exist multiple parameters that define a spot. The hallmark feature of a spot is its close assembly to a circle with strong staining in the center and fading staining in the periphery. This feature is driven by the diffusion of the cytokine away from the cell that is secreting it. Most cytokine is captured by the coating antibody in close proximity of the cell, hence the dark center of a spot.

Important spot parameters are illustrated in Fig. 11. Perhaps the two most commonly used parameters are the spot size and the spot intensity. Both are first and most of all driven by the actual protocol choices made, e.g., a high amount of coating antibody leads to smaller, denser (hence more intense) spots due to the fact that secreted cytokine is captured immediately after being secreted, in contrast to instances when lower amounts of capture antibody are used for coating which leads to larger and less intense spots because the cytokine has to diffuse further away from the cell in order to be captured. The amount of capture antibody bound to the membrane is also dependent on the membrane type used (PVDF membranes tend to bind capture antibody more efficiently than nitrocellulose membranes). Prewetting the PVDF membrane further influences how well the capture antibody binds; hence how well defined the spots are (*see* **Note 10**). In addition, the longer the incubation of cells, the larger the spots will be, since the spot size reflects the total amount of cytokine secreted over time by a cell. But even the incubation length with substrate influences the final size of spots. It becomes obvious that standardization of protocols applied for a study is essential to permit comparability of results obtained from different experiments.

Once the protocol has been standardized, the spot size and intensity can be a direct measure of the amount of cytokine secreted. Generally the larger a spot, the more cytokine was secreted. Reader systems typically provide a size readout for spots that were counted, which can usually be correlated with their staining intensity measures (also provided by most reader systems).

The spot color, shape, and measures of the degree of color fading from the spot center to its periphery are excellent tools to distinguish spots from artifacts (see Fig. 11). An extensive review of possible artifacts with examples of well images is contained in separate publications [24, 25]. They can typically be divided into artifacts caused by

1. The Sample (see Fig. 6) or

2. Outside interference

The rule of thumb is that the purer and healthier the sample is that is added to the Elispot plate, the cleaner the Elispot well. The most common artifacts are caused by dying cells, which produce especially in IFNγ assays small speckles that can accumulate in the well periphery and form a typical artifact ring (Fig. 6). As a matter of fact, an artifact ring consisting of small speckles is such a strong indication for cell death, that the sample's viability and degree of apoptosis prior to plating out should be re-checked. Adjusting spot

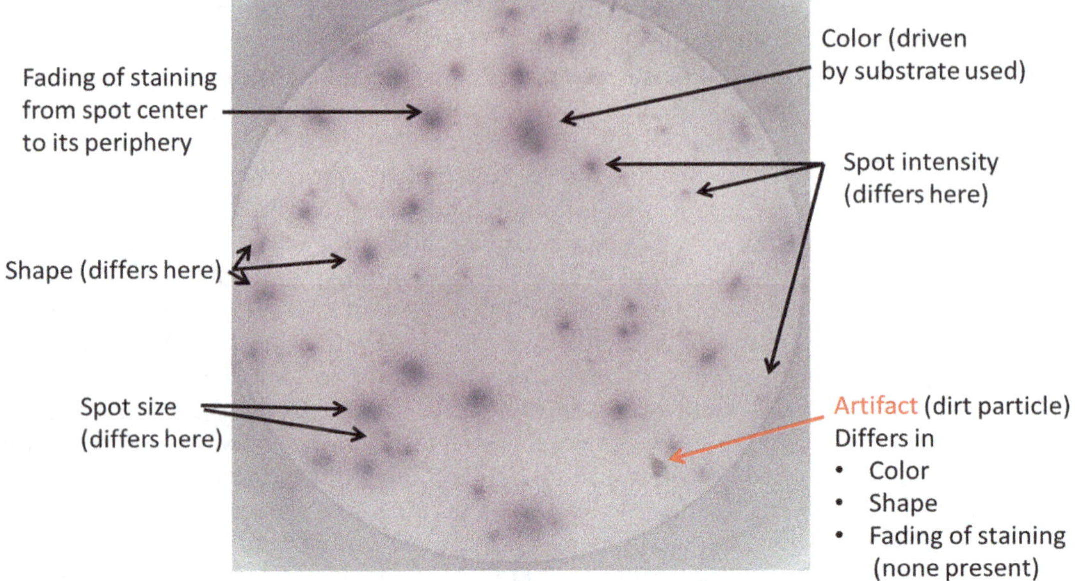

Fig. 11 Spot parameters. A spot is defined by its size, color, intensity, shape, and fading of staining from the spot center to its periphery, among others (e.g., saturation). A fine-tuning of these parameters allows the discrimination of meaningful spots from nonmeaningful spots and from artifacts

size and intensity can be helpful to exclude those artifacts, as can be decreasing the AOI.

There are other artifacts caused by the sample that indicate that an issue is present. Figure 12 demonstrates a netlike artifact across the well that indicates cell death during thawing which leads to DNA release by dying cells which serves as a highly sticky matrix and creates clumps in the cell sample that cannot be resuspended. It is extremely difficult to exclude these artifacts from not being counted. Shape and intensity settings can be helpful. It is recommended to avoid such artifacts by adding DNase during the thawing procedure.

Perhaps one of the most neglected artifacts that are often seen in PBMC samples are white ghost spots that may be so dominant that they disintegrate spots and make their accurate enumeration almost impossible. Such ghost spots are caused by granulocytes that are bound to the capture antibody via their Fc receptor. Granulocytes can be isolated together with PBMC when the time frame between blood draw and PBMC isolation extends 8 h. During that time, granulocytes get activated and change their buoyancy profile in a way that they cannot be effectively separated during Ficolling. While most granulocytes die during the freezing and thawing process, they still disturb the spot formation due to the mechanism described above, and they dilute the sample. The scenario is demonstrated in Fig. 13. Evidence of granulocyte contamination in Elispot wells should trigger the investigation of how

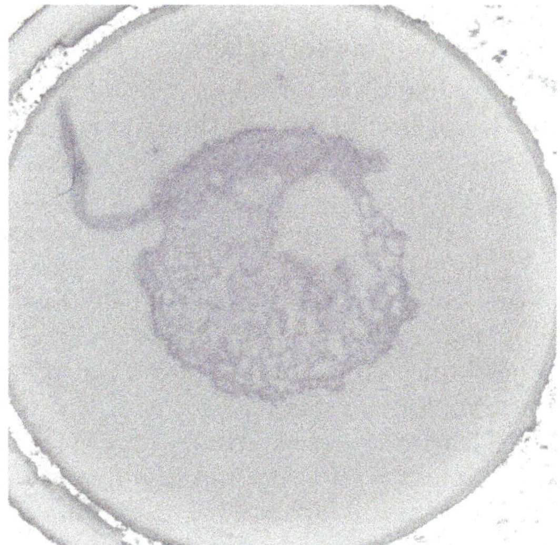

Fig. 12 DNA precipitates. The well image contains a large netlike artifact that was caused by a DNA precipitate. Two blue spots can also be seen above the artifact. The image was taken with a KS Elispot reader system (Carl Zeiss, Inc., Thornwood, NY)

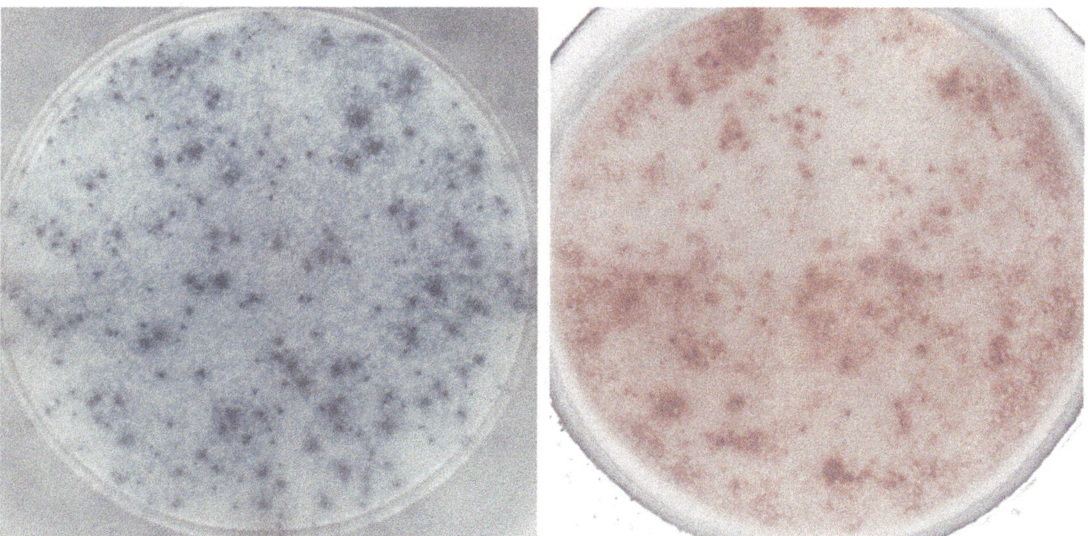

Fig. 13 Granulocyte contamination. Two well images are presented (left image developed with TMB, right image developed with AEC) from PBMC testing. High levels of white ghost spots can be recognized in both wells, and spot disintegration is evident. It is very challenging to adjust parameters to obtain accurate spot counts. It is recommended to set the algorithm with focus on large spots, in order to allow the software to "repair" some of the spot disintegration and to avoid multiple counts for the same spot. The images were taken by a KS Elispot reader system (Carl Zeiss, Inc., Thornwood, NY)

blood samples were obtained and how fast PBMC were isolated. It is likely that PBMC isolation occurred after 8 h of time lapse. During that time, granulocytes will have asserted their suppression on T-cell functionality, as shown previously [26–30].

Other artifacts can be caused by insufficient removal of cells after incubation (*see* **Note 11**), what leads to white spot centers due to the occupation of the membrane site by sticking cells and inhibition of efficient binding of the secondary antibody (Fig. 14). Those white spots are only contained within a spot, and they do not disintegrate spots from the periphery, as shown in Fig. 13. Algorithm settings focusing on larger spots can help accomplishing accurate spot counts.

Other artifacts like tissue remains, membrane cracks, dirt particles, pipette tip impressions, and so on can best be excludes by adapting a combination of parameters, led by the spot shape. Features in reader programs exist that allow removing counts manually which were caused by artifacts. The plate file needs to be annotated with such actions taken and specific software features are available to help accomplishing that.

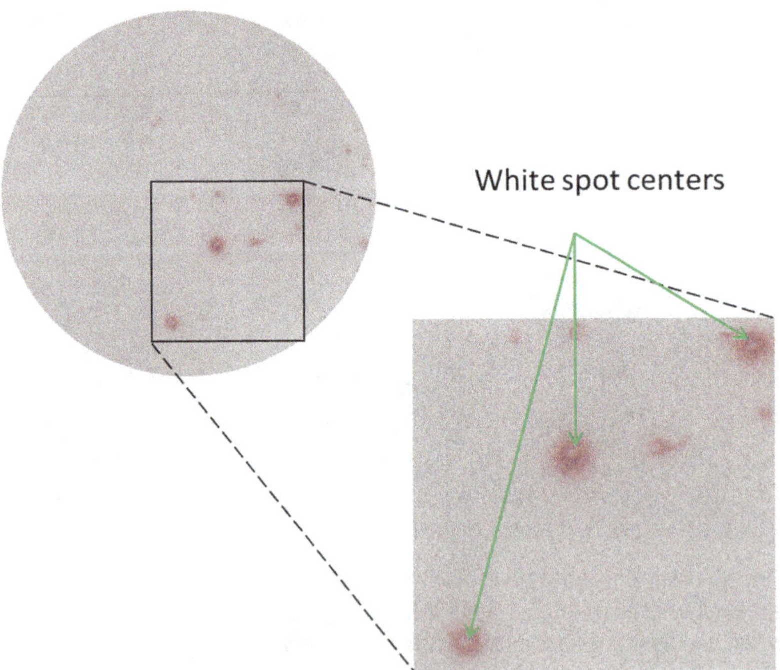

Fig. 14 White spot centers. A zoomed in well area is depicted (the original well image is shown in the left upper corner). Spots have a white spot center. Importantly, spots are otherwise not further disintegrated, especially not from the periphery. This feature is essential to distinguish the underlying mechanism from granulocyte contamination

A flow chart with each step and decision to be made including logistics behind those decisions during the evaluation process has been created in a large and field-spanning consensus process and is available in Nature Protocols [24].

The most important aspect of reading an Elispot plate is the acceptance of the following rule:

Algorithms and parameters are set assuming that all wells that are evaluated with them present themselves with similar conditions (this is the working hypothesis). Such conditions pertain to spot definition, background reactivity levels, background (membrane) staining, amount and appearance of artifacts, and spot crowdedness. It is recommended to set algorithms and spot parameters checking experimental wells that contain well-separated spots, and comparing them with the negative control wells (typically cells plus medium only). Often a fine-tuning of parameters is necessary by going back and forth between negative control and experimental wells. Each subject tested in an experiment should be tested for the applicability of the established set of reading parameters. It may be necessary to establish a new set of parameters for certain subjects, e.g., in case of high nonspecific background reactivity or evidence of cell death or granulocyte contamination.

Parameters must not be changed within a subject if conditions (as listed above) remain similar. However, this may not hold true through the entire experiment. As already elaborated on earlier, certain conditions can present with such high spot counts that algorithms and/or spot parameters have to be adjusted to allow efficient spot recognition. Not only does the overall background staining increases in crowded wells, but spot separation may be hampered, and even the average spot size may decrease. Such lowering in observed spot size can be caused by the high cytokine concentration within a well with an overwhelming number of responder cells, which inhibits fast diffusion of cytokine away from the cell that secretes it, hence spots may become smaller. The operator has to be aware though that adjusted parameter sets for crowded wells are typically not applicable for the remaining, "normal" wells and would lead to false high counts. It is hence advised to consider working with two parameter sets, one for wells falling under the working hypothesis, and one for wells that follow different rules, e.g., wells from mitogenic stimulation of cells and hence with very high spot numbers.

Certain circumstances require changes of applied parameters just for one well or a set of wells, e.g., when sporadic artifacts occur (e.g., crack in membrane, DNA precipitates). Wells should be annotated with the changes made and why changes were made.

An interesting phenomenon can occur in cases of suboptimal cell health that leads to an accumulation of small speckle artifacts due to ongoing cell death during incubation as described above. It may be possible that certain stimulation conditions activate enough cells early on within the plated sample that a flood of multiple cytokines is produced that promotes cell health. Such wells typically lack indications of cell death (artifacts) and instead present an abundance of well defined spots. Such scenario is demonstrated in Fig. 15.

Countless examples exists for "out of the norm" appearances of wells. Just a few have been shown here, and more examples can be found in previously referred to publications [24, 25]. The reader is advised to neglect existing and circulating dogmas to establish a reading parameter set once, and never change it again for the sake of consistency. Not one biological sample is exactly the same as another one. This is reflected in responder status to antigenic stimulation, in the number of cells secreting cytokines without the appropriate antigenic stimulation, in signs of bystander activation or lack thereof, in activation of NK cells, suppression, granulocyte contamination, degree of apoptosis, and so on. While creating a working set of algorithms and spot parameters for the evaluation of a specific set of plates run under the same Standard Operating Procedure (SOP), each sample requires to be checked for the applicability of the established reading parameters. Adjustments may be necessary to allow reliable evaluation of a specific sample. Annotations have to be made which and why certain adjustments to the parameters were made. Well conditions that do not follow the original working hypothesis (e.g., positive control wells) may require an own set of reading parameters. The Elispot evaluation process of biological samples should be guided by plausibility and transparency.

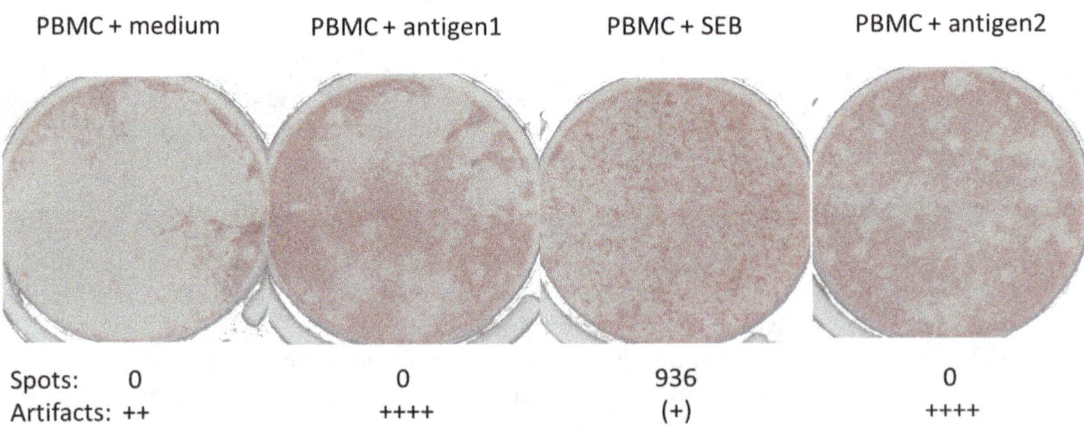

Fig. 15 Changing amount of artifacts within a sample. Four well images present different stimulation conditions for the same PBMC sample in an IFNγ Elispot. There are high amount of artifacts present in the negative control as well as in two different stimulations with peptide antigen. When cells are stimulated with SEB, the amount of artifacts decreases dramatically, and many well-defined spots are visible. The images were taken with a KS Elispot reader system (Carl Zeiss, Inc., Thornwood, NY)

4   Notes

1. For further guidance, it is recommended to use the Nature Protocols Guidelines on Elispot plate evaluation [24], and the recently published book addressing all three steps of Elispot [25].

2. Wet plates lead to the reflection of light during the scanning/evaluation process and artificially distorted well images. It is recommended to leave plates to dry in a dark place over night before evaluation.

3. Enzymatically developed Elispot plates produce spots that are stable for a prolonged time, typically weeks to months. Hence, it is acceptable if plates are evaluated after a reasonable delay.

4. The currently leading manufacturers of Elispot reader systems are A-ELIVS (http://www.aelvis.net/), AID (http://www.elispot.com/), Biosys (http://www.biosys.us/), and CTL (http://www.immunospot.com/). Various Zeiss imaging systems are also on the market, but the company has ceased their production. Each of the providers offers a range of different machines, covering basic enzymatic plate evaluation, evaluation of Fluorospot plates, different plate formats in addition to the standard 96-well plates (e.g., 24-well or 384-well plates), and other assays (e.g., viral plaque assays), as well as automation with robotic features for continuous loading capabilities of plates.

5. The Elispot reader should be checked and maintained by a representative of the manufacturer. Companies offer and provide various servicing plans for that. A yearly maintenance service will suffice for most users.

6. Elispot software should be continuously upgraded. It is recommended to use software that is compliant with 21 CFR Part 11, referring to the Code of Federal Regulations that defines the criteria under which electronic records and electronic signatures are considered to be trustworthy, reliable and equivalent to paper records. The capability of a program to log all activities taken once the software is started provides transparency to the evaluation approach.

7. The accurate representation of an Elispot plate is even more important in the light of the fact, that in large studies plates may be discarded, and that over time spots will start to fade away. Accuracy, trustworthiness and transparency come to mind as important guidance parameters especially for clinical studies.

8. Old and newer format Elispot plates from Millipore can be differentiated by the first two letters. Older plates start with a "MA" (e.g., MAHA or MAIP), while newer plates start with a "MS" (e.g., MSHA or MSIP). The actual membranes perform comparably. In addition to a straightened membrane, newer

format MS plates have an improved frame that reduces the temperature gradient within a plate, what leads to lower variability in spot counts from well to well, and permits automation compatibility.

9. There are various ways to deal with spot confluence. It is advisable to determine the Upper Limit of Quantitation (ULOQ) for an assay, which describes the highest spot number in a well that can be reliably distinguished. The ULOQ depends most of all on the average spot size. However, as shown before, the algorithm and spot parameters have to be optimized for spot discrimination. If well areas have spot confluence and are spared from evaluation, an option is to report that that well has more spots than the spot number determined to be the ULOQ. Various reader software programs let the user determine a degree of spot confluence that will be reported as TMTC = too many to count. It is also possible to obtain an estimate of the confluent area and to report the percentage of confluence that occurred in a well. Lastly, using that percentage, a total spot count for that well can be estimated by using an equation that assumes that the confluent area of a well contains at least double as many spots compared to the nonconfluent area. It is important to realize that an accurate spot count cannot be achieved for confluent wells, and even when extrapolating spot counts using such equation, the overall spot count is an estimate or approximation.

10. PVDF membranes are very hydrophobic. It is recommended to prewet PVDF plates before coating with a low amount (15–20 µl) of 70% Ethanol (pure). Higher volumes of Ethanol will promote leakage. The plate has to be taped for even distribution of the Ethanol, which can be recognized by the membranes turning entirely dark gray. The Ethanol needs to be washed out with PBS (three washes) before coating, which has to follow immediately in order to prevent wells to dry out, what would reset them to their initial hydrophobic state.

11. Efficient removal of cells after incubation is achieved with repeated (six times) rigorous washing with PBS/0.05% Tween 20. The washing step after cell incubation is the most important washing step in the entire protocol. Using a squirt bottle with the spout tip cut off for high volume flow suffices.

References

1. Czerkinsky CC, Nilsson LA, Nygren H, Ouchterlony O, Tarkowski A (1983) A solid-phase enzyme-linked immunospot (ELISPOT) assay for enumeration of specific antibody-secreting cells. J Immunol Methods 65: 109–121

2. Weiss AJ (2005) Membranes and membrane plates used in ELISPOT. Methods Mol Biol 302:33–50

3. Weiss AJ (2012) Overview of membranes and membrane plates used in research and diagnostic ELISPOT assays. Methods Mol Biol 792:243–256

4. Janetzki S, Panageas KS, Ben-Porat L, Boyer J, Britten CM, Clay TM, Kalos M, Maecker HT, Romero P, Yuan J, Kast WM, Hoos A (2008) Results and harmonization guidelines from two large-scale international Elispot proficiency panels conducted by the Cancer Vaccine Consortium (CVC/SVI). Cancer Immunol Immunother 57:303–315

5. Britten CM, Gouttefangeas C, Welters MJ, Pawelec G, Koch S, Ottensmeier C, Mander A, Walter S, Paschen A, Muller-Berghaus J, Haas I, Mackensen A, Kollgaard T, thor Straten P, Schmitt M, Giannopoulos K, Maier R, Veelken H, Bertinetti C, Konur A, Huber C, Stevanovic S, Wolfel T, van der Burg SH (2008) The CIMT-monitoring panel: a two-step approach to harmonize the enumeration of antigen-specific CD8+ T lymphocytes by structural and functional assays. Cancer Immunol Immunother 57:289–302

6. Mallone R, Mannering SI, Brooks-Worrell BM, Durinovic-Bello I, Cilio CM, Wong FS, Schloot NC (2011) Isolation and preservation of peripheral blood mononuclear cells for analysis of islet antigen-reactive T cell responses: position statement of the T-Cell Workshop Committee of the Immunology of Diabetes Society. Clin Exp Immunol 163:33–49

7. Janetzki S, Britten CM (2012) The impact of harmonization on ELISPOT assay performance. Methods Mol Biol 792:25–36

8. Cox JH, Ferrari G, Kalams SA, Lopaczynski W, Oden N, D'Souza M (2005) Results of an ELISPOT proficiency panel conducted in 11 laboratories participating in international human immunodeficiency virus type 1 vaccine trials. AIDS Res Hum Retrovir 21:68–81

9. Rountree W, Berrong M, Sanchez AM, Denny TN, Ferrari G (2016) Variability of the IFN-gamma ELISpot assay in the context of proficiency testing and bridging studies. J Immunol Methods 433:69–76

10. Janetzki S, Price L, Britten CM, van der Burg SH, Caterini J, Currier JR, Ferrari G, Gouttefangeas C, Hayes P, Kaempgen E, Lennerz V, Nihlmark K, Souza V, Hoos A (2010) Performance of serum-supplemented and serum-free media in IFNgamma Elispot Assays for human T cells. Cancer Immunol Immunother 59:609–618

11. van der Burg SH, Kalos M, Gouttefangeas C, Janetzki S, Ottensmeier C, Welters MJ, Romero P, Britten CM, Hoos A (2011) Harmonization of immune biomarker assays for clinical studies. Sci Transl Med 3:108ps144

12. ICH (1996.) I. C. o. H. Guidance for Industry: Q2B Validation of Analytical Procedures: Methodology

13. Tuomela M, Stanescu I, Krohn K (2005) Validation overview of bio-analytical methods. Gene Ther 12(Suppl 1):S131–S138

14. Janetzki S, Cox JH, Oden N, Ferrari G (2005) Standardization and validation issues of the ELISPOT assay. Methods Mol Biol 302:51–86

15. Mander A, Chowdhury F, Low L, Ottensmeier CH (2009) Fit for purpose? A case study: validation of immunological endpoint assays for the detection of cellular and humoral responses to anti-tumour DNA fusion vaccines. Cancer Immunol Immunother 58:789–800

16. Smith JG, Liu X, Kaufhold RM, Clair J, Caulfield MJ (2001) Development and validation of a gamma interferon ELISPOT assay for quantitation of cellular immune responses to varicella-zoster virus. Clin Diagn Lab Immunol 8:871–879

17. Patton K, Aslam S, Lin J, Yu L, Lambert S, Dawes G, Esser MT, Woo J, Janetzki S, Cherukuri A (2014) Enzyme-linked immunospot assay for detection of human respiratory syncytial virus f protein-specific gamma interferon-producing T cells. Clin Vaccine Immunol 21:628–635

18. Sahin U, Derhovanessian E, Miller M, Kloke BP, Simon P, Lower M, Bukur V, Tadmor AD, Luxemburger U, Schrors B, Omokoko T, Vormehr M, Albrecht C, Paruzynski A, Kuhn AN, Buck J, Heesch S, Schreeb KH, Muller F, Ortseifer I, Vogler I, Godehardt E, Attig S, Rae R, Breitkreuz A, Tolliver C, Suchan M, Martic G, Hohberger A, Sorn P, Diekmann J, Ciesla J, Waksmann O, Bruck AK, Witt M, Zillgen M, Rothermel A, Kasemann B, Langer D, Bolte S, Diken M, Kreiter S, Nemecek R, Gebhardt C, Grabbe S, Holler C, Utikal J, Huber C, Loquai C, Tureci O (2017) Personalized RNA mutanome vaccines mobilize poly-specific therapeutic immunity against cancer. Nature 547:222–226

19. Bestard O, Crespo E, Stein M, Lucia M, Roelen DL, de Vaal YJ, Hernandez-Fuentes MP, Chatenoud L, Wood KJ, Claas FH, Cruzado JM, Grinyo JM, Volk HD, Reinke P (2013) Cross-validation of IFN-gamma Elispot assay for measuring alloreactive memory/effector T cell responses in renal transplant recipients. Am J Transplant 13:1880–1890

20. Tureci O, Vormehr M, Diken M, Kreiter S, Huber C, Sahin U (2016) Targeting the hetero-

geneity of cancer with individualized neoepitope vaccines. Clin Cancer Res 22:1885–1896

21. Meier T, Eulenbruch HP, Wrighton-Smith P, Enders G, Regnath T (2005) Sensitivity of a new commercial enzyme-linked immunospot assay (T SPOT-TB) for diagnosis of tuberculosis in clinical practice. Eur J Clin Microbiol Infect Dis 24:529–536

22. Viklicky O, Hruba P, Tomiuk S, Schmitz S, Gerstmayer B, Sawitzki B, Miqueu P, Mrazova P, Tycova I, Svobodova E, Honsova E, Janssen U, Volk HD, Reinke P (2017) Sequential targeting of CD52 and TNF allows early minimization therapy in kidney transplantation: from a biomarker to targeting in a proof-of-concept trial. PLoS One 12:e0169624

23. Janetzki S, Schaed S, Blachere NE, Ben-Porat L, Houghton AN, Panageas KS (2004) Evaluation of Elispot assays: influence of method and operator on variability of results. J Immunol Methods 291:175–183

24. Janetzki S, Price L, Schroeder H, Britten CM, Welters MJ, Hoos A (2015) Guidelines for the automated evaluation of Elispot assays. Nat Protoc 10:1098–1115

25. Janetzki S (2016) Elispot for Rookies (And Experts Too). In: Kalyuzhny AE (ed) Techniques in life sciences and biomedicine for the non-expert. Springer, Cham, Switzerland

26. Schmielau J, Finn OJ (2001) Activated granulocytes and granulocyte-derived hydrogen peroxide are the underlying mechanism of suppression of t-cell function in advanced cancer patients. Cancer Res 61:4756–4760

27. De Rose R, Taylor EL, Law MG, van der Meide PH, Kent SJ (2005) Granulocyte contamination dramatically inhibits spot formation in AIDS virus-specific ELISpot assays: analysis and strategies to ameliorate. J Immunol Methods 297:177–186

28. McKenna KC, Beatty KM, Vicetti Miguel R, Bilonick RA (2009) Delayed processing of blood increases the frequency of activated CD11b+ CD15+ granulocytes which inhibit T cell function. J Immunol Methods 341:68–75

29. Bull M, Lee D, Stucky J, Chiu YL, Rubin A, Horton H, McElrath MJ (2007) Defining blood processing parameters for optimal detection of cryopreserved antigen-specific responses for HIV vaccine trials. J Immunol Methods 322:57–69

30. Kierstead LS, Dubey S, Meyer B, Tobery TW, Mogg R, Fernandez VR, Long R, Guan L, Gaunt C, Collins K, Sykes KJ, Mehrotra DV, Chirmule N, Shiver JW, Casimiro DR (2007) Enhanced rates and magnitude of immune responses detected against an HIV vaccine: effect of using an optimized process for isolating PBMC. AIDS Res Hum Retrovir 23:86–92

31. Janetzki S, Rabin R (2015) Enzyme-linked immunospot (elispot) for single-cell analysis. Methods Mol Biol 1346:27–46

32. Janetzki S, Rueger M, Dillenbeck T (2014) Stepping up ELISpot: multi-level analysis in fluorospot assays. Cell 3:1102–1115

33. Moodie Z, Price L, Gouttefangeas C, Mander A, Janetzki S, Lower M, Welters MJ, Ottensmeier C, van der Burg SH, Britten CM (2010) Response definition criteria for ELISPOT assays revisited. Cancer Immunol Immunother 59:1489–1501

34. Moodie Z, Price L, Janetzki S, Britten CM (2012) Response determination criteria for ELISPOT: toward a standard that can be applied across laboratories. Methods Mol Biol 792:185–196

Chapter 3

Essential Controls for ELISpot Assay

Jodi Hagen and Alexander E. Kalyuzhny

Abstract

Nonspecific staining in ELISpot assay is a major obstacle in accurate quantification of experimental data. The appearance of nonspecific spots may be caused by different factors including cell- and immunoassay-related issues. In our study, we have shown that nonspecific spots can result from either cells or their debris sticking to the membranes in ELISpot plates, as well as by impurities in wash buffers and precipitation of aggregated detection antibodies. Although there is a growing interest in using Fluorospot assays allowing for simultaneous detection of multiple cell-secreted proteins, it appears that these fluorescence assays are more susceptible to developing nonspecific profiles resembling specific spots. In this chapter, we outline necessary ELISpot controls that need to be employed to tell the difference between bona fide spots vs. stained artifacts.

Key words ELISpot, Mitogens, Nonspecific spots, Positive control, Negative control

1 Introduction

ELISpot assay represents a combination of both bioassay and immunoassay components [1–5]. It belongs to bioassays because it analyzes the protein secretion capacity of live cells, and maintaining the viability and physiology of these cells is extremely critical for obtaining accurate and reliable data. Chemistry-wise, ELISpot belongs—like ELISA—to sandwich immunoassay, utilizing capture and detection antibodies as its key components [3, 6]. The end-point of ELISpot assay is colored spots of different sizes (2–70 μm) scattered on the surface of the PVDF membranes backing the 96-well plates [4]. Based on spectral characteristic of the spots, there are two types of ELISpot assays: chromogenic bright-field and fluorescence dark-field (e.g., Fluorospots) [4, 7–11]. Spot formation in chromogenic assays is based on the conversion of colorless substrate (e.g., AEC and BCIP/NBT) by enzymes (e.g., HRP and alkaline phosphatase) into colored precipitate. Fluorospots are based on using detection antibodies directly conjugated to fluorescent probes and do not utilize any enzymatic

Alexander E. Kalyuzhny (ed.), *Handbook of ELISPOT: Methods and Protocols*, Methods in Molecular Biology, vol. 1808, https://doi.org/10.1007/978-1-4939-8567-8_3, © Springer Science+Business Media, LLC, part of Springer Nature 2018

conversion of substrates [11]. Regardless of the type of ELISpot assay, resulting spots may be either specific (depicting bona fide cell-secreted protein) or nonspecific (unrelated to secreted proteins). Specific and nonspecific spots may have comparable size and morphology, which makes it difficult or even impossible to separate one from the other when counting using ELISpot readers built around machine-vision detection algorithms. This situation becomes even more dramatic when doing large-scale ELISpot runs with tens or hundreds of plates and it is not practical for the operator to analyze each well for specific vs. nonspecific spots.

There are several reasons for the appearance of nonspecific spots:

(a) Staining of cells sticking to the bottom of the wells

(b) Precipitation of chromogenic substrates

(c) Precipitation of detection antibodies

(d) Contaminants in the culture medium

(e) Debris of dead cells

(f) Contaminants in wash buffers

(g) Dust from lab coats and paper towels (these are particularly problematic in Fluorospots because they autofluoresce)

In this chapter, we outline controls that can be performed for side-by-side comparison with experimental data. For the sake of example, we show data obtained using human IFN gamma ELISpot assay, but the same principles apply to ELISpot assays analyzing the secretion of other proteins.

2 Materials

2.1 Cell Preparation

1. Cell separation media: Ficoll-Paque ™ PLUS.

2. PBS: 50 mM phosphate-buffered saline, pH 7.2.

3. Red blood cell lysing solution: 155 mM NH_4Cl, 10 mM $NaHCO_3$, and 0.1 mM EDTA.

4. Culture media: RPMI 1640 media supplemented with 50 mL of heat-inactivated fetal bovine serum, 1× Penicillin/Streptomycin (*see* **Note 1**).

5. Centrifuge for spinning 50 mL culture tubes at $500 \times g$.

6. Hemacytometer to count human PBMCs under the microscope to determine cell dilution.

7. Trypan Blue Dye for the staining of dead cells.

8. Upright bright-field microscope equipped with phase-contrast illumination.

2.2 ELISpot Assay

1. Commercially available, ELISpot ready-to-use kits to measure secretion of Human IFNγ (R&D Systems, Inc., Catalog #EL285).

2. PBS: 137 mM NaCl, 2.7 mM KCl; 8.1 mM Na_2HPO_4; 1.5 mM KH_2PO_4; pH 7.2–7.4. Sterile filtered through 0.2 μm filter.

3. Mitogens to stimulate release of cytokines from human PBMCs: Calcium Ionomycin (CaI) and phorbol 12-myristate 13-acetate (PMA).

4. CEF peptide pool to stimulate CD8+ T-cells (Anaspec; Freemont, CA).

5. Hand-held Nunc-Immuno™ 12-plate washer.

6. ELISpot plate reader QuantiHub (http://www.mvspacific.com).

3 Methods

3.1 Cell Preparation

1. Obtain samples of fresh blood from donors.

2. Using density centrifugation separation, layer 10 mL of leukocyte concentrated blood from donor mixed with 15 mL of 1× PBS on 20 mL of Ficoll-Paque ™ PLUS at 25 °C and centrifuge at $500 \times g$ for 30 min (*see* **Note 2**).

3. Discard the top layer after centrifugation and transfer PBMCs (buffy coat layer) into sterile 50 mL tube.

4. Resuspend isolated PBMCs in 45 mL of sterile PBS and centrifuged for 5 min at $500 \times g$.

5. Discard the supernatant, rack tube and resuspend the pellet in 10 mL of red blood cell lysing solution and incubate for 10 min at room temperature.

6. After lysing, add sterile PBS to reach 50 mL graduation mark on the tube to resuspend PBMCs.

7. Centrifuge tubes for 5 min at $500 \times g$.

8. Discard supernatants and add 40–50 mL of RPMI complete to the tubes with PBMCs (*see* **Note 3**).

9. Mix a small sample of cells 1:2 with trypan blue dye and pipette 10 μL of this mixture into each side of a hemacytometer under a coverslip. Count cells under the microscope using 20× lens and phase-contrast condenser (*see* **Note 4**).

3.2 ELISpot Assay

1. Plate PBMCs (100 μL/well) into the ELISpot plates at cell concentrations of 1×10^5 cells/mL and 5×10^5 cells/mL (*see* **Notes 5** and **6**).

2. Add RPMI cell culture media without addition of PBMCs (background control), unstimulated PBMCs (unstimulated/negative

control), and reconstituted recombinant protein (positive control) to plate and then stimulate PBMCs with 0.5 μg/mL CaI and 50 ng/mL PMA or 1 μg/mL of CEF peptide pool added directly to cells in ELISpot plates and incubated in a humidified CO_2 incubator at 37 °C for 18 h (*see* **Note 7**).

3. After finishing the incubations, aspirate cells from the plates and wash the plate by rinsing wells four times with ELISpot wash buffer (*see* **Note 8**).

4. Add dilution buffer 1 to some wells of the plate for detection antibody control. Make working solutions of detection antibodies by diluting concentrated detection antibody 1:120 in dilution buffer 1.

5. Add 100 μL of detection antibody working solution into each well and incubate ELISpot plates overnight at 4 °C.

6. Wash plates three times with the wash buffer (*see* **Note 9**).

7. Prepare working solution of streptavidin-alkaline phosphatase by mixing the concentrated stock solution 1:120 with dilution buffer 2.

8. Add 100 μL of streptavidin-alkaline phosphatase working solution into each well and incubate for 2 h at room temperature.

9. Wash plates three times with wash buffer.

10. Add 100 μL of ready-to-use BCIP/NBT substrate into each well and incubate for 30–60 min at room temperature in a place protected from direct light.

11. Wash plates three times with distilled water and let them dry completely (*see* **Note 10**).

12. Quantify spots using automated ELISpot reader.

3.3 ELISpot Assay Controls

Figure 1 illustrates a cross section through a typical specific spot developed with alkaline phosphatase substrate BCIP/NBT, which labels cytokine spreading around the cell from which it was secreted. It is clearly shown that diffusion of the cytokines mostly occurs in the lateral rather than vertical direction of the PVDF membrane. A major advantage of PVDF membrane is its high porosity that provides a large surface area for the immobilization of capture antibodies, which is critical for ELISpot assay sensitivity. The density of spots depends on the number of plated cells (Fig. 2), and if the number of cells is too high (in ELISpot jargon, the "plate is overloaded") it will cause the production of an excessive number of spots merging into large-size blobs that are difficult or impossible to analyze. In addition to being an excellent material for the immobilization of capture antibodies, PVDF membrane has a strong tendency to "capture" cells, aggregated antibodies, and impurities from reagents it contacts during assay development. Artifacts may be counted by ELISpot readers as specific spots, thereby contributing to erroneous data

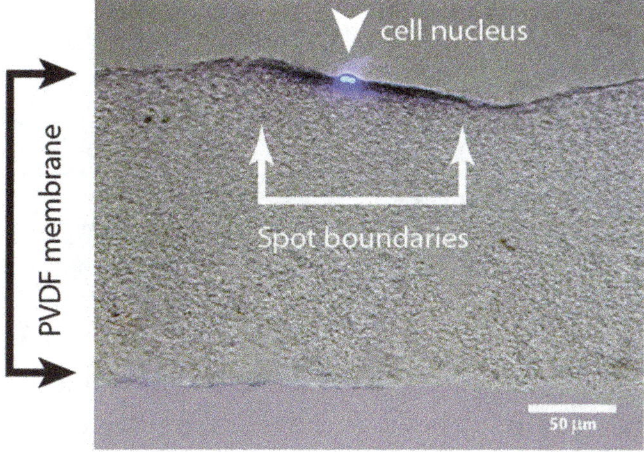

Fig. 1 Anatomy of a typical spot. After finishing the ELISpot assay developed with BCIP/NBT chromogen and immobilizing cells to the PVDF membrane, the membrane was removed from the plate and sectioned on the cryostat in a perpendicular direction. DAPI was used to counterstain the nuclei of immobilized cells (arrowhead). Spot boundaries indicate that cell-secreted proteins can migrate away from the cell in distances that exceed the size of the cell 3–5 times

analysis. Figure 3 shows a high magnification of the PVDF membrane from the developed ELISpot assay with chromogenic dye depicting cells and their debris sticking to the membrane. Many of these profiles resemble specific spots, which would most likely be counted by ELISpot readers. The situation becomes even more dramatic when using fluorescent tags for detection in Fluorospot: dust particles from clothing, lab coats, and air can easily stick to the PVDF membrane and either autofluoresce or reflect epifluorescent light, mimicking specific fluorescent spots (Fig. 4).

It is advisable to optimize assay conditions to minimize the appearance of nonspecific spots, which can be accomplished by employing different types of controls.

1. Cell-based controls.

    These are negative controls intended to determine whether formed spots are a product of cultured cells or artifacts caused by precipitation of reagents.

    (a) No-detection antibody control: ELISpot is performed as usual but with the addition of detection antibodies. Specific spots are not supposed to form and the membrane is expected to look like Fig. 5. The appearance of spots indicates the precipitation of reagents, and the simplest way to troubleshoot this would be the filtration of reagents before adding them to ELISpot plate.

    (b) No-cell stimulation control: ELISpot is performed as usual, but cells are not stimulated with reagents that stim-

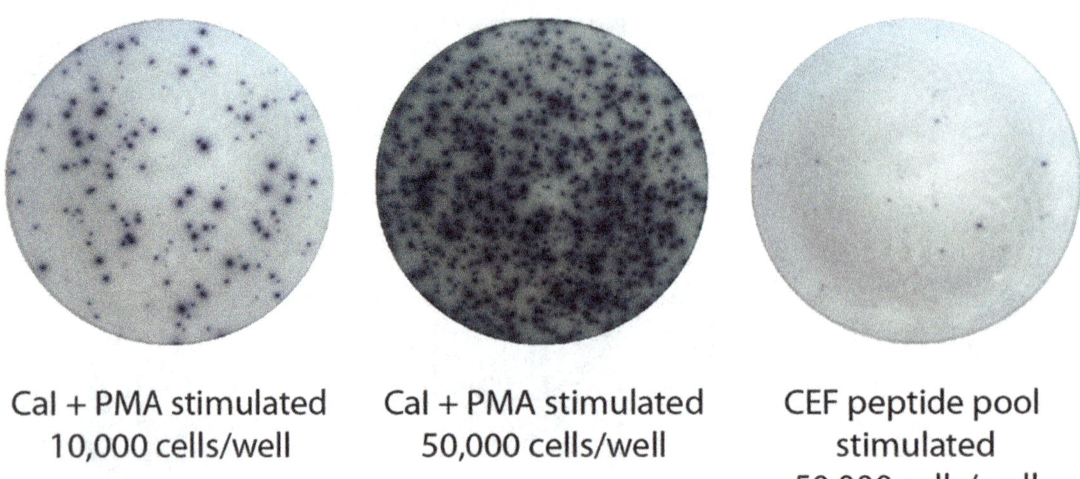

Fig. 2 Specific spots generated by treating cells with different mitogens. The number of spots can vary significantly depending on the number of cells per well and on mitogens used. Note the dramatic difference in the number of spots produced by the same number of cells treated with either Cal + PMA or CEF peptide pool. These images are examples of what appear to be specific spots

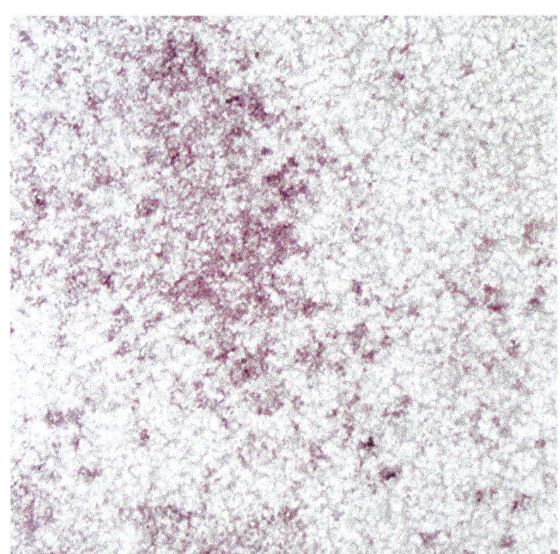

Fig. 3 Example of nonspecific spots generated by cells sticking to PVDF membrane in the ELISpot plate. Cells sticking to the PVDF membrane in the ELISpot plate can be the source of a signal that resembles spots formed by cell-secreting proteins. This image illustrates nonspecific spots using HRP-AEC chromogenic detection (red color)

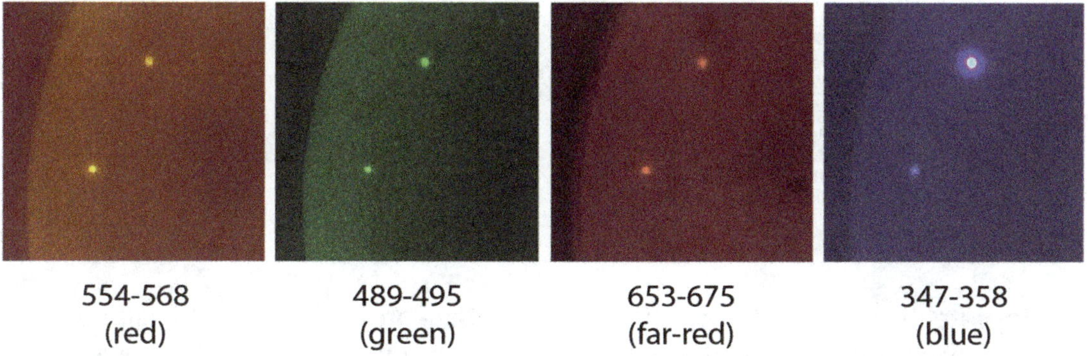

Emission (nanometers and color range)

Fig. 4 Nonspecific spots in FluoroSpot assays. Nonspecific spots are frequently observed in Fluorospot assays. Unlike specific spots detected using a fluorophore with a known emission spectrum (e.g., either red or green), nonspecific spots fluoresce within a broad spectral range (*see* **Note 11**)

ulate the secretion of proteins from cells. The appearance of spots indicates either the precipitation of reagents and/ or the cells stuck to the PVDF membrane, which absorb developing reagents nonspecifically and become stained, resembling spots. The way to troubleshoot this would be to filter the reagents before adding them to the ELISpot plate and checking the viability of plated cells, because dying cells are sticky. We have found that dead cells can adhere more strongly to the membrane than live cells, and with a high number of dead cells (30–50% or more) the density of nonspecific spots may be quite profound. Therefore, it is of critical importance to determine the percentage of dead cells before plating them to the ELISpot plate. If the appearance of nonspecific spots is due to stained cells that have stuck to the membrane, it may be advisable to use cell removal reagents [12].

2. Immunoassay controls.

Because ELISpot is a combination of bioassay and immunoassay [3], it is necessary to find out whether reagents are working properly and are suitable to perform the assay.

(a) No-cell control: This is a negative control when ELISpot assay is performed as usual but cells are not added to the plate. Figure 5 illustrates what would be considered an acceptable no-cell control. If spots are developing, this indicates the aggregation of antibodies and impurities in staining regents and the wash buffer. Filtration should help to get rid of contaminants.

(b) Positive control: ELISpot assay is run as usual, but a matching recombinant protein is added instead of cells (e.g., in IFNγ ELISpot add recombinant IFNγ). If the

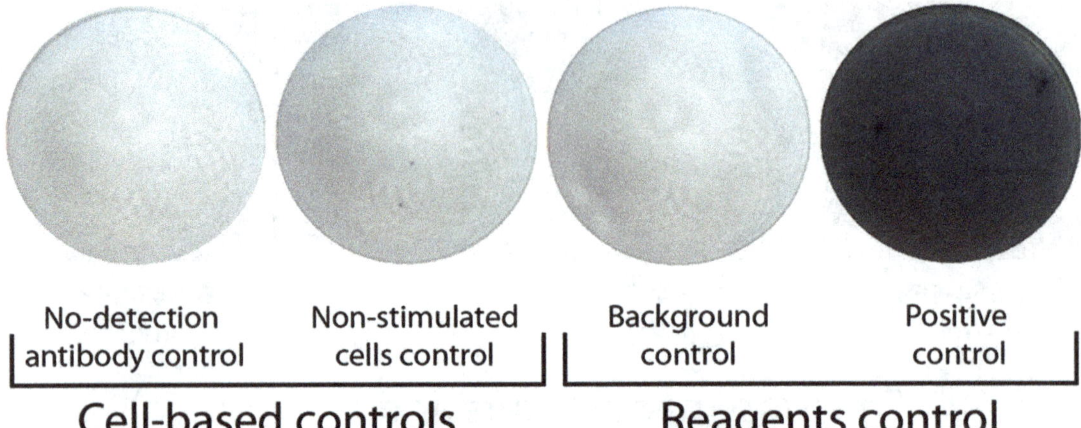

Fig. 5 Controls recommended for running side by side with experimental groups. Several controls are recommended to make sure that experimental conditions and reagents are not causing the formation of nonspecific spots: (1) Background control—complete ELISpot development with no cells added to wells; (2) No-detection antibody control—cells are added to the wells but ELISpot development omits adding detection antibodies; (3) Non-stimulated cells control—complete ELISpot development using non-stimulated cells (*see* **Note 12**); and (4) Immunoassay control—complete ELISpot development adding a corresponding recombinant protein rather than stimulated cells

reagents are working properly, then the entire well will become stained as shown in Fig. 5. This is an important control because it provides confidence that the immunoassay is working properly.

4   Notes

1. When using fetal calf serum, it is important to heat-inactivate the serum at 56 °C for 30 min. After heat inactivation, the serum should be filtered.

2. Be sure to turn off the brake for the initial centrifugation with Ficoll so that the layers of blood and Ficoll do not mix while the centrifuge is coming to a stop.

3. Sterilize RPMI-complete culture medium and filter reagents that will be used to separate out the white blood cells through a 0.2 μm sterile filter.

4. Overfilling the hemacytometer with cell solution may result in inaccurate cell quantification. When counting cells on a hemacytometer, first locate the middle square that contains 25 smaller squares and count cells in 5 of them. Calculate the average, multiply by 25 (total number of squares in that area), then multiply by 2 (cell dilution factor), and then multiply by 10,000 to determine the number of cells in 1 mL of the original cell suspension. The resulting number should be used for

calculating serial dilutions of PBMCs. To avoid counting cells more than once, pick two sides of each of the squares on the hemacytometer that you will be counting and keep that consistent throughout the rest of the count.

5. Making serial dilutions of cells allows the user to avoid over-development of the ELISpot plate and obtain a quantifiable number of spots that can be counted either manually or by using an automated ELISpot reader. The intensity of the staining depends on the number of cells plated into the well—the addition of an excessive number of cells per well may result in over-staining due to a specific background (see above). Since the secretion capacity of cells is not known in advance, it is always recommended to test the serial dilution of cells from each individual donor (e.g., 10^3, 10^4, 10^5, 10^6 cells per well) in the same ELISPOT plate. This ensures having enough data points to choose from in case over- or under-development occurs. Using cells of unknown secretion capacity requires dedicating many wells in the plate for cell optimization rather than for experimental groups. The solution to this problem is to preserve cell suspensions, freeze them, and store them in liquid nitrogen.

6. For better well-to-well reproducibility, cells need to be mixed thoroughly before adding them into the wells. This may require systematically shaking the tube with cells after filling every four wells in the ELISpot plate. Adding aluminum foil to the bottom of the plate allows for even heat distribution and can help prevent the "edge effect" of the plate in which the cells migrate to the side wells of the plate where the plastic is warmer. Multiple washes ensure that cells are removed from the plate eliminating wells from being developed with a "sand" effect on the membrane caused by cells sticking to it. It is also acceptable to have a brief incubation (5 min) with a cell dissociation media to ensure the complete removal of cells. Wrapping ELISPOT plates into aluminum foil reduces background staining and improves contrast. It also produces a more uniform distribution of specific spots across the filter membrane [13]. In addition, the application of foil appears to improve well-to-well reproducibility. The reason aluminum foil reduces background staining is not known, but it is tempting to speculate that aluminum foil facilitates even distribution of heat over the bottom of ELISPOT plate during its incubation in the CO_2 incubator.

7. Shelves in the CO_2 incubator must be leveled to avoid having cells drift toward one side of the well. This may produce either under- or over-developed parts of the well and hinder the quantification of spots. It is also important to avoid disturbing cultured cells (e.g., by slamming the door of the incubator)

during incubation, which may cause the development of weakly stained fuzzy spots.

8. Filter the wash buffer through a 0.45 μm filter to exclude impurities from the sorption to the PVDF membranes in the ELISpot plates. Microparticles sticking to the membrane may become stained and mistakenly counted by the ELISpot analyzer as specific spots.

9. Multiple washes ensure that cells are removed from the plate, eliminating wells from being developed with a "sand" effect on the membrane caused by cells sticking to it. It is also acceptable to have a brief incubation (5 min) with a cell dissociation media to ensure the complete removal of cells. Make sure that the height of the prongs in the hand-held plate washer is properly adjusted so the prongs do not touch the membranes on the bottom of the ELISpot plate. The PVDF membranes on the ELISpot plate are fragile and can be easily punctured by protruding prongs.

10. When the PVDF membranes in the ELISpot plate are wet, they will look completely dark, which may create the impression of overstaining. Before counting spots, plates need to be completely dry. Wells that have not dried completely will give inaccurate spot counts and spots will appear fuzzy or not well defined.

11. To make sure fluorescent spots are specific rather than artifactual, it is helpful to analyze staining under different filters. Unlike specific spots, nonspecific ones will fluoresce under different filters emitting different colors. However, the technique of changing filters is not very helpful when analyzing cells co-secreting different cytokines detected with fluorescent dyes of different colors.

12. Some cytokines, like TNF-alpha and Granzyme B, are secreted from unstimulated cells. Therefore, no-stimulation cell controls are not helpful when analyzing secretion of these proteins.

References

1. Sedgwick JD, Holt PG (1983) A solid-phase immunoenzymatic technique for the enumeration of specific antibody-secreting cells. J Immunol Methods 57(1–3):301–309

2. Czerkinsky CC, Nilsson LA, Nygren H et al (1983) A solid-phase enzyme-linked immunospot (ELISPOT) assay for enumeration of specific antibody-secreting cells. J Immunol Methods 65(1–2):109–121

3. Kalyuzhny AE (2005) Chemistry and biology of the ELISPOT assay. Methods Mol Biol 302:15–31

4. Kalyuzhny AE (2009) ELISPOT assay on membrane microplates. Methods Mol Biol 536:355–365

5. Czerkinsky C, Moldoveanu Z, Mestecky J, Nilsson LA, Ouchterlony O (1988) A novel two colour ELISPOT assay. I. Simultaneous

    detection of distinct types of antibody-secreting cells. J Immunol Methods 115(1):31–37

6. Kemeny DM (1997) Enzyme-linked immunoassays. In: Johnstone AP, Turner MW (eds) Immunochemistry 1. Oxford University Press, Oxford, pp 147–175

7. Kalyuzhny AE (2015) Membrane microplates for one- and two-color ELISPOT and FLUOROSPOT assays. Methods Mol Biol 1312:435–437

8. Gazagne A, Claret E, Wijdenes J et al (2003) A FluoroSpot assay to detect single T lymphocytes simultaneously producing multiple cytokines. J Immunol Methods 283(1–2):91–98

9. Gazagne A, Malkusch W, Vingert B et al (2005) FluoroSpot assay: methodological analysis. Methods Mol Biol 302:289–296

10. Rebhahn JA, Bishop C, Divekar AA et al (2008) Automated analysis of two- and three-color fluorescent ELISpot (FluoroSpot) assays for cytokine secretion. Comput Methods Prog Biomed 92(1):54–65

11. Ahlborg N, Axelsson B (2012) Dual- and triple-color FluoroSpot. Methods Mol Biol 792:77–85

12. Grant A, Palzer S, Hartnett C et al (2005) A cell-detachment solution can reduce background staining in the ELISPOT assay. Methods Mol Biol 302:87–94

13. Kalyuzhny A, Stark S (2001) A simple method to reduce the background and improve well-to-well reproducibility of staining in ELISPOT assays. J Immunol Methods 257:93–97

Chapter 4

Automatic Search of Spots and Color Classification in ELISPOT Assay

Sergey S. Zadorozhny and Nikolai N. Martynov

Abstract

Accuracy of spot detection and classification plays a critical role in the analysis of ELISPOT data. Differences in staining intensities of spots and their morphological variations make it difficult developing a reliable software application. An image recognition method allowing the automatic detection and classification of round objects (spots) on ELISPOT images independently of the registration conditions was developed. The emphasis is done on objects of elliptical shape, which is typical for a wide range of spots. It can be analyzed by both monochrome and a dual-color version of our software. The method of subdivision of objects into groups is also described which is based on color attributes of spots.

Key words ELISPOT, Image analysis, Spot recognition, Spot detection, Mathematical algorithm, Dual-color ELISPOT

---

1 Introduction

Accuracy of spot detection and quantification plays a critical role in the analysis of ELISPOT data. Differences in staining intensities of spots make it difficult developing a reliable software application, especially for ELISPOT with two spot types.

It is well known that identical objects can look dramatically different depending on illumination conditions and optical characteristics of illuminated objects. This hinders the analysis and interpretation of the objects in the field of view when image processing must be independent of its registration conditions. For solving such problems, morphological image analysis methods were designed and they proved their efficiency [1, 2].

Mathematical notion of the form comprises the foundation of such methods. The form (e.g., profile or shape of the spot) is the maximum invariant of image transformations that take place under various registration conditions using different cameras and so on [1]. That is why the form is defined not only by the analyzed object and by the scene it is on, but is also connected with the model of

Alexander E. Kalyuzhny (ed.), *Handbook of ELISPOT: Methods and Protocols*, Methods in Molecular Biology, vol. 1808,
https://doi.org/10.1007/978-1-4939-8567-8_4, © Springer Science+Business Media, LLC, part of Springer Nature 2018

scene (or object) registration being the fundamental part of morphological analysis.

In some practical cases, the profiles of objects are predefined. For example, the spots in ELISPOT assay (including dual-color ELISPOT assays) are either round or have a concentric profile. This makes it possible to solve a variety of application problems related to detecting and classifying such objects.

The method of image recognition allowing automatic detection and counting of spots on ELISPOT images with two spot types, independently of the registration conditions, is proposed.

2   Materials

1. Standard IBM-PC compatible personal computer was used running under Microsoft Windows 10 operating system.

2. Microsoft C++ compiler was used to compile the software described in this chapter.

3. Test images, captured using color industrial Unibrain Fire-i 785c video camera (www.unibrain.com), were collected by MVS Pacific, LLC (www.mvspacific.com).

3   Methods

3.1   Algorithm

1. *Image form construction.*

   Image form construction is a substantial part of the morphological analysis. The quality of form construction greatly influences the ultimate result of morphological analysis. For example, the round objects can be described in terms of a set of concentric circles, whereas the image composed of linear object can be described in terms of a set of narrow parallel bars and so on.

2. *Objects comparison based on image form.*

   Let us define the image form by defining the sets of constant brightness in the visual field X. Let set V_f be the set of all images with forms what is not more compound than the form of image f.

   From this set to choose the image having the best approximation of image g, we need to solve the following extreme problem:

   $$\| P_f g - g \|^2 = \inf \left\{ \| f' - g \| \big| f' \in V_f \right\}. \qquad (1)$$

   where operator P_f is the orthogonal projector on the linear image space with forms not more complicated than the form of image f:

$$P_f g = \sum_i \frac{\left(\chi_i\left(x,y\right)g\right)}{\|\chi_i\left(x,y\right)\|^2}\,\chi_i\left(x,y\right) = \sum_i C_i \chi_i\left(x,y\right) \qquad (2)$$

Here $\chi_i(x,y)$ is the indicating function of i field of image f. It is equal to one in inner i field dots and equal to zero in other dots, C_i—the brightness of i field of the chosen image.

Not more complicated than f image constructed by means of combination of brightness levels C_i.

So, $P_f g$ is the best approximation for image g by images with forms not more complicated than the form of image f.

Consequently, the image $P_f g - g$ represents all form distinctions between image f and image g and it called the "residual image." Functional $\|P_f g - g\|$ could be used as the measure of form difference between image g and image f. However, this algorithm for low-contrast images is error-prone because any low-contrast image is similar to any other image (brightness levels coincide). That is why the measure of the similarity by form is defined as the following ratio:

$$t_f g = \frac{\|P_f g - g\|}{\|P_f g - P_0 g\|}, \qquad (3)$$

where P_0 is the projector of image g on constant image $P_0 g = \dfrac{\left(\chi_X g\right)}{\|\chi_X\|^2}\,\chi_X$ (indicating function χ_X c is equal to one in the whole view angle X).

Let us state the obvious features of the functional Eq. 3. The less the value of the functional, the more the similarity between the image g and the image f and the farther it is from constant. In real situations, if the image g is close to constant, then the denominator of the fraction is small and is comparable to the nominator of the fraction. If the image g is not more complicated than the image f by form and is not a constant, then the fraction equals zero. At last, if the image g is not similar to image f by form and differs from the constant, then the numerator and denominator of the fraction are approximately equal to each other.

3.2 Morphological Approach to Search for Objects

According to this theory, the problem of searching for objects formulated as follows:

1. Let g be the image with some objects inside.

2. Let f be the ideal image defined on some subspace of the view field X.

3. The problem is to find positions of all objects on image g with forms close to ideal image f.

When objects are spots of a circular profile, then we may choose an ideal image as decomposition of a view field into rings with 1–2 pixels width.

As a result, a search process reduced to the following procedure:

1. Define the window over the given image with dimensions equal to dimensions of the ideal image. This window scans the image progressively meanwhile processing the part of the given image under the window.

2. The fragment of the given image under the window compared to the ideal image according to the criterion defined by functional (Eq. 3).

3. Local minimums retrieved after calculating the value of the functional in each pixel inside the image. All points (pixels) with minimum values less than some threshold are associated with centers of the spots.

Figure 1 shows the typical results of the search process based on described morphological method. Figure 1a illustrates an even illumination situation (background is almost uniform), whereas Fig. 1b shows the example of a no uniform illumination.

As it comes from these examples, sharp round spots are easily detected, whereas blurred spots of uncertain shape remained not detected.

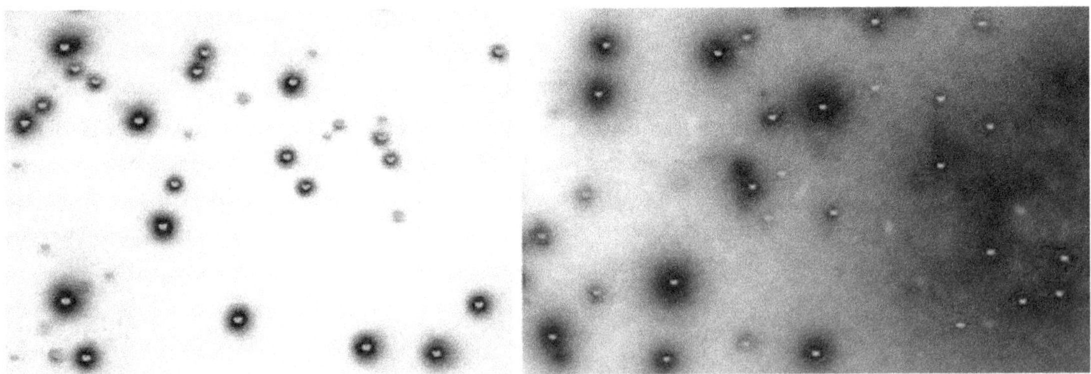

Fig. 1 Effects of illumination conditions on the results of the automated search process. (**a**) Field of view in bottom of the ELISPOT well is evenly illuminated which results in almost a uniform background. (**b**) Illumination is uneven and as a result, the software easily detects sharp round spots, whereas blurry spots that have irregular form may remain undetected

3.3 Classification of Color Spots

There are situations when detecting the correct color of the spot is important for accurate diagnostics: in dual-color ELISPOT assays, the color of the spot not only provides means for recognizing spots, but also serves as a marker of the type of a secreted cytokine. The problem of color classification is well known and can be solved by image analysis algorithms for spot detection cluster analysis [3] which subdivides sets of objects by associating them with some classes based on the mathematical criterion of classification quality. This criterion must reflect somehow the following no formal demands:

1. Inside the groups, objects are closely connected to each other.
2. Objects of different groups are quite distant from each other.

The central point in cluster analysis is the choice of metrics (measure of proximity of objects to each other). The choice of metrics greatly influences the ultimate result of subdivision of objects into groups according to a given algorithm of the dividing process. This choice is closely correlated with main goals of the research in whole, with physical and statistical nature of utilized information, etc.

Another important feature of cluster analysis is the measure of proximity between groups of objects (*see* **Note 1**).

Cluster analysis algorithms vary significantly. For example, these may be algorithms targeting a linear search of either object combinations or random division of object set. The majority of such algorithms consist of two groups. The first group is intended for initial (possibly, artificial or arbitrary) subdivision of objects set into classes and a certain criterion of the quality of automatic classification is defined. The second group of algorithms intended for objects that interchanged between classes until the value of criterion quits refining.

Let's go over the most popular proximity measures characterizing mutual disposition of groups of objects.

Let WI is the i-th group of objects, N_i—the number of objects in the group w_i, vector μ_i—arithmetic mean of objects in w_i, and $q(w_n, w_m)$— the distance between groups w_n and w_m.

The nearest neighbor distance is the distance between the closest objects of the clusters:

$$q_{\min}\left(w_n, w_m\right) = \min_{x_i \in w_n, x_j \in w_m} d\left(x_i, x_j\right) \tag{4}$$

The farthest neighbor distance is the distance between the farthest objects of the clusters:

$$q_{\max}\left(w_n, w_m\right) = \max_{x_i \in w_n, x_j \in w_m} d\left(x_i, x_j\right) \tag{5}$$

The centroid distance is the distance between the central points of the clusters:

$$q\left(w_1, w_m\right) = d\left(\mu_1, \mu_m\right) \tag{6}$$

The choice of the measure of the distance between the clusters affects the outline of the geometrical groups of objects generated by cluster analysis algorithms in the feature space. Those algorithms based on the nearest neighbor distance are adequate in a specific case of groups have complicated chain structure. On the other hand, the algorithms based on determining the farthest neighbor distance are suitable for spheroid clouds in a feature space. The centroid distance algorithms occupy the intermediate position and satisfy the specific case of objects with ellipsoid shape (*see* **Note 2**).

Problem of grouping ELISPOT spots based on their color features easily solved because typically it contains no more than two groups.

First, the farthest spots from the whole set of detected spots are determined. If there are only two clusters, then these spots must belong to different clusters and proximity measure according to Eq. 5.

Then, the iteration continues for all other spots and they are associated with either first or a second cluster corresponding to their distance from the earlier-found farthest spots.

Finally, Eqs. 4 and 6 used as a proximity criterion for clusters. If the distance calculated according to above formulas is less than some critical value, then the subdivision of two clusters is not valid: there are more than two clusters in the set of objects.

Figure 2 illustrates a color subdivision of spots in dual-color ELISPOT images.

3.4 Practical Application of the Method

The described methods are a useful mathematical foundation of software application for counting spots in ELISPOT assays [4]. However, a mathematical method is not sufficient itself for obtaining accurate and reliable quantification results (*see* **Note 3**).

It is impossible to correctly interpret whether the spots are too small or too big. It has to point out that the information about the mean value of spots dimensions and a mean value of their deviations has a critical importance (*see* **Note 4**).

That is why many other systems need precise manual adjustments to compensate for different image capture conditions. Using algorithms described above, we have developed a QuantiHub software (distributed by MVS Pacific LLC, http://www.mvspacific.com) which utilizes a different approach: adjustments for fixed image capture conditions are done beforehand.

QuantiHub software is capable of automatic processing of the images captured from the ELISPOT plates (including dual-analyze ELISPOT assays) in 1–2–3–4 predefined spot-counting modes.

QuantiHub version for single-color ELISPOT assays (Versions 3.6 or less) was released in 2002 and completely redeveloped in 2017 (Version 6.1) allowing quantification of both single-analyze (single-color detection) and two-analyze (dual-color detection) ELISPOT assays. The system utilizes Unibrain Fire-i 785c camera

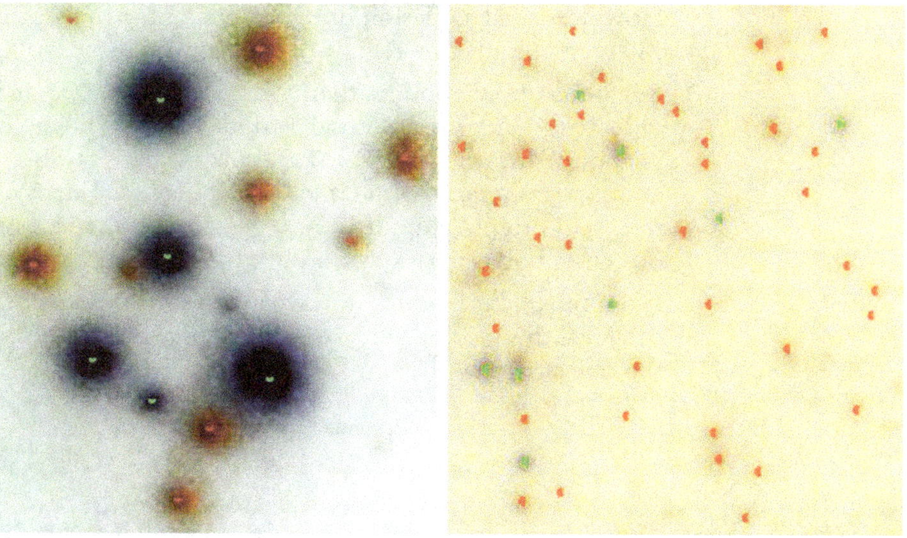

Fig. 2 Spots color subdivision for ELISPOT images. Left panel—the image with large dark blue spots and small red spots. Five blue and eight red spots were selected. Right panel—image with small brown and gray spots. Eight gray and 40 brown spots were selected

(http://www.unibrain.com) and allows for accurate quantification results without the necessity of manual adjustments of the system during image acquisition at different illumination conditions.

QuantiHub Version 6.1 developed for Windows 10 (64 bit) operating system. It has four predefined counting modes. The first mode allows to count very small spots, the second used for count all spots except too large spots, the third allows to count all spots except very small, and the last counts all spots (small and large).

4   Notes

1. Cluster analysis algorithms can vary significantly. For example, these may be algorithms targeting a linear search of either objects combinations or random division of objects set. The majority of such algorithms consist of two groups. The first group is intended for initial (possibly artificial or arbitrary) subdivision of objects set into classes and a certain criterion of the quality of automatic classification is defined. The second group of algorithms is intended for objects which are interchanged between classes until the value of criterion quits refining.

2. Any image with the profile which is not more complicated than f can be constructed by combination of brightness levels C_i. Therefore, the construction of image form is reduced to definition of indicating functions. For simplicity, the entire interval of images' brightness may be divided into n equal intervals.

However, such a division does not guarantee that each interval will contain only one region of constant brightness of image f.

3. Regardless how good mathematical algorithms are, it's impossible to get uniformly good results with all possible sets of images of the wells in ELISPOT plates. This is observed, for example, on images with either inadequate (too dark) or excessive (too bright) illumination, when the differences in object-object and object-background brightness are not profound.

4. From the physical point of view, dimensions of spots depend on the focal distance of the lens and the distance from the lens to the object which can vary significantly.

References

1. Pyt'ev YP (1993) Morphological image analysis. Pattern Recognit Image Anal 1:19–28
2. Zadorozhny SS, Pyt'ev YP, Chulichkov AI (2000) Morphological methods in automatic recognition of cars' license plates from their video-images. Pattern Recognit Image Anal 2:288–292
3. Zhuravlev YI (1998) An algebraic approach to recognition or classifications problems. Pattern Recognit Image Anal 1:59–100
4. Zadorozhny SS, Martynov NN (2011) Mathematical algorithms for automatic search, recognition, and detection of spots in ELISPOT assay. In: Kalyuzhny AE (ed) Handbook of ELISPOT: methods and protocols, Methods in molecular biology, vol 792. Springer Science & Business Media, New York

Chapter 5

Four Color ImmunoSpot® Assays for Identification of Effector T-Cell Lineages

Jodi Hanson, Diana R. Roen, and Paul V. Lehmann

Abstract

Single color IFN-γ ELISPOT assays have evolved as a highly sensitive T cell immune monitoring platform. By detecting individual T cells that secrete IFN-γ in response to antigen exposure, these assays permit the measurement of the frequency of antigen-specific T cells among white blood cells. These assays therefore are well suited to assess clonal expansions, that is, whether a (Th1) T cell response has been induced to an antigen in a test subject. Single color IFN-γ ELISPOT assays are not suited, however, to provide information on the Th2/Th17 quality of the T cell response, nor do they provide insights into the differentiation state of CD8 cells. Recently it has been established that co-expression profiles of IL-2, TNF-α, and granzyme B along with IFN-γ permit to identify CD8 cell subpopulations. Naïve CD8 cells, central CD8 memory cells, CD8 terminal effector cells, polyfunctional CD8 cells, stem-cell like CD8 memory cells, dysfunctional- and senescent CD8 cells all differ in the extent they produce these molecules upon antigen re-encounter. We therefore have developed, and introduce here, a four color T cell ELISPOT assay in which the co-expression levels of IFN-γ, IL-2, TNF-α, and granzyme B can be established for individual antigen-specific CD8 cells, thereby identifying the activation/differentiation state of these cells.

Key words Central CD8 memory cells, CD8 terminal effector cells, Polyfunctional CD8 cells, Stem-cell like CD8 memory cells, Dysfunctional CD8 cell, Senescent CD8 cell, IFN-γ, IL-2, TNF-α, Granzyme B, Co-expression, ELISPOT, Multiplexing, Tumor immunity, Autoimmunity, Immune monitoring

---

1 Introduction

The immune system protects from various infections and tumors, but can also cause allergies, autoimmunity, and transplant rejection. Over the last decades, it has become clear that in each of these cases different types of effector T cell lineages play a role, the major ones for CD4 cells being Th1, Th2, and Th17 [1]. Th1 cells operate via the secretion of IFN-γ that shuts down viral replication in infected cells and induces MHC expression on such cells preparing them for T cell recognition. Th2 cells produce IL-4 that is involved in the regulation of immune globulin class switching, and a sub-lineage of Th2 cells is central to anti-parasite defense by activation of eosino-

Alexander E. Kalyuzhny (ed.), *Handbook of ELISPOT: Methods and Protocols*, Methods in Molecular Biology, vol. 1808, https://doi.org/10.1007/978-1-4939-8567-8_5, © Springer Science+Business Media, LLC, part of Springer Nature 2018

phils via the secretion of IL-5. Finally, the Th17 cell type mediates DTH (delayed type hypersensitivity) by secreting IL-17 [2]. In DTH, macrophages are attracted and activated to protect against intracellular pathogens.

The Th1, Th2, and Th17 effector cell lineages emerge through instructed differentiation [3–6]. Once this differentiation is completed, the cytokine profiles of these cells are imprinted to be mutually exclusive [7]. Upon antigen re-encounter, Th1 cells will produce IFN-γ (but no IL-4 nor IL-17), Th2 cells will secrete IL-4 or IL-5 (but no IFN-γ and no IL-17), and Th17 cells will produce IL-17 in the absence of IFN-γ, IL-4, or IL-5 [8, 9]. The relative frequency of Th1/Th2/Th17 cells within the antigen-specific CD4 cell repertoire defines the quality of the immune response, that is, whether it is suitable for the different types of antigen encounters. Therefore, unambiguous measurements of Th1, Th2, and Th17 cell frequencies are critical for immune monitoring.

Antigen-specific Th1, Th2, and Th17 cells can be readily detected in ELISPOT assays that measure the cytokines that these cells produce after antigen stimulation. While IFN-γ release by CD4 cells peaks at 24 h after T cell receptor stimulation, IL-17 secretion by Th17 cells does not even start within 48 h, and peaks at 96 h [10]. It takes Th2 cells 48 h to engage in maximal IL-4 production, and their IL-5 secretion does not reach maximal levels until 96 h after antigen encounter [11]. Due to these fundamentally different secretion kinetics of TH1-, Th2- and TH17 cytokines, the CD4 effector lineages are best studied in single color ELISPOT assays that account for the optimal time point for each cytokine. While an ELISPOT test kit for the simultaneous detection of IFN-γ/IL-4/IL-17 can be readily manufactured, due to the underlying CD4 cell biology, such an IFN-γ/IL-4/IL-17 multiplex assay could provide inaccurate and false negative frequency measurements for antigen-specific Th1, Th2, and Th17 cells.

Like CD4 cells, also CD8 cells can differentiate into sublineages that produce IL-4 (Tc2) or IL-17 (Tc17), or function as regulatory cells [12]. The unique contribution of CD8 cells to host defense is, however, the ability to kill infected target cells. Naïve CD8 cells neither kill nor produce cytokine (Fig. 1A), but within 5 days after having been engaged in an immune response, they will develop into terminal effector CD8 cells that express high levels of perforin and granzyme B enabling them to kill target cells [13]. Terminal effector CD8 cells excel in the secretion of IFN-γ and TNF-α, but they produce little to no IL-2 (Fig. 1B) [14]. If the antigen is successfully eliminated, the effector cells return to a quiescent state in which they are called central memory cells. In the absence of antigen, it takes approximately 3 weeks for the terminal effector cell to become a resting memory cell [15]. Central CD8 memory cells will secrete IFN-γ within 24 h of re-antigen encounter, but they have lost their ability to secrete instantly granzyme B and perforin, and they will

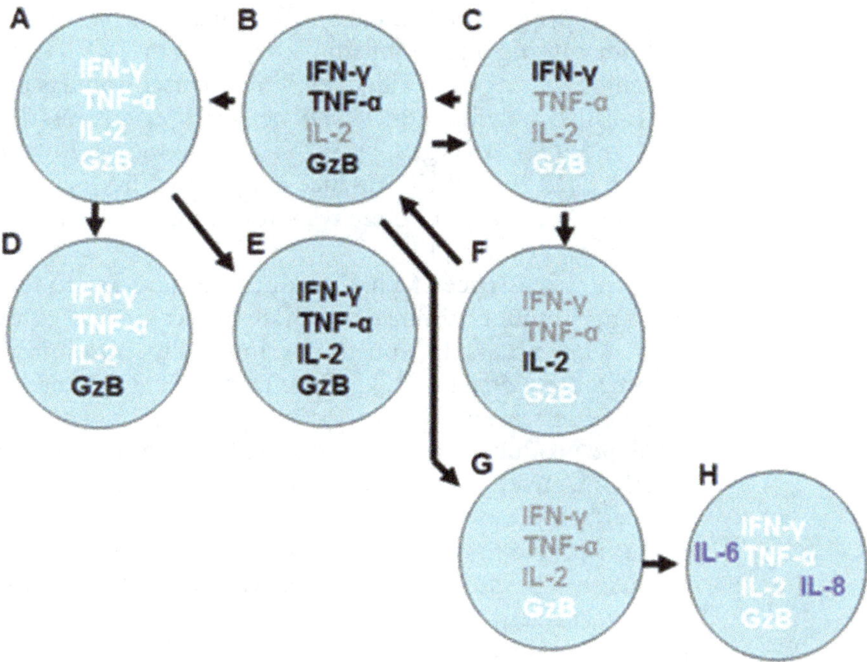

Fig. 1 CD8 cell activation and differentiation states can be identified via their expression pattern of IFN-γ, TNF-α, IL-2, and GzB. (A): Naïve CD8 cell, (B): Terminal effector CD8 cell, (C): Central CD8 memory cell, (D): Silent CD8 killer cell, (E): Polyfunctional CD8 cell, (F): Stem-cell like CD8 memory cell, T_{SCM}, (G): Dysfunctional CD8 cell, (H): Senescent CD8 cell. The phenotypes shown here correspond to the consensus nomenclature for CD8 T cell phenotypes established in 2015 [14]. Here we focus on the analyte secretion patterns of these subsets. The corresponding cell surface markers that can be established by flow cytometry are summarized in that publication

secrete little to no TNF-α or IL-2 (Fig. 1C) but within 3–4 days after antigen-re-encounter resting memory cells can convert again into terminal effector cells [16].

Recently, a CD8 memory cell type has drawn attention that is called "stem-cell like CD8 memory cells," T_{SCM} [17]. T_{SCM} secrete low levels of IFN-γ and TNF-α, no GzB, but they produce abundant IL-2 (Fig. 1F) [14]. In the field of adoptive cancer therapy, it was observed that—counter to initial expectations—injections of fully differentiated CD8 terminal effector cells cause less tumor clearance than the infusion of less differentiated CD8 cells. These T_{SCM} have the property, much like naïve CD8 cells, to re-engage in extensive proliferative responses upon re-encounter of the antigen, a property that terminal effector cells increasingly loose with repeated antigen stimulation. Due to their self-renewing potential, and longevity, T_{SCM} enable us to come up with high numbers of terminal effector cells when repeated antigen encounters call for a sustained CD8 cell attack.

There is a lineage of cytotoxic CD8 cells that does not produce IFN-γ (Fig. 1D) [15]. Such effector cells are granzyme B (and perforin) positive, and their cytolytic activity in a tissue is exerted without causing a local inflammatory reaction [2]. Therefore they are called "Silent CD8 killer cell." Much attention has been drawn to so-called polyfunctional CD8 cells that co-express IFN-γ with IL-2 and TNF-α (Fig. 1E). While representing a low percentage among CD8 cells, their presence in increased frequencies has been linked to successful immune responses mounted against infectious diseases and cancer [14].

With persistence of a high antigen burden, due to the resulting ongoing immune stimulation, CD8 cells can undergo exhaustion [18]. This occurs in anti-tumor immunity, autoimmunity, and chronic infections. First, "dysfunctional" CD8 cells arise that have lost their self-renewing and cytolytic potential, and display reduced cytokine producing ability (Fig. 1F) [14]. These cells are not completely inactive, as their name might suggest, but exhibit attenuated effector functions as needed to prevent excessive collateral damage on the tissue in which the antigen persists and from which it could not be cleared by the initial vigorous CD8 cell attack. With further antigen persistence, CD8 cells eventually burn out, and become "senescent" (Fig. 1H) Senescent CD8 cells do not secrete IFN-γ, TNF-α, or IL-2 [14]. While void of direct cytolytic or pro-inflammatory cytokine function, senescent cells are still not completely inactive, but secrete IL-6 and IL-8 [14]. The latter cytokines primarily serve tissue repair, but in the case of tumors, this translated to promoting tumor growth [19].

As summarized in Fig. 1, subpopulations of CD8 cells can be identified by their respective profiles of IFN-γ, TNF-α, IL-2, and GzB production. We therefore developed a four color ELISPOT assay in which these analytes can be measured simultaneously, and which will be described in the following. For the accurate identification of the distinct CD8 subpopulations, the following general principles of multicolor ELISPOT analysis need to be considered. First, it is critical that each of the analytes is detected without the cross-bleeding of color. This is accomplished by using combinations of fluorochromes that would cross-bleed if excited broadly, but by selecting narrow excitation wavelengths and emission filters for each color, these can be completely separated, and each color plane analyzed, without the need for compensation, essentially as a single color ELISPOT assay. An example for this type of unambiguous detection of colors is provided in Fig. 1 of a chapter on seven color analysis in this book [20]. In the next step, the images containing the "spots" for the different color planes are superimposed to identify cells that co-express analytes. This cannot be just done by simple matching of centers of masses for the individual spots because T cells migrate from APC to APC during the ELISPOT assay's capture phase that lasts 24 h, or more. Thus, tolerances need to be accommodated as we describe in detail in a chapter dedicated to the experimental validation of multicolor analysis [21]. If these tolerance values are set accurately, serial dilution of the T cells will show a linear relationship between analyte co-expressers and cell numbers plated; however, the same percentage of cells will be co-expressers irrespective of the total cell number plated per well. In contrast, the chance for random overlays of single positive spots occurring will drop exponentially as fewer cells are plated. In that chapter [21], these principles have been verified subjecting CD8 cells and B cells to multicolor ELISPOT analysis. With CD8 cells, analyte co-expressers can be expected, while with B cells any multi-positive spot must result from chance overlays of single positive cells as a single B cell can produce only one class or subclass of antibody at a time. Once single vs. multiple analyte producing cells are identified, which is done automatically by the ImmunoSpot® software, the data is converted automatically in flow cytometry standard (FCS format), from where on standard flow cytometry software can be used to analyze the co-expression levels and patterns. The step by step process of multicolor ELISPOT analysis is described in a dedicated chapter in this book [22]. Here we focus on performing the wet lab part of the four color fluorescent ELISPOT assay to measure the antigen-triggered secretion of IFN-γ, TNF-α, IL-2, and GzB. The results of a representative four color assay in which these analytes have been detected are shown in Fig. 2.

2   Materials

2.1   Instrumentation and Software

1. ImmunoSpot® Series 6 Ultimate Analyzer (CTL, Shaker Heights, OH USA, cat# S6UTM12).

2. ImmunoSpot® 7.0 Software (CTL, cat. IPS01).

3. Cell counting 1.4 software (CTL, cat. LDA01).

2.2   ImmunoSpot Kits

1. IFNγ-IL2-TNFα-GrzB 4 Color Capture kit (CTL, cat. hT4001F).

2. IFNγ Detection kit (CTL, cat. hT02).

3. TNFα Detection kit (CTL, cat. hT13).

4. IL2 Detection kit (CTL, cat. hT56).

5. GrzB Detection kit (CTL, cat. hT59).

6. Live/dead Cell Counting kit (CTL, cat. CTL-LD-100).

2.3   Media

1. Anti-Aggregate (CTL, cat. CTL-AA-005).

2. CTL-TEST serum-free medium (CTL, cat. CTLT-005).

3. L-Glutamine (Gibco, cat. 25030-081).

4. RPMI-1600 (Lonza, cat. BW12167Q).

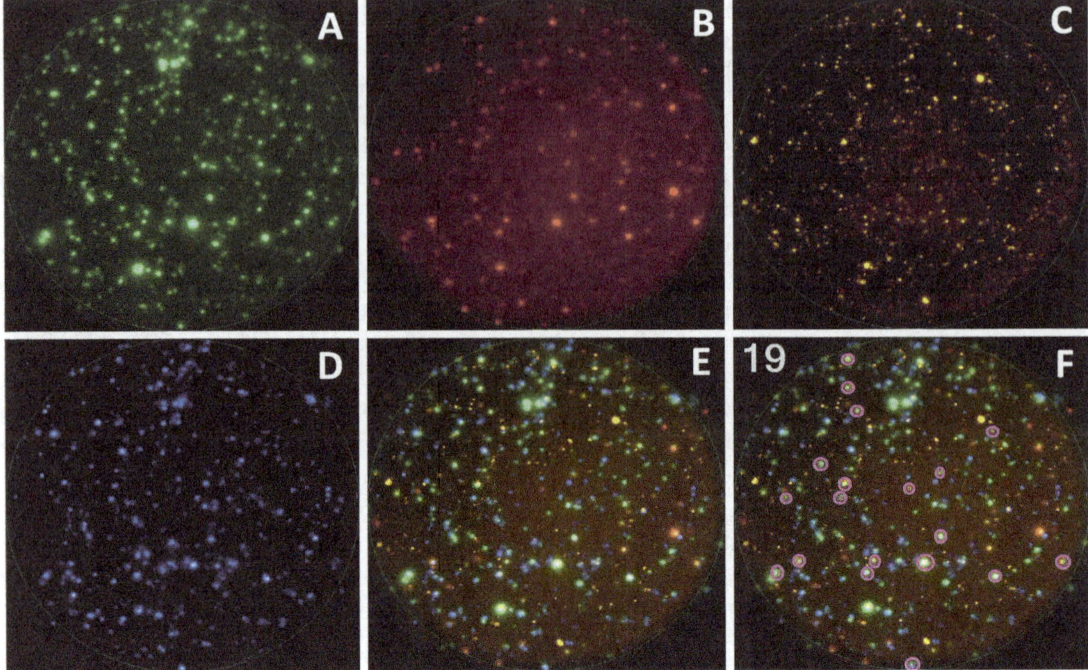

Fig. 2 Four color ImmunoSpot® results measuring IFN-γ, TNF-α, IL-2, and GzB. The four color assay was performed as described here testing CEF-peptide-reactive CD8 cells. For each analyte, a separate channel was established permitting detection of that analyte without cross-bleeding of color. Panel (**a**) shows the IFN-γ channel in green (**b**) the IL-2 channel in red, (**c**) the TNF-α channel in yellow, and (**d**) the GzB channel in blue. The overlay of the four color planes is shown in (**e**). Polyfunctional CD8 cells positive for all four analytes have been counted in (**f**). The fact that these cells are indeed quadruple positive, as opposed to resulting from random overlays was established by serial dilution of the cells

2.4 Miscellaneous

1. CEF plus pool (CTL, cat. CTL-CEF-002).
2. 50 mL conical centrifuge tubes (Falcon, cat. 352070).
3. Sterile gauze (Covidien, cat. 8044).
4. Reservoir (Denville, cat. P8826-ST).
5. Ethyl alcohol, 190 proof (Sigma, cat. 493511).
6. Parafilm "M" (Hach, cat. PM-996).
7. Vacuum Manifold (Millipore, cat. MSVMHTS00).
8. 10 mL syringe Lluer Lok tip (BD 309604).
9. 0.1 μm syringe filter (Millipore, cat. SLVV033RS).
10. Distilled water (Millipore, cat. 6442-85).
11. Tween-20, to make 0.05% Tween-PBS wash buffer (Sigma, cat. P1379).
12. 1× Sterile DPBS, Ca-Mg free (Hyclone, cat. SH30028-02).
13. 25 cm² sterile culture flasks (Corning, cat. 430639).

14. Wide-orifice tips for plating cells (Rainin, 17007101).

15. Frozen PBMC (CTL, cat. CTL-CP1) http://www.immunospot.com/ImmunoSpot-ePBMC

---

3 Methods

3.1 Thawing and Stimulation of PBMC

PBMC were used with known IFN-γ reactivity from the ePBMC database. Cells were stored in liquid nitrogen vapor phase until use.

1. Thaw cryopreserved PBMC by warming them in a 37 °C metal bead bath for 15 min. Wipe vial with 70% EtOH to sterile and invert twice to mix cells.

2. Transfer vial contents into a 50 mL conical tube. Rinse the cryovial with 1 mL of warm (37 °C) anti-aggregate solution and add this slowly in a dropwise fashion to the conical tube. Continue to add warm anti-aggregate solution while swirling the cells until the volume reaches 10 mL per vial (*see* **Note 1**).

3. Centrifuge cells at 300 × g for 10 min at room temperature with maximum break.

4. Decant the supernatant and resuspend the pellet by flicking the bottom of the conical tube. Add 10 mL of anti-aggregate solution.

5. Take 20 µL of cell suspension and mix it with 20 µL of Live/Dead Cell Counting Dye. Load 15 µL of the mixed solution into a hemocytometer and count the live and dead cells on the ImmunoSpot Series 6 Ultimate Analyzer using the ImmunoSpot® LDA 1.4 Software.

6. Centrifuge cells at 300 × g for 10 min at room temperature with maximum break.

7. Decant supernatant and resuspend cells at five million live cells/mL in warm (37 °C) CTL-TEST Medium.

8. Add 0.5 µg/mL of CEF peptide pool plus to the cell suspension.

9. Transfer the contents of the conical tube to a sterile 25 cm² cell culture flask and incubate at 37 °C with 5% CO_2 for 72 h (*see* **Note 2**).

3.2 Coating of the ELISPOT Plates

Forty eight hours after stimulation of PBMC with CEF peptide pool, a 96 well PVDF membrane plate with low auto-fluorescence needs to be coated for the four color fluorescent ELISPOT assay.

1. Prepare Capture Solution contained in the kit for the four color fluorescent ELISPOT assay according to manufacture protocol.

2. Remove the underdrain carefully and add 15 µL of freshly prepared 70% ethanol to each well using a multi-channel pipette (*see* **Note 3**).

3. Immediately add 150 µL of sterile DPBS to each well (*see* **Note 4**).

4. Decant and wash the plate two more times with 150 µL/well of sterile DPBS.

5. Decant the final wash, tap on sterile gauze to remove access liquid.

6. Replace the underdrain and quickly add 80 µL Capture Solution to each well. Wrap the plate in parafilm and store at 4 °C overnight.

3.3 Counting PBMC

1. Seventy two hours after the beginning of the stimulation, take cells from cell culture flask and add them to a 50 mL conical tube.

2. Add 40 mL of CTL-TEST Medium, centrifuge at $300 \times g$ for 10 min at room temperature with maximum break.

3. Decant supernatant and resuspend by tapping the bottom of the tube.

4. Add CTL-TEST Medium for cell counting, approximately 5×10^6/mL.

5. Take 20 µL of the cell suspension and mix it with 20 µL of Live/Dead Cell Counting Dye. Load 15 µL of the mixed solution into a hemacytometer and establish the number of live and dead cells using an ImmunoSpot® Series 6 Ultimate Analyzer using ImmunoSpot® LDA 1.4 Software.

6. Centrifuge cells at $300 \times g$ for 10 min at room temperature with maximum break.

7. Decant the supernatant and resuspend the cells according to the live count.

3.4 Plating of Antigen and PBMC

1. Remove the coated ELISPOT plate from 4 °C and unwrap the parafilm.

2. Decant the Capture Solution and wash the plate with 150 µL/well sterile DPBS.

3. Decant the DPBS and tap the plate on sterile gauze to remove any excess liquid.

4. Quickly add 100 µL/well of CEF peptide pool plus solution at 1 µg/mL in CTL-Test Medium using a multi-channel pipette and sterile reservoirs (*see* **Note 5**).

5. Add 100 µL of the counted stimulated cells in serial dilution using wide-orifice tips (*see* **Note 6**).

6. Tap the plate gently before storing it in an incubator at 37 °C, 5% CO_2 overnight (*see* **Note 7**).

3.5 Multicolor ELISPOT Detection

1. Prepare the Detection Solution according to the manufacturer's protocol specified in the kit, and pass through a 0.1 μm syringe filter.

2. After an overnight incubation, remove the plate from the incubator and decant antigen and cells (*see* **Note 8**).

3. Decant and wash the plate twice with PBS and twice with 0.05% Tween-PBS, 150 μL/well.

4. Tap the plate on paper towels to remove excess liquid.

5. Add 80 μL of Detection Antibody Solution and incubate the plate for 2 h at room temperature, protected from light.

6. Prepare the Tertiary Solution according to the protocol and pass through a 0.1 μm syringe filter.

7. Decant the plate, wash 3× with 150 μL/well 0.05% Tween-PBS and tap to remove excess liquid.

8. Add 80 μL/mL of Tertiary Solution and incubate for 1 h at room temperature, protected from light.

9. Decant the plate, wash 3× with 150 μL of distilled water. Remove the underdrain and wash the plate upside down on a vacuum manifold with distilled water to remove excess fluorochrome.

10. Let plate dry completely, protected from light under a laminar flow hood, before scanning.

3.6 Data Capture and Analysis

1. The ELISPOT plate is to be scanned using the CTL Series 6 Ultimate Analyzer using fixed exposure. Each filter and corresponding excitation LED was used in order to avoid cross-bleeding of colors (*see* **Note 9**). The theoretical and practical aspects of accurate multicolor ELISPOT analysis are respectively described in chapters [21, 22].

2. ImmunoSpot 7.0 was used to enumerate spots. Each filter had individual parameters set for accurate counting; gates were set using positive wells and negative wells and the algorithm for pairing was set.

3. Excel spreadsheets are made from every counted plate by ImmunoSpot® Software 7.0 and those were used to make graphs with their corresponding R values to calculate linearity, average R value 0.98726 (data not shown).

4. Once the linearity was confirmed, the percent analyte of the co-expressing cells was calculated by dividing the number of SFU counted by the number of cells plated; the percent quadruple co-expressing cells was 0.005% (data not shown).

4   Notes

1. Adding warm media slowly helps minimize the osmotic gradient between the interior and exterior of the cells as the concentration of DMSO drops with dilution in the exterior. One can add the content of up to five cryovials of the same PBMC donor to one 50 mL conical tube.

2. CEF-peptide-reactive CD8 cells typically are resting memory cells in healthy donors, and thus have no pre-formed GzB stored. To detect GzB production by CEF-specific CD8 cells, addition to IFN-γ and TNF-α, a 3 day pre-stimulation culture is required during which central memory cells transform into terminal effector cells. If antigen exposure triggers GzB production in CD8 cells ex vivo that indicates that in vivo the antigen-specific CD8 cells had been in an activated state, being terminal effector cells.

3. For multicolor ELISPOT assays, it is important to activate the PVDF membrane with ethanol pre-wetting in order to increase its binding capacity. It happens instantaneously after the addition of ethanol, and can be seen as the graying of the membrane. Washing afterwards should be done as quickly as possible to avoid leakage of the membrane.

4. Once the plate has been activated with ethanol, for all subsequent steps, the plate membrane should never dry until completion of the assay.

5. We highly recommend the use of CTL Serum-Free Media for freezing, washing, and testing of PBMC. Even brief exposure to mitogenic serum can cause high background while other sera can have suppressive effects.

6. CTL recommends using wide-orifice tips to reduce sheer forces while pipetting cells.

7. Do not stack plates in the incubator and do not allow the incubator or the plates to be disturbed during incubation. Doing so will cause the cells within the wells to roll which will interfere with co-expression analysis.

8. After the incubation of cells on the ELISPOT plate, a large percentage of the cells are still viable and, except for antigen stimulation, largely unaffected by the test procedure. Instead of discarding the cells, they can be used for subsequent analysis, including ELISPOT and flow cytometric analysis.

9. For unambiguous detection of individual analytes using fluorochrome combinations, a setup is needed in which the dyes do not cross-bleed among the detection channels. Each chan-

nel is defined by a narrow excitation wavelength combined with a narrow emission filter and can be selected from an array of channels preinstalled on CTL fluorescent readers. Please consult CTL customer support for the selection of channels suitable for the fluorochrome combinations of choice.

References

1. Steinman L (2007) A brief history of T(H)17, the first major revision in the T(H)1/T(H)2 hypothesis of T cell-mediated tissue damage. Nat Med 13(2):139–145. https://doi.org/10.1038/nm1551

2. Tigno-Aranjuez JT, Lehmann PV, Tary-Lehmann M (2009) Dissociated induction of cytotoxicity and DTH by CFA and CpG. J Immunother 32(4):389–398. https://doi.org/10.1097/CJI.0b013e31819d79a7

3. Bettelli E, Carrier Y, Gao W, Korn T, Strom TB, Oukka M, Weiner HL, Kuchroo VK (2006) Reciprocal developmental pathways for the generation of pathogenic effector TH17 and regulatory T cells. Nature 441(7090):235–238. https://doi.org/10.1038/nature04753

4. Hsieh CS, Macatonia SE, Tripp CS, Wolf SF, O'Garra A, Murphy KM (1993) Development of TH1 CD4+ T cells through IL-12 produced by Listeria-induced macrophages. Science 260(5107):547–549

5. Macatonia SE, Hosken NA, Litton M, Vieira P, Hsieh CS, Culpepper JA, Wysocka M, Trinchieri G, Murphy KM, O'Garra A (1995) Dendritic cells produce IL-12 and direct the development of Th1 cells from naive CD4+ T cells. J Immunol 154(10):5071–5079

6. Seki N, Miyazaki M, Suzuki W, Hayashi K, Arima K, Myburgh E, Izuhara K, Brombacher F, Kubo M (2004) IL-4-induced GATA-3 expression is a time-restricted instruction switch for Th2 cell differentiation. J Immunol 172(10):6158–6166

7. Szabo SJ, Kim ST, Costa GL, Zhang X, Fathman CG, Glimcher LH (2000) A novel transcription factor, T-bet, directs Th1 lineage commitment. Cell 100(6):655–669

8. Karulin AY, Hesse MD, Tary-Lehmann M, Lehmann PV (2000) Single-cytokine-producing CD4 memory cells predominate in type 1 and type 2 immunity. J Immunol 164(4):1862–1872

9. Kuerten S, Rottlaender A, Rodi M, Velasco VB Jr, Schroeter M, Kaiser C, Addicks K, Tary-Lehmann M, Lehmann PV (2010) The clinical course of EAE is reflected by the dynamics of the neuroantigen-specific T cell compartment in the blood. Clin Immunol 137(3):422–432. https://doi.org/10.1016/j.clim.2010.09.004

10. Wunsch M, Zhang W, Hanson J, Caspell R, Karulin AY, Recks MS, Kuerten S, Sundararaman S, Lehmann PV (2015) Characterization of the HCMV-specific CD4 T cell responses that are associated with protective immunity. Viruses 7(8):4414–4437. https://doi.org/10.3390/v7082828

11. Duechting A, Przybyla A, Kuerten S, Lehmann PV (2017) Delayed activation kinetics of Th2 and Th17 vs. Th1 cells. Cells. https://doi.org/10.3390/cells6030029

12. Kaech SM, Wherry EJ, Ahmed R (2002) Effector and memory T-cell differentiation: implications for vaccine development. Nat Rev Immunol 2(4):251–262. https://doi.org/10.1038/nri778

13. Wherry EJ, Teichgraber V, Becker TC, Masopust D, Kaech SM, Antia R, von Andrian UH, Ahmed R (2003) Lineage relationship and protective immunity of memory CD8 T cell subsets. Nat Immunol 4(3):225–234. https://doi.org/10.1038/ni889

14. Apetoh L, Smyth MJ, Drake CG, Abastado JP, Apte RN, Ayyoub M, Blay JY, Bonneville M, Butterfield LH, Caignard A, Castelli C, Cavallo F, Celis E, Chen L, Colombo MP, Comin-Anduix B, Coukos G, Dhodapkar MV, Dranoff G, Frazer IH, Fridman WH, Gabrilovich DI, Gilboa E, Gnjatic S, Jager D, Kalinski P, Kaufman HL, Kiessling R, Kirkwood J, Knuth A, Liblau R, Lotze MT, Lugli E, Marincola F, Melero I, Melief CJ, Mempel TR, Mittendorf EA, Odun K, Overwijk WW, Palucka AK, Parmiani G, Ribas A, Romero P, Schreiber RD, Schuler G, Srivastava PK, Tartour E, Valmori D, van der Burg SH, van der Bruggen P, van den Eynde BJ, Wang E, Zou W, Whiteside TL, Speiser DE, Pardoll DM, Restifo NP, Anderson AC (2015) Consensus nomenclature for CD8+ T cell phenotypes in cancer. Oncoimmunology 4(4):e998538. https://doi.org/10.1080/2162402X.2014.998538

15. Schlingmann TR, Shive CL, Targoni OS, Tary-Lehmann M, Lehmann PV (2009) Increased per cell IFN-gamma productivity indicates

recent in vivo activation of T cells. Cell Immunol 258(2):131–137. https://doi.org/10.1016/j.cellimm.2009.04.002

16. Nowacki TM, Kuerten S, Zhang W, Shive CL, Kreher CR, Boehm BO, Lehmann PV, Tary-Lehmann M (2007) Granzyme B production distinguishes recently activated CD8(+) memory cells from resting memory cells. Cell Immunol 247(1):36–48. https://doi.org/10.1016/j.cellimm.2007.07.004

17. Lugli E, Dominguez MH, Gattinoni L, Chattopadhyay PK, Bolton DL, Song K, Klatt NR, Brenchley JM, Vaccari M, Gostick E, Price DA, Waldmann TA, Restifo NP, Franchini G, Roederer M (2013) Superior T memory stem cell persistence supports long-lived T cell memory. J Clin Invest 123(2):594–599. https://doi.org/10.1172/JCI66327

18. Wherry EJ (2011) T cell exhaustion. Nat Immunol 12(6):492–499

19. Naugler WE, Karin M (2008) The wolf in sheep's clothing: the role of interleukin-6 in immunity, inflammation and cancer. Trends Mol Med 14(3):109–119. https://doi.org/10.1016/j.molmed.2007.12.007

20. Caspell R, Lehmann PV (2018) Detecting all immunoglobulin classes and subclases in a multiplex 7 color immunospot assay. In: Kalyuzhny AE (ed) Handbook of ELISPOT, Methods in molecular biology, 3rd edn. Springer, New York pp 85–94

21. Karulin AY, Megyesi Z, Caspell R, Hanson J, Lehmann PV (2018) Multiplexing T- and B-Cell FLUOROSPOT Assays: Experimental Validation of the Multi-color ImmunoSpot® Software Based on Center of Mass Distance Algorithm. In: Kalyuzhny AE (ed.), Handbook of ELISPOT, Methods in Molecular Biology, 3rd ed. Springer, New York. pp 95–113

22. Megyesi Z, Lehmann PV, Karulin AY (2018) Multi-Color FLUOROSPOT Counting Using ImmunoSpot® Fluoro-X™ Suite. In: Kalyuzhny AE (ed) Handbook of ELISPOT, Methods in Molecular Biology, 3rd ed. Springer, New York. pp 115–131

Chapter 6

Detection of Cross-Reactive B Cells Using the FluoroSpot Assay

Peter Jahnmatz and Niklas Ahlborg

Abstract

B cell ELISpot enables a sensitive analysis of antigen-specific B cells at the single cell level but is limited to the analysis of reactivity with a single antigen. By reversing the B cell ELISpot and using anti-IgG capture antibodies instead of coated antigen, the specificity of antibodies secreted by B cells can be defined using soluble tagged antigen for detection. When combining this approach with fluorescent detection of the antigen in a B cell FluoroSpot assay, reactivity with multiple antigens can be defined. In the protocol described herein, splenocytes from a mouse immunized with an antigen were analyzed for their reactivity with the antigen used for immunization and for cross-reactivity with a different but structurally related antigen. Using this assay, we found that at least 15% of the B cells displayed detectable cross-reactivity. B cell FluoroSpot utilizing multiple antigens provides a tool for a single-cell analysis of B cell cross-reactivity, for example, with variable and polymorphic antigens found in various pathogens; or analysis of other types of immune responses where analysis of cross-reactivity is of interest. It is also possible to simultaneously analyze B cell reactivity to completely different antigens.

Key words Antibody, B cell, Cross-reactivity, ELISpot, FluoroSpot, Peptide tag

1 Introduction

The B cell ELISpot assay is a sensitive tool for studies on B cells. Using ELISpot, antibodies secreted by single B cells can be analyzed for their antigen specificity and/or their isotype and subclass. The antigen specificity of antibodies, derived from single B cells, is usually analyzed in plates with antigen-coated wells in which the cells are cultured. The antibodies bind to the antigen in close proximity to the location of the cell and are commonly detected using an enzyme-labeled anti-immunoglobulin (Ig) antibody and a precipitating substrate. This generates spots on the membrane, each spot being the secretory footprint of a single antigen-specific B cell [1]. B cell ELISpot has been used by researchers for over three decades for studies on B cells in various fields including vaccine development, HIV, malaria, influenza, and fundamental immunology [2–5].

Alexander E. Kalyuzhny (ed.), *Handbook of ELISPOT: Methods and Protocols*, Methods in Molecular Biology, vol. 1808, https://doi.org/10.1007/978-1-4939-8567-8_6, © Springer Science+Business Media, LLC, part of Springer Nature 2018

Being restricted to the analysis of only one analyte has always been a limitation of the ELISpot assay. By dual color ELISpot, two analytes can actually be analyzed simultaneously utilizing separate detection systems with different enzymes and sequential development with different substrates [6], but various technical and analytical difficulties have limited the usefulness of the method [7]. The FluoroSpot assay, described by Gazagne et al. in 2003, overcomes these limitations by the use of fluorescent detection systems allowing simultaneous analysis of two or more analytes in the same well. As the FluoroSpot reader exposes the well to light, fluorophores get excited and emit light at different wavelengths, which in turn allows separate analysis of each fluorophore using wavelength-specific filters [8]. FluoroSpot was initially developed for the study of cytokine secretion and co-expression by T cells, but the assay has also been adapted to studies on B cells for the simultaneous measurement of, for example, antigen-specific IgG- and IgA-producing B cells [9, 10]. However, neither dual color ELISpot nor the regular B cell FluoroSpot approach makes it possible to analyze reactivity to more than one antigen per well.

In 2009, Dosenovic et al. described a reversed assay format for B cell ELISpot. Rather than coating with antigen, wells were coated with anti-IgG antibodies that captured IgG secreted by B cells. The specificity of the secreted IgG was then analyzed with a biotinylated antigen and enzyme-labeled streptavidin (SA) followed by substrate development. The new assay format not only resulted in better spot quality but also reduced the amount of antigen needed [11]. The combination of the reversed ELISpot with fluorescent-based detection opened up for the possibility to use multiple antigens in a B cell FluoroSpot assay, thereby facilitating the study of multiple B cell specificities in one well [12]. Assessment of multiple antigen specificities simultaneously takes the B cell FluoroSpot toward a multiplex functionality and facilitates its use in a broad field of applications. The assay may for instance be a suitable tool for evaluation of B cell responses to multi-valent or multi-component vaccines. By studying multiple B cell populations, with specificity for different antigens, the dynamics of the humoral response and immune memory can be analyzed. Furthermore, the multiplex approach reduces time, cost, and materials needed for the analysis.

The new assay format also makes it possible to study B cell cross-reactivity. Studies on cross-reactivity can be of great value in various fields such as the development of immunity to malaria and other pathogens that have allelic and polymorphic antigen variants, or vaccination against HIV where broadly neutralizing antibodies directed against variable antigens are of potential protective value. It is also possible to combine the analysis of the antigen specificity displayed by B cells with other parameters such as the isotype/

subclass of the secreted antibodies. IgG subclasses differ in their effector function and such analyses may provide detailed insights to the immune response.

In order to detect reactivity with multiple antigens, each antigen has to be labeled with different tags that in turn are recognized by fluorophore-labeled anti-tag reagents. In addition to using biotin together with SA, a variety of peptide tags to which specific monoclonal antibodies (mAb) have been raised provide complementary tag systems. Biotin can be coupled to the antigens chemically. Also peptide tags can be chemically conjugated by coupling maleimide to the antigen; the maleimide is then used to covalently bind a peptide tag with a terminal cysteine. For smaller antigens, with a limited number of epitopes, the addition of a tag could potentially interfere with the antibody's epitope recognition. Thus it may be preferable to insert the tag N- or C-terminally in the antigen recombinantly, or even make two antigen variants that are tagged in different termini. Recombinant antigens with tags also have the advantage that they can be used without having to be purified. Another approach is to use antigen-specific antibodies for detection, but for smaller antigens there is a potential risk that antibodies secreted by B cells and the detection antibody compete for overlapping epitopes [13].

The protocol herein describes the use of FluoroSpot for the analysis of B cell cross-reactivity at the single cell level (Fig. 1). Splenocytes from mice immunized with an antigen are analyzed for reactivity with that same antigen, and for cross-reactivity with a different but structurally related antigen. After capture of the antibodies secreted by splenocyte B cells, the two antigens, labeled with different tags, are added and bound antigens are detected with anti-tag reagents labeled with two different fluorophores. Antibodies reactive only with the antigen used for immunization will then give rise to single-colored spots only, whereas cross-reactive antibodies having bound both antigens will generate double-positive spots (Fig. 2). If desired, additional antigens, anti-tag systems, and fluorophores can be used. So far the use of four different tag systems/fluorophores simultaneously has been described [12].

2　Materials

1. FluoroSpot plates: 96-well Immobilon™-FL polyvinylidene difluoride (PVDF) membrane plates with low autofluorescence (Millipore, Bedford, MA, USA).

2. EtOH pre-wetting solution: 35% EtOH in sterile water.

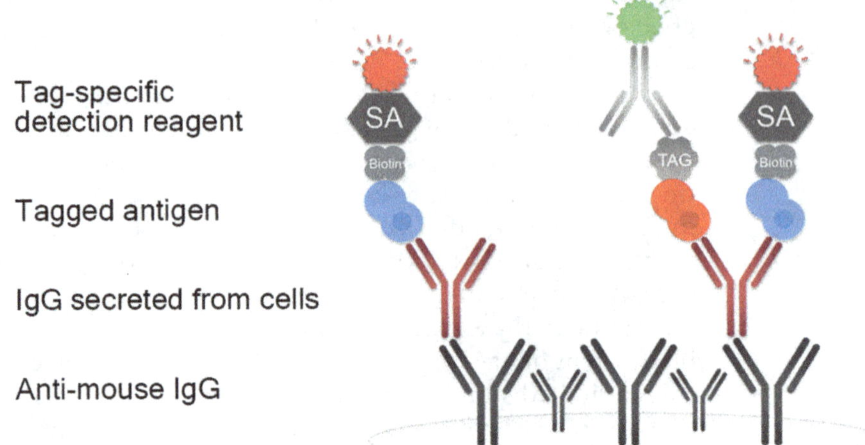

Fig. 1 Assay principle of the B cell FluoroSpot used for the analysis of cross-reactive B cells. Immobilized anti-mouse IgG antibodies were used to capture IgG secreted by splenocytes from a mouse immunized with cat interferon gamma (IFN-γ). IgG secreted by B cells was allowed to bind two structurally similar antigens, tagged with biotin (cat IFN-γ; blue antigen) or a peptide tag (dog IFN-γ; red antigen), respectively. By using fluorescently labeled detection systems, i.e., streptavidin (SA) with red fluorophore and anti-tag antibody with green fluorophore, respectively, cross-reactivity of IgG antibodies from single B cells was analyzed. Antibodies having bound only one of the antigens were detected by only one detection system while cross-reactive antibodies were identified by their binding of both tagged antigens

3. Capture antibody: Polyclonal goat IgG anti-mouse IgG (Mabtech, Nacka Strand, Sweden).

4. Blocking solution after coating and culture medium: Dulbecco's modified Eagle's medium (DMEM) supplemented with 10% fetal calf serum (FCS), 100 U/mL penicillin, and 100 µg/mL streptomycin (culture medium). All reagents from Invitrogen Life Technologies, Carlsbad, CA, USA.

5. Cells: Splenocytes from a mouse immunized with recombinant cat interferon gamma (IFN-γ) suspended in culture medium. For the production of recombinant cat IFN-γ, HEK293/T17 cells (American Type Culture Collection, Manassas, VA, USA) were transiently transfected with a pcDNA3.1/Zeo(-) plasmid containing DNA encoding a mouse IgG kappa leader followed by the sequence for cat IFN-γ (Uniprot accession number P42161) [14]. The mouse was immunized on three occasions with 75 µg/mL cat IFN-γ and 25 µg/mL G3-VAXSAP adjuvant (MOREINX AB, Uppsala, Sweden) in 200 µL sterile phosphate-buffered saline (PBS). Cat IFN-γ in PBS was used to boost the mouse four days prior to removal of the spleen. To obtain spleen cells, the spleen was passed through a cell strainer followed by several washing steps of the splenocytes in culture medium.

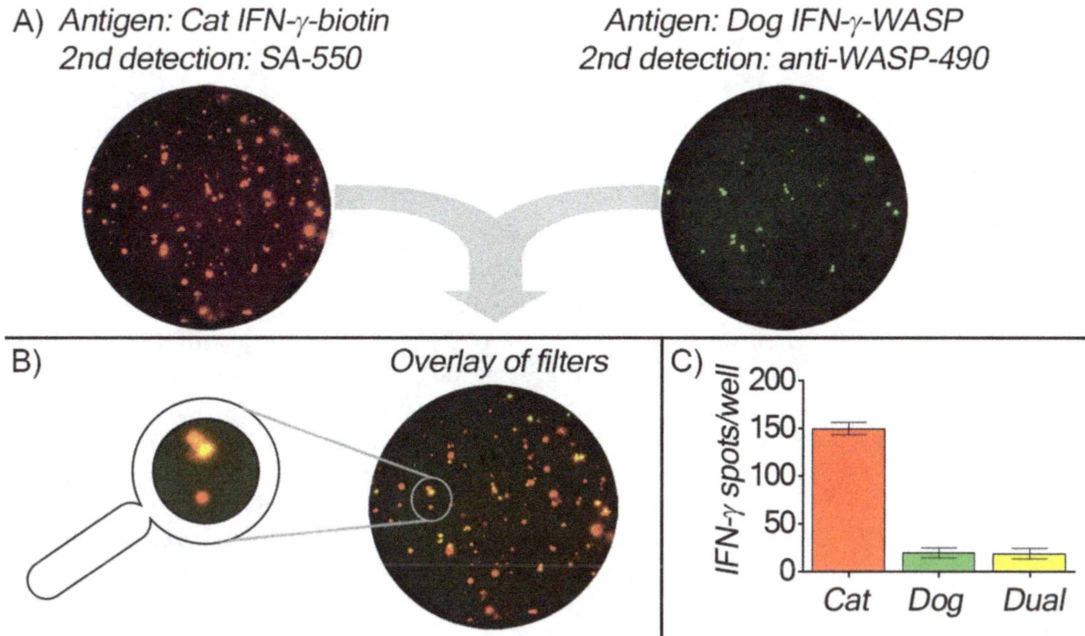

Fig. 2 FluoroSpot analysis of anti-cat interferon gamma (IFN-γ)-reactive B cells, potentially cross-reactive with dog IFN-γ. (**a**) Separate images from wells demonstrating splenocyte reactivity with cat (left) and dog IFN-γ (right) using tagged antigens and fluorescently labeled detection systems. (**b**) Computerized overlay of the two separate well images enables the identification of co-localized spots, i.e., cross-reactive splenocytes. The magnified image displays a single-positive spot (red) and two double-stained co-localized spots (yellow). (**c**) Number of spots in the separate images. All green spots represent cross-reactive B cells (co-localized spots)

6. Blocking reagent after cell culture: PBS supplemented with 20% mouse serum (Innovative research, Novi, MI, USA).

7. Dilution buffer for antigens and secondary reagents: PBS supplemented with 0.1% bovine serum albumin (BSA).

8. Antigens used in assay: biotinylated recombinant cat IFN-γ (RnD Systems, Minneapolis, MN, USA) and recombinant dog IFN-γ. Biotinylation of cat IFN-γ was performed using long-chain biotinyl-N-hydroxysuccinimide ester sulfonic acid (Thermo Fisher Scientific, Rockford, IL, USA) according to the manufacturer's instructions. Dog IFN-γ was produced as cat IFN-γ described above (Uniprot accession number P42161) but the peptide tag WASP was included C-terminally [12].

9. Secondary reagents for detection: SA labeled with a fluorophore absorbing and emitting light at 550/570 nm (SA-550), and mouse mAb anti-WASP labeled with a fluorophore absorbing and emitting light at 490/520 nm (WASP-490; both reagents from Mabtech).

10. Fluorescence enhancer II: a solution used to increase the fluorescent signal (Mabtech).

11. FluoroSpot reader: ELISpot/FluoroSpot reader system (*i*Spot Spectrum, AID, Strassberg, Germany), with software version 7.0 (build 14790).

3   Methods

The FluoroSpot assay protocol herein describes a model system for assessment of B cell cross-reactivity. The assay is based on the capture of mouse IgG antibodies from single B cells, followed by the determination of the antibody specificity using different antigens for detection. In the assay described, splenocytes from a mouse immunized with cat IFN-γ were analyzed. The same antigen, as well as a structurally related antigen (dog IFN-γ with 87% amino acid homology to cat IFN-γ), were used to define the reactivity with cat IFN-γ, and the potential cross-reactivity with dog IFN-γ, displayed by the B cells. The method can also be adapted to analyze multiple and completely different antigens where antibodies do not cross-react.

3.1 Reversed B cell FluoroSpot assay for the analysis of cross-reactivity

1. Add 20 μL of 35% EtOH to a sterile 96-well PVDF plate for 1 min at room temperature. Following pre-wetting, wash the plate five times with 200 μL sterile water per well (*see* **Note 1**).

2. Dilute goat anti-mouse IgG to 15 μg/mL in sterile PBS and add 100 μL to each well. Wrap the plate with aluminum foil to prevent evaporation. Incubate overnight at +4–8 °C.

3. Empty the plate and wash the wells five times with sterile PBS (200 μL/well).

4. To block the PVDF membrane, empty the plate again and add culture medium (200 μL/well). Block for 30 min.

5. Suspend the cells in culture medium to a suitable concentration. Add 100 μL of cell suspension to each well (*see* **Note 2**). In this experiment, 500,000 cells per well were used.

6. Incubate the plate overnight in a humidified atmosphere at +37 °C and 5% CO_2. In order to minimize evaporation of the cell suspension, wrap the plate in aluminum foil before incubation. Do not move the plate during the incubation.

7. Empty and wash each well five times with PBS (200 μL/well) by hand or in an automated plate washer adjusted for ELISpot/FluoroSpot plates. Discard remaining wash buffer before next step, but make sure the wells do not dry.

8. Block potentially remaining binding sites on the capture antibody for 1 h using PBS with 20% mouse serum (200 μL/well) at room temperature (*see* **Note 3**).

9. Wash the plate again as described in **step 7**.

10. In the same tube, dilute the two tagged antigens in PBS supplemented with 0.1% BSA, and then add 100 μL/well. Incubate 1 h at room temperature. Working concentrations of each antigen have to be optimized prior to setting up the assay (*see* **Note 4**).

11. Wash again as described in **step 7**.

12. In the same tube, dilute anti-WASP-490 and SA-550 in PBS supplemented with 0.1% BSA. Working concentration was 1 μg/mL for anti-WASP-490 and 0.25 μg/mL for SA-550. Add 100 μL/well of the cocktail and incubate 1 h at room temperature in the dark.

13. Wash as **step 7**.

14. Empty the plate and add Fluorescence enhancer II (50 μL/well) and incubate in the dark for 15 min at room temperature.

15. Discard the enhancer and carefully remove the soft plastic underdrain before gently tapping the plate against dry tissue paper to remove excess enhancer. Let the plate dry in the dark.

3.2 Analysis of spots

1. Before reading the plate, make sure that the plate is completely dry. The analysis of the plate is preferably made in an automated reader for FluoroSpot. The reader should be equipped with wavelength-specific filters for the separate analysis of fluorophores that absorb and emit light at 490/520 nm and 550/570 nm, respectively (*see* **Note 5**).

2. Spots of different colors are identified separately. B cells producing antibodies reactive with cat IFN-γ will yield red spots. B cells producing antibodies that cross-react with dog IFN-γ will yield green spots in the single filter analysis. Double-positive spots, i.e., spots derived from cross-reactive antibodies, are identified as being co-positioned in a computerized image overlay and will visually appear as yellow spots.

3. The plate can be stored for several days without loss of fluorescent signal. However, in order to obtain the best results, it is recommended to store the plate in the dark and perform the analysis within the following days.

4　Notes

1. EtOH treatment of plates: Pre-wetting of wells with EtOH prior to addition of coating antibody is highly recommended. The EtOH treatment maximizes the capacity of the membrane to bind proteins. After EtOH treatment, wells should be washed extensively with water in order to remove remaining EtOH. The well membrane has to remain wet during the coating process. If

the membrane dries before the capture antibody is added, EtOH treatment and washes have to be repeated before coating antibody is added.

2. Cells: In contrast to serological analyses, where circulating antibodies are examined, B cell analysis by ELISpot or FluoroSpot requires the presence of antibody-secreting B cells. Analysis of circulating memory B cells requires in vitro activation before the analysis in order to differentiate them into antibody-secreting cells. Both mouse and human memory B cells can be pre-activated with a mix of R848 and IL-2. In contrast, in vivo-activated plasmablasts can be analyzed directly, without pre-activation, but often just shortly after their in vivo activation. The cells used herein were not pre-activated since the splenocytes were activated in vivo via immunization using a potent adjuvant. The number of splenocytes added to each well has to be adjusted according to the expected number of spots. The frequency of antigen-specific B cells can be relatively low even after multiple immunizations. Therefore it is recommended to use 250–500,000 cells per well in settings similar to the experiment described herein.

3. Blocking of capture antibody: In order to avoid binding of the detection mAb (anti-WASP which originates from mouse) by the goat anti-mouse IgG capture antibodies, free binding sites on the capture antibodies have to be blocked. This blocking can be performed by addition of a blocking solution (PBS supplemented with 20% mouse serum) to wells prior to the addition of the detection mAb. When human B cells or B cells from animals other than mouse are analyzed, this step is not necessary as long as detection antibodies used are not recognized by the capture antibody.

4. Tag/anti-tag systems for detection: If using antigens labeled with multiple tags for detection, it is important to use tags that will not be recognized by memory B cells present in the animal assessed in the assay. If this happens, the spots derived from such B cells will represent tag-reactive B cells rather than antigen-specific B cells. If antigens used in the assay only have a single tag, this will not be an issue.

5. Analysis: Fluorescent spots were counted using separate wavelength-specific filters for each fluorophore, i.e., 490/520 nm and 550/570 nm, respectively. Wavelength-specific filters with narrow bandwidth minimize the possibility of "bleeding over" effects between filters. As a consequence, detection of green spots with a red filter and vice versa should not result in any detectable spots. This can be verified using control wells with only one of the antigens added.

The FluoroSpot reader software analyzes the position of the spots in each filter image. The fluorophores used in this experiment emit light that generates red or green spots. In the computerized overlay of filter images, the double-positive spots will be observed as spots with a mixed color (yellow).

To be defined as a spot by the software, the spot must have reached a certain size and intensity threshold. When assessing cross-reactive B cells, several parameters will affect the intensity of the colors of a double-positive spot. Compared to a single-positive red spot, a double-positive spot can display lower red color intensity because the cross-reactive B cell-derived antibodies bind two antigens. The intensity of the two colors will also depend on the amount of antibody secreted by single B cells, the antibody affinity as well as the degree of cross-reactivity. In the case of cross-reactive antibodies, B cells with a high degree of cross-reactivity can bind comparable amounts of two antigens compared to a B cell that cross-reacts less and bind more of one antigen and less of the other. Also other parameters will influence the spot intensity such as the functionality of the tag/anti-tag system used and the intrinsic properties of the fluorophores used.

Acknowledgment

The authors would like to thank Kajsa Prokopec, Bernt Axelsson, and Gun Kesa for critical reading of the manuscript. Peter Jahnmatz is a graduate student financed by The Swedish Foundation for Strategic Research (ID14-0070) and Mabtech.

References

1. Czerkinsky CC, Nilsson LA, Nygren H et al (1983) A solid-phase enzyme-linked immunospot (ELISPOT) assay for enumeration of specific antibody-secreting cells. J Immunol Methods 65(1–2):109–121. https://doi.org/10.1016/0022-1759(83)90308-3

2. Ellebedy AH, Krammer F, Li GM et al (2014) Induction of broadly cross-reactive antibody responses to the influenza HA stem region following H5N1 vaccination in humans. Proc Natl Acad Sci U S A 111(36):13133–13138. https://doi.org/10.1073/pnas.1414070111

3. Amanna IJ, Carlson NE, Slifka MK (2007) Duration of humoral immunity to common viral and vaccine antigens. N Engl J Med 357(19):1903–1915. https://doi.org/10.1056/NEJMoa066092

4. Ndungu FM, Lundblom K, Rono J et al (2013) Long-lived Plasmodium falciparum specific memory B cells in naturally exposed Swedish travelers. Eur J Immunol 43(11):2919–2929. https://doi.org/10.1002/eji.201343630

5. Walsh PN, Friedrich DP, Williams JA et al (2013) Optimization and qualification of a memory B-cell ELISpot for the detection of vaccine-induced memory responses in HIV vaccine trials. J Immunol Methods 394(1–2):84–93. https://doi.org/10.1016/j.jim.2013.05.007

6. Okamoto Y, Abe T, Niwa T et al (1998) Development of a dual color enzyme-linked immunospot assay for simultaneous detection of murine T helper type 1- and T helper type 2-cells. Immunopharmacology 39(2):107–116. https://doi.org/10.1016/s0162-3109(98)00007-1

7. Janetzki S, Rueger M, Dillenbeck T (2014) Stepping up ELISpot: multi-level analysis in FluoroSpot assays. Cell 3(4):1102–1115. https://doi.org/10.3390/cells3041102

8. Gazagne A, Claret E, Wijdenes J et al (2003) A Fluorospot assay to detect single T lymphocytes simultaneously producing multiple cytokines. J Immunol Methods 283(1–2):91–98. https://doi.org/10.1016/j.jim.2003.08.013

9. Kesa G, Larsson PH, Ahlborg N et al (2012) Comparison of ELISpot and FluoroSpot in the analysis of swine flu-specific IgG and IgA secretion by in vivo activated human B cells. Cell 1(2):27–34. https://doi.org/10.3390/cells1020027

10. Weinberg A, Muresan P, Richardson KM et al (2015) Determinants of vaccine immunogenicity in HIV-infected pregnant women: analysis of B and T cell responses to pandemic H1N1 monovalent vaccine. PLoS One 10(4):e0122431. https://doi.org/10.1371/journal.pone.0122431

11. Dosenovic P, Chakrabarti B, Soldemo M et al (2009) Selective expansion of HIV-1 envelope glycoprotein-specific B cell subsets recognizing distinct structural elements following immunization. J Immunol 183(5):3373–3382. https://doi.org/10.4049/jimmunol.0900407

12. Jahnmatz P, Bengtsson T, Zuber B et al (2016) An antigen-specific, four-color, B-cell FluoroSpot assay utilizing tagged antigens for detection. J Immunol Methods 433:23–30. https://doi.org/10.1016/j.jim.2016.02.020

13. Hadjilaou A, Green AM, Coloma J et al (2015) Single-cell analysis of B cell/antibody cross-reactivity using a novel multicolor FluoroSpot assay. J Immunol 195(7):3490–3496. https://doi.org/10.4049/jimmunol.1500918

14. Areström I, Zuber B, Bengtsson T et al (2012) Measurement of human latent transforming growth factor-beta1 using a latency associated protein-reactive ELISA. J Immunol Methods 379(1–2):23–29. https://doi.org/10.1016/j.jim.2012.02.016

Chapter 7

Multiplex ImmunoSpot® Assays for the Study of Functional B Cell Subpopulations

Diana R. Roen, Jodi Hanson, and Paul V. Lehmann

Abstract

B cells mediate humoral immunity by producing antibody molecules, but they also participate in innate and acquired immune functions via the secretion of effector molecules such as cytokines, chemokines, and granzyme. B cell subpopulations releasing such effector molecules have been implicated in immunobiology and a number of diseases.

Unlike antigen-specific T cells that can be identified by multimer staining, and then counter-stained to define T cell subpopulations, antigen-specific B cells cannot be detected by flow cytometry. Staining antigen-specific B cells with labeled antigen, in large, has been unsuccessful. Instead, antigen-specific B cells can be and are commonly studied by ELISPOT. In the ELISPOT approach, the B cell is identified via the antibody that it secretes being captured on a membrane by the antigen itself. Should it be feasible to measure simultaneously antibody production and the secretion of other secretory B cell products, it would then be possible to identify B cell subpopulations that co-express effector molecules. Here we introduce multiplex ELISPOT assays in which measurements of antibody secretion are combined with the detection of Granzyme B, IL-6, IL-10, IFN-γ, and TNF-α. Such multiplex assays will help define effector B cell subpopulations, as well as the understanding of their role in health and disease.

Key words ELISPOT, Fluorospot, B cell subpopulation, Effector B cell, Multiplexing, Granzyme B, B-reg, IL-10, Co-expression, Antibodies, Polyfunctional B cells, IL-10, IL-6, TNF-α, IFN-γ, Immune monitoring, Antigen-specific B cell, Be-1, Be-2, Effector plasma cells, Cytokine, Chemokine

1 Introduction

Each B cell has a unique antigen specificity endowed by its antigen receptor, a membrane-anchored immunoglobulin molecule. When a B cell engages in an immune response, its progeny, plasma cells, will secrete immunoglobulins with the same hypervariable region, that is, with the same antigen specificity. These hypervariable regions, however, will be combined with different constant regions defining the antibody class and subclass [1]. While each B cell can secrete only one class/subclass of antibody, the different classes/subclasses mediate various effector functions due to

Alexander E. Kalyuzhny (ed.), *Handbook of ELISPOT: Methods and Protocols*, Methods in Molecular Biology, vol. 1808,
https://doi.org/10.1007/978-1-4939-8567-8_7, © Springer Science+Business Media, LLC, part of Springer Nature 2018

their differential ability to neutralize antigen, activate complement, promote phagocytosis, bind to mast cells, and be exported to mucosal surfaces [2]. When defining antibody-mediated B cell effector functions, therefore, mainstream interest has focused on the delineation of the class and subclass of the antigen-specific B cell repertoire. This can be readily done in the ELISPOT format (but not by flow cytometry) when seeding B cells over antigen-coated membranes [3]. If a B cell is specific for the test antigen, the antibody it secretes will bind to the antigen-coated membrane around the secreting B cell and will be retained as an antibody "spot." This type of membrane-bound antibody "spot" can then be identified by using immune globulin class- and subclass-specific detection reagents. In this way, not only the frequency of antigen-specific B cells within peripheral blood mononuclear cells (PBMC) can be established, that is, the clonal size/magnitude of B cell memory, but also its quality, as the frequencies of B cells will be determined for each immunoglobulin class and subclass. Multiplex ELISPOT assays permitting measurement of all antibody classes and subclasses simultaneously are described in a dedicated chapter of this book [4].

An alternative method for detecting antigen-specific B cells begins with coating the membrane with immunoglobulin-specific capture antibody, for example, antibodies specific for the κ/λ light chains. When B cells secrete antibodies, they first will be captured, irrespective of their antigen specificity. However, the addition of labeled antigen in a second step permits to identify those "spots" formed by B cells that produced antigen-specific antibodies [5].

In addition to secreting antibodies, B cells also exert immune functions via the secretion of cytokines, chemokines, and Granzyme B [6]. While antigen-specific B cells can be reliably detected in ELISPOT assays, as described above, they cannot be readily identified by flow cytometry. Unlike T cells, which can be stained with antigen-containing multimers [7], antigen-specific B cells typically do not stain with labeled antigen. Therefore, while the definition of functional T cell subpopulations can be achieved by counter-staining of multimer-positive T cells for other markers, defining subclasses of antigen-specific B cells cannot be done by flow cytometry. The point of reference for the multiplex B cell ELISPOT assays described here for identifying functional B cell subpopulations is therefore the identification of the antigen-specific B cell via the antibody it produces. B cells that secrete effector molecules other than that antibody will produce a double positive ELISPOT in an assay that captures both the antibody and the effector molecule of interest [8]. Such assays can be multiplexed by introducing an increasing number of analytes, presently up to six, next to the antibody to be captured as the seventh color. The principle of 7 color B cell ELISPOT assays is described in a chapter [4], and that of multicolor ELISPOT analysis in another chapter [9] of this book.

In this chapter, we focus on the detection of Granzyme B, IL-6, IL-10, IFN-γ, and TNF-α co-secretion along with immunoglobulin. Although, in essence, any secretory product of B cells should be measurable taking this approach, we narrowed in on these analytes because they have been the primary ones implicated in B cell biology and immune pathology [6]. Due to the extensive literature published on this topic, we provide just a few examples here illustrating the significance of studying B cell subpopulations in health and disease.

B cells that produce cytokines can be further subdivided into regulatory and effector subsets. The regulatory subset, B-regs, produce IL-10 and/or TGF-β, whereas the Be-1 effector subset secretes IFN-γ, IL-12, and TNF-α, and Be-2 cells produce IL-2, IL-4, and IL-6 [10]. In addition, B cells can engage in Granzyme B (GzB) production following stimulation with IL-21 alone, or with the combination of IL-4 and IL-10 (but not other cytokines) [11]. Additionally, B cell receptor triggering can result in Granzyme B secretion within less than 24 h. These B cells however do not secrete Perforin, Granzyme A, or TRAIL. The selective GzB response occurs simultaneously with the upregulation of antigen presentation on the B cell, including MHC class II and adhesion molecule (CD54) expression. It is not yet known what the physiological role of Granzyme B production by B cells is, in particular because it happens in the absence of Perforin and FAS secretion, but recent findings suggest it may play a role in early antiviral immunity, the regulation of autoimmunity, and in cancer immunosurveillance [12]. Increased Granzyme B secretion by B cells has also been linked with recent vaccination [11] and infectious disease [13].

B cells of patients with multiple sclerosis (MS) have been reported to secrete high levels of IL-6 [14], and this cytokine, when produced by B cells, aggravated disease severity in the animal model of MS, experimental allergic encephalomyelitis, EAE [15]. IL-15 production by B cells was also elevated in MS, and was linked to the ability of B cells to penetrate the blood brain barrier [14]. GM-CSF and IL-10 production by B cells was shown to be reciprocally regulated in MS patients [16], and B cell-derived IL-10 has been implied in controlling EAE [15].

In systemic lupus erythematosus (SLE), B cells produce increased amounts of IL-1α, IL-4, and IL-6 [6], and in B cell chronic lymphocytic leukemia, IL-8 production by B cells has been linked with disease progression [6]. B cell-derived TNF-α is required for lymphoid structure development, and for sustained antibody production [6]. IL-17 production by B cells was shown to exert a protective role in the immune control of the parasite *Trypanosoma cruzi* [17].

Much remains to be elucidated regarding the biological significance of B cell subsets in health and disease, but it has become clear that these subsets exert major contributions to immunity and provide valuable biomarkers for disease and pathology. Multiplex B cell ELISPOT assays that detect the co-secretion of various effector molecules along with antibodies may facilitate substantial progress in this field.

2 Materials

2.1 Instrumentation and Software

1. ImmunoSpot® Series 6 Ultimate Analyzer (Cellular Technology Limited (CTL), Cat # S6UTM12).

2. ImmunoSpot® 7.0 Software, (CTL, Cat # IPS01).

3. ImmunoSpot® LDA 1.4 Software (CTL, Cat # LDA01).

2.2 ImmunoSpot® Kits (See Notes 1 and 2)

Human Granzyme B Detection Kit (CTL, Cat # hT59).

Human IL-10 Detection Kit (CTL, Cat # hT24).

Human IL-6 Detection Kit (CTL, Cat # hT62).

Human IFN-γ Detection Kit (CTL, Cat # hT03).

Human TNF-α Detection Kit (CTL, Cat # hT12).

Human IgG Detection Kit (CTL, Cat # hB09).

Human IgA Detection Kit (CTL, Cat # hB17).

Human IgM Detection Kit (CTL, Cat # hB01).

Human Granzyme B/IgG/IgA Three-Color FluoroSpot Capture Kit (CTL, Cat # hCA3002F).

Human Granzyme B/IgG/IgM Three-Color FluoroSpot Capture Kit (CTL, Cat # hCA3003F).

Human IL-10/IgG/IgA Three-Color FluoroSpot Capture Kit (CTL, Cat # hCA3004F).

Human IL-10/IgG/IgM Three-Color FluoroSpot Capture Kit (CTL, Cat # hCA3005F).

Human IL-6/IgG/IgA Three-Color FluoroSpot Capture Kit (CTL, Cat # hCA3006F).

Human IL-6/IgG/IgM Three-Color FluoroSpot Capture Kit (CTL, Cat # hCA3007F).

Human IFN-γ/IgG/IgA Three-Color FluoroSpot Capture Kit (CTL, Cat # hCA3000F).

Human IFN-γ/IgG/IgM Three-Color FluoroSpot Capture Kit (CTL, Cat # hCA3001F).

Human TNF-α/IgG/IgA Three-Color FluoroSpot Capture Kit (CTL, Cat # hCA3008F).

Human TNF-α/IgG/IgM Three-Color FluoroSpot Capture Kit (CTL, Cat # hCA3009F).

2.3 Media	1. CTL-Test Medium (CTL, Cat # CTLT-005).
	2. CTL-Anti-Aggregate Wash Supplement (CTL, Cat # CTL-AA-005).
	3. RPMI-1640 (Lonza, Cat # BW12167Q).
	4. L-Glutamine (Gibco, Cat # 25030-081).
2.4 Cells, Cell Separation, and Cell Counting	1. Cryopreserved human PBMC, (CTL, ePBMC, http://www.immunospot.com/ImmunoSpot-ePBMC).
	2. Human B cell Isolation Kit, by negative selection (Stemcell Technologies, Cat # 17954) *or* EasySep Release Human CD19 Positive Selection Kit (Stemcell Technologies, Cat # 17754).
	3. EasySep Buffer (Stemcell Technologies, Cat # 20144).
	4. Live-Dead Cell Counting kit with hemocytometers (CTL, Cat # CTL-LD-100).
2.5 Miscellaneous	1. B-Poly-S (CTL, Cat # CTL-hBPOLYS-200).
	2. Lipopolysaccharide (LPS) (Sigma, Cat # L 4391).
	3. Phosphate-buffered saline, PBS (Hyclone, Cat # SH30028-02).
	4. Tween-20 (Sigma, Cat # P1379) to prepare 0.05% Tween-PBS.
	5. Distilled water (Millipore, USA).
	6. Ethyl alcohol, EtOH, 190 proof (Sigma, Cat # 493511).
	7. Wide-orifice tips for plating cells (Rainin, Cat # 17007101).
	8. 5 mL Round-Bottom Tube, 12 × 75 mm style, with cap (Falcon, Cat # 352003).
	9. 25 cm² sterile culture flasks (Corning, Cat # 430639).
	10. 50 mL conical centrifuge tubes (Falcon, Cat # 352070).
	11. Sterile Gauze (Covidien, Cat # 8044).
	12. Cell Reservoir (Denville, Cat # P8826-ST).
	13. Parafilm "M" (Hach, Cat # PM-996).
	14. Vacuum Manifold (Millipore, USA).
	15. 10 mL syringe Luer Lok tip (BD, Cat # 309604).
	16. 0.1 µm syringe filters, low protein binding (Millipore, Cat # SLVV033RS).

---

3   Methods

3.1 Preparation and Stimulation of PBMC	1. Thaw cryopreserved PBMC by placing them in a 37 °C metal bead bath for 15 min. Wipe vial with 70% EtOH to sterilize, and invert twice to mix.

2. Transfer contents of cryovial to a 50 mL conical polypropylene tube. Rinse cryovial with 1 mL warm (37 °C) Anti-Aggregate solution to recover remainder of cells, and add these to the conical tube. Slowly add dropwise, while swirling, an additional 9 mL warm Anti-Aggregate solution to minimize osmotic gradient as DMSO gets diluted.

3. Centrifuge cells at 300 × g for 10 min at room temperature (RT) with max brake.

4. Decant supernatant. Resuspend pellet by flicking the bottom of the tube. Add 10 mL Anti-Aggregate solution.

5. Take 20 µL of cell suspension for counting, and mix well with 20 µL Live/Dead Cell Counting dye. Load into hemocytometer and count live and dead cells on ImmunoSpot® Series 6 Ultimate Analyzer using ImmunoSpot® LDA 1.4 Software.

6. Centrifuge cells at 300 × g for 10 min at RT with maximal brake.

7. Decant supernatant and resuspend cells at five million live cells per milliliter in warm (37 °C) CTL-Test Medium.

8. Transfer cells to a sterile 25 cm² cell culture flask. Add B-Poly-S to the flask at 1 µL/mL final concentration. *See* also **Note 3**. Incubate at 37 °C with 9% CO_2 for 72 h.

3.2 Preparation of ELISPOT Plate

1. Remove underdrain of IPFL plate contained in ImmunoSpot® kit—this plate has a PVDF membrane that has been modified for low autofluorescence.

2. Pre-wet with 15 µL/well freshly prepared 70% EtOH and immediately wash with 150 µL PBS per well (*see* **Note 4**). Decant and repeat PBS wash two more times.

3. Blot plate on sterile gauze, replace the underdrain, and add 80 µL Capture Solution to each well. The Capture Solution contains the κ/λ capture antibodies as well as capture antibodies specific for each analyte to be detected in the multiplex assay, whereby each capture antibody is present at an optimized concentration. Cover plate and incubate overnight in a humidified chamber at 4 °C.

3.3 Isolation of CD19+ B Cells

1. Harvest the PBMC after 72 h polyclonal stimulation (continued from Subheading 3.1) transferring the cells from the culture flask to a sterile 50 mL conical tube. Wash with an excess of warm (37 °C) CTL-Test Medium by centrifugation at 300 × g for 10 min with max brake.

2. Decant supernatant. Resuspend pellet by flicking the bottom of the tube. Add 10 mL CTL-Test Medium.

3. Take 20 µL of cell suspension for counting, and mix well with 20 µL Live/Dead Cell Counting dye. Load into hemocytometer and count on CTL analyzer using Cell Counting software.

4. Centrifuge cells at $300 \times g$ for 10 min at room temperature with max brake.

5. Decant supernatant and resuspend cells in EasySep Buffer at the concentration suggested in the manufacturer's protocol for the desired isolation kit. (In the following, we describe obtaining purified B cells by negative selection; *see* **Note 2** for positive selection). For negative selection, resuspend cells at a final concentration of 5×10^7 cells/mL.

6. Transfer cell suspension to a sterile 5 mL round-bottom tube. Follow manufacturer's protocol for isolation of CD19+ B cells from the pre-stimulated whole PBMC.

7. Add 50 μL/mL Cocktail Enhancer to sample.

8. Add 50 μL/mL Isolation Cocktail to sample. Mix and incubate at room temperature for 5 min.

9. Vortex RapidSpheres and add 50 μL/mL to sample. Mix well.

10. Add EasySep buffer to a final volume of 2.5 mL. Cap tube and invert gently to mix.

11. Place tube into EasySep magnet and remove lid. Incubate for 3 min. Do not agitate tube during incubation.

12. Pick up magnet and invert both magnet and tube to decant liquid into a new sterile 5 mL round-bottom tube. Do not tap or shake off any droplets that remain hanging from the tube.

13. Remove tube from the magnet and replace it with the new tube. Incubate a second time for 1 min within the magnet. Do not agitate tube during incubation.

14. Pick up magnet and invert both magnet and tube to decant liquid into a new sterile 15 mL conical tube. This is the isolated fraction.

15. Wash isolated fraction in CTL-Test Medium by centrifugation at $300 \times g$ for 10 min at room temperature with max brake to remove traces of isolation buffer.

16. Decant supernatant. Resuspend pellet by flicking the bottom of the tube. Add 10 mL CTL-Test Medium per 10 million cells.

17. Take 20 μL of cell suspension for counting, and mix well with 20 μL Live/Dead Cell Counting dye. Load into hemocytometer and count on CTL analyzer using Cell Counting software.

18. Centrifuge cells at $300 \times g$ for 10 min at room temperature with max brake.

19. Decant supernatant and flick tube to resuspend cell pellet. Adjust B cells to 1×10^6/mL in CTL-Test medium, and store in incubator at 37 °C until the cells are plated into the assay.

3.4 Plating of B Cells

1. Remove coated plate from humidified chamber (continued from Subheading 3.2). Decant coating solution and wash one time with 150 μL PBS/well. Decant PBS and blot.

2. If additional stimulation of B cells is required, plate stimulant in 100 μL CTL-Test at 2× final concentration (*see* **Note 3**). If no stimulant is required, add 100 μL CTL-Test to each well.

3. Using wide-orifice tips, add 100 μL per well isolated CD19+ B cells in serial titration (*see* **Note 5**).

4. Cover plate and tap gently on all sides to ensure even distribution of cells.

5. Incubate plate at 37 °C with 9% CO_2 for 24 h (*see* **Note 6**).

3.5 Detection of Antigen-Specific B Cells and Secretory Products

1. Prepare Detection Solution per manufacturer's protocol, containing all the detection antibodies specific for each analyte to be detected at an optimized concentration. If antigen-specific B cells are to be identified in addition, add labeled antigen as described in [5].

2. Filter Detection Solution through a low protein binding 0.1 μm syringe filter.

3. Remove plate from the incubator and decant. Wash 2× with 150 μL PBS, and 2× with 150 μL 0.05% Tween-PBS. Blot to remove residual liquid from the wells (*see* **Notes 7** and **8**).

4. Add 80 μL/well Detection Solution and cover plate. Incubate at room temperature for 2 h, protected from light.

5. Prepare Tertiary Detection solution per manufacturer's protocol. Filter through a low protein binding 0.1 μm syringe filter.

6. Decant plate and wash 3× with 150 μL/well 0.05% Tween-PBS. Blot to remove excess liquid from wells.

7. Add 80 μL/well Tertiary Detection solution and cover plate. Incubate at room temperature for 1 h, protected from light.

8. Decant plate and wash 3× with 150 μL/well distilled water. Remove underdrain and wash upside-down on a vacuum manifold 3× with distilled water to remove any excess fluorochrome.

9. Let plate dry completely, protected from light, before scanning and analysis.

3.6 Data Capture and Analysis

The plate is to be scanned and analyzed on a CTL Series 6 Ultimate Analyzer, or other compatible CTL fluorescent ELISPOT reader that is customized to avoid cross-bleeding of colors (Fig. 1) across detection channels (*see* **Note 1**). The theoretical and practical aspects of accurate multicolor ELISPOT analysis are described in dedicated chapters in this book [9, 18], respectively.

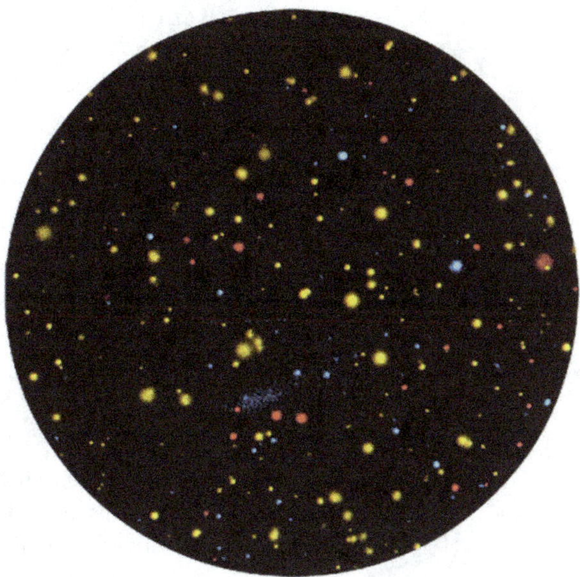

Fig. 1 Example of multicolor ImmunoSpot assay in which measurements of immunoglobulins are multiplexed with detection of cytokine. In this assay, IL-6 (in blue) was detected along with IgG (in yellow) and IgA (in red). The test procedure is detailed in the body of this chapter

---

4 Notes

1. For unambiguous detection of individual analytes using fluorochrome combinations, a setup is needed in which the dyes do not cross-bleed among the detection channels. Each channel is defined by a narrow excitation wavelength combined with a narrow emission filter and can be selected from an array of channels preinstalled on CTL fluorescent readers. Please consult CTL customer support for the selection of channels suitable for the fluorochrome combinations of choice.

2. To isolate CD19+ B cells by positive selection, the EasySep Release Human CD19 Positive Selection Kit can be used. Begin by resuspending whole PBMC at a final concentration of 1×10^8 cells/mL. Transfer cell suspension to a sterile 5 mL round-bottom tube and follow manufacturer's protocol for isolation of CD19+ B cells from the pre-stimulated whole PBMC.

3. For detection of several analytes, including Granzyme B, pre-stimulation may be necessary. The duration of pre-stimulation is dependent upon both the nature of the stimulatory agent and the donor's underlying state of immunobiology/pathology—it can last up to 1 week. With the need for pro-

longed activation, it is advised to add the stimulatory agent along with B-Poly-S at stage 3.1 of the protocol. Alternatively, add stimulant at Subheading 3.4, **step 3** of the protocol.

4. Activation of the membrane with ethanol is instantaneous and can be seen visually as a graying of the membrane. Ethanol should be washed off as quickly as possible following activation to avoid leakage of wells.

5. Numbers of analyte co-expressing B cell subpopulations vary largely and will depend upon the specific combination of analytes being detected, as well as the underlying immunobiology/immune pathology state of the donor. Therefore, titrations of cell concentration are very helpful in determining the optimal starting concentration for the assay.

6. Do not stack plates in the incubator, and do not allow incubator or plates to be disturbed during incubation. Doing so will cause cells within the wells to roll, and spots will become blurred and less distinct, resulting in increased difficulty detecting co-expression of analytes.

7. Do not allow membrane to dry at any point during the analyte detection process described in Subheading 3.5 until the plate is ready to be scanned in **step 9**.

8. Plate washes may be performed manually or with a suitable automated plate washer with adjusted pin length and flow rate, so that membranes and spots are not damaged (CTL recommends the CTL 405LSR).

Acknowledgements

The authors thank Dr. Alexey Karulin and Zoltan Megyesi for developing the software tools for multicolor ELISPOT analysis. Thanks are due also to Richard Caspell and Edith Karacsony for expert technical assistance.

References

1. Xu Z, Zan H, Pone EJ, Mai T, Casali P (2012) Immunoglobulin class-switch DNA recombination: induction, targeting and beyond. Nat Rev Immunol 12(7):517–531. https://doi.org/10.1038/nri3216

2. Abbas AK, Lichtman AH, Pillai S (2014) Cellular and molecular immunology, 8th edn. Elsevier, Amsterdam. pp viii, 535 pages

3. Czerkinsky CC, Nilsson LA, Nygren H, Ouchterlony O, Tarkowski A (1983) A solid-phase enzyme-linked immunospot (ELISPOT) assay for enumeration of specific antibody-secreting cells. J Immunol Methods 65(1–2):109–121

4. Caspell R, Lehmann PV (2018) Detecting all immunoglobulin classes and subclases in a multiplex 7 color ImmunoSpot assay. In: Kalyuzhny AE (ed) Handbook of ELISPOT, Methods in molecular biology, 3rd edn. Springer, New York. pp 85–94

5. Jahnmatz P, Bengtsson T, Zuber B, Farnert A, Ahlborg N (2016) An antigen-specific, four-color, B-cell FluoroSpot assay utilizing tagged antigens for detection. J Immunol Methods

433:23–30. https://doi.org/10.1016/j.jim.2016.02.020

6. Bao Y, Cao X (2014) The immune potential and immunopathology of cytokine-producing B cell subsets: a comprehensive review. J Autoimmun 55:10–23. https://doi.org/10.1016/j.jaut.2014.04.001

7. Altman JD, Moss PA, Goulder PJ, Barouch DH, McHeyzer-Williams MG, Bell JI, McMichael AJ, Davis MM (1996) Phenotypic analysis of antigen-specific T lymphocytes. Science 274(5284):94–96

8. Karulin AY, Hesse MD, Tary-Lehmann M, Lehmann PV (2000) Single-cytokine-producing CD4 memory cells predominate in type 1 and type 2 immunity. J Immunol 164(4):1862–1872

9. Karulin AY, Megyesi Z, Caspell R, Hanson J, Lehmann PV (2018) Multiplexing T- and B-Cell FLUOROSPOT Assays: Experimental Validation of the Multi-color ImmunoSpot® Software Based on Center of Mass Distance Algorithm. In: Kalyuzhny AE (ed.), Handbook of ELISPOT, Methods in Molecular Biology, 3rd ed. Springer, New York. pp 95–113.

10. Lund FE (2008) Cytokine-producing B lymphocytes-key regulators of immunity. Curr Opin Immunol 20(3):332–338. https://doi.org/10.1016/j.coi.2008.03.003

11. Hagn M, Schwesinger E, Ebel V, Sontheimer K, Maier J, Beyer T, Syrovets T, Laumonnier Y, Fabricius D, Simmet T, Jahrsdorfer B (2009) Human B cells secrete granzyme B when recognizing viral antigens in the context of the acute phase cytokine IL-21. J Immunol 183(3):1838–1845. https://doi.org/10.4049/jimmunol.0901066

12. Hagn M, Jahrsdorfer B (2012) Why do human B cells secrete granzyme B? Insights into a novel B-cell differentiation pathway. Oncoimmunology 1(8):1368–1375. https://doi.org/10.4161/onci.22354

13. Hagn M, Panikkar A, Smith C, Balfour HH Jr, Khanna R, Voskoboinik I, Trapani JA (2015) B cell-derived circulating granzyme B is a feature of acute infectious mononucleosis. Clin Transl Immunol 4(6):e38. https://doi.org/10.1038/cti.2015.10

14. Li R, Rezk A, Healy LM, Muirhead G, Prat A, Gommerman JL, Bar-Or A, Team MCBciM (2015) Cytokine-defined B cell responses as therapeutic targets in multiple sclerosis. Front Immunol 6:626. https://doi.org/10.3389/fimmu.2015.00626

15. Nielsen CH, Bornsen L, Sellebjerg F, Brimnes MK (2016) Myelin basic protein-induced production of tumor necrosis factor-alpha and Interleukin-6, and presentation of the immunodominant peptide MBP85-99 by B cells from patients with relapsing-remitting multiple sclerosis. PLoS One 11(1):e0146971. https://doi.org/10.1371/journal.pone.0146971

16. Li R, Rezk A, Miyazaki Y, Hilgenberg E, Touil H, Shen P, Moore CS, Michel L, Althekair F, Rajasekharan S, Gommerman JL, Prat A, Fillatreau S, Bar-Or A, Canadian BMST (2015) Proinflammatory GM-CSF-producing B cells in multiple sclerosis and B cell depletion therapy. Sci Transl Med 7(310):310ra166. https://doi.org/10.1126/scitranslmed.aab4176

17. Dang VD, Hilgenberg E, Ries S, Shen P, Fillatreau S (2014) From the regulatory functions of B cells to the identification of cytokine-producing plasma cell subsets. Curr Opin Immunol 28:77–83. https://doi.org/10.1016/j.coi.2014.02.009

18. Megyesi Z, Lehmann PV, Karulin AY (2018) Multi-Color FLUOROSPOT Counting Using ImmunoSpot® Fluoro-X™ Suite. In: Kalyuzhny AE (ed) Handbook of ELISPOT, Methods in Molecular Biology, 3rd ed. Springer, New York. pp 115–131

Chapter 8

Detecting all Immunoglobulin Classes and Subclasses in a Multiplex 7 Color ImmunoSpot® Assay

Richard Caspell and Paul V. Lehmann

Abstract

Antibody molecules in peripheral blood have a relatively short half-life of roughly 20 days, and therefore their persistence in the serum depends on continuous replenishment by plasma cells. Serum antibody titers are thus indirect and unreliable indicators of immunological memory. In contrast, memory B cells persist in peripheral blood for decades, and enumerating these cells provides direct evidence of having developed an immune response to a given antigen. ELISPOT is an ideal research tool for enumerating antigen-specific memory B cells. Traditionally, B cell ELISPOT assays have been performed for detecting a single class of immunoglobulin (Ig), using a single colorimetric substrate. For comprehensive monitoring of B cell memory, however, all immunoglobulin classes and subclasses need to be assessed. Thus, seven single color assays would need to be performed to measure the numbers of antigen-specific B cells producing IgM, IgA, IgE, IgG_1, IgG_2, IgG_3, and IgG_4. We report here the development of a multiplex seven color B cell ImmunoSpot® assay in which the number of antigen-specific B cells can be established simultaneously for all major antibody classes and subclasses, requiring the PBMC, antigen, and labor corresponding to a single color assay.

Key words Immune monitoring, B cell, Humoral immunity, Antibody, ELISPOT, Fluorospot, Multiplexing

1 Introduction

For over a century, the detection of serum antibodies has served as the gold standard for the assessment of exposure to, and development of, immunity to an antigen. Indeed, in many instances serum antibodies can be detected even decades after an infection, as seen for example with influenza [1]. In other cases however, antibody titers wane over time, and booster immunizations are required to maintain protective antibody titers, as exemplified by tetanus, and many other vaccines [2]. An increasing number of recent findings show that seronegative individuals can develop strong T-cell immunity, as was seen in subsets of HIV- and HCMV-exposed individuals [3–7]. In the majority of multiple sclerosis patients, neuroantigen-specific memory B cells were detected in peripheral blood, demonstrating that an

Alexander E. Kalyuzhny (ed.), *Handbook of ELISPOT: Methods and Protocols*, Methods in Molecular Biology, vol. 1808,
https://doi.org/10.1007/978-1-4939-8567-8_8, © Springer Science+Business Media, LLC, part of Springer Nature 2018

autoimmune response had occurred, while titers of serum antibodies specific for neuroantigens were not elevated [8]. Limitations of serologic tests are also well known in other fields. Thus, the interpretation of serological testing results remains inconclusive for subjects who have received transfusions of blood or blood products due to the transfer of donor antibodies. This also applies to children less than 12 months of age, while the mother's antibodies continue to be detectable [9, 10].

The reason for the above limitations of serodiagnostics becomes evident by taking a closer look at the relevant immunobiology. Antibody molecules in serum have a relatively short half-life, in the range of days to weeks, and therefore their presence in serum depends on ongoing production by B cell-derived plasma cells [11]. During the course of an immune response, naïve antigen-specific B-cells become activated by the antigen and through interactions with antigen-specific CD4 T-helper cells. As a consequence of activation, these B cells differentiate into plasma cells that produce antibodies. At the same time, long-lived memory B-cells also develop. These memory cells can give rise to new generations of plasma cells in the presence of persisting/reappearing antigen and T-cell-help, or in the absence of antigen, long-lived plasma cells can continue to spontaneously secrete antibody [1]. In either case, the presence of antibodies in serum of individuals results from an active, ongoing antibody synthesis process, which may or may not truthfully reflect previous antigen exposure. As antigen itself rarely persists to drive the continuous production of antibodies, it is now assumed that non-antigen-specific polyclonal stimuli maintain serological memory [12].

Serum antibodies are, therefore, indirect indicators of immunity that arise from complex and sometimes even random cellular reactions. Subsequently, it has become a mainstream effort to go directly to the source, and assess B cell memory itself. Memory B cells are long lived and persist for decades while recirculating in the blood [13]. Unlike antigen-specific T cells that can be stained with antigen-embedding multimers of MHC molecules (tetramers, pentamers, dextramers) [14], efforts to directly stain B cells with labeled antigen so far have failed in large. Instead, the detection of antigen-specific B cells is enabled by the ELISPOT technique [15]. In brief, 96 well plates with a special PVDF membrane on the bottom of each well are coated with the test antigen. When PBMC (which contain B cells) or purified B cells are plated into such wells, antibodies produced by the B cells that are specific for the test antigen will be captured on the membrane around the secreting B cell. These plate-bound antibodies can then be visualized by adding labeled detection antibodies. In this way, each antigen-specific B cell will produce a "spot," and counting the numbers of these Spot Forming Units (SFU) permits one to establish the frequency of antigen-specific B cells among all cells plated. Increased numbers of antigen-specific B cells detected in PBMC ex vivo prove that these B cells have undergone clonal expansions in vivo. Importantly, antigen-specific B cell ELISPOT assays also provide insight into the affinity of the antibody that each B cell produces. Antibodies secreted by B cells that have high affinity for antigen will bind faster and stronger to the antigen on the membrane than low affinity antibodies, resulting in dense ELISPOTs for high affinity B cells, and diffuse spots for low affinity B cells [16]. By studying the morphology of spots produced by a high number of antigen-specific B cells within a test subject, one therefore can gain insights into the affinity distribution of the B cell/antibody repertoire within that individual (*see* **Note 1**).

Antibodies occur in different classes and subclasses, and each differ in their ability to precipitate antigen, neutralize, activate complement, promote phagocytosis, migrate to mucosal surfaces, or sensitize mast cells (reviewed in [17]). All B cells initially produce IgM, but in the course of an immune response, undergo class switching to secrete other types of immunoglobulins, whereby the mature plasma B cells will each secrete only one class/subclass of antibody. Immunoglobulin class switching is under tight control by CD4 T cells and cytokines, as the engagement of the appropriate class and subclass of antibody critically defines successful immune defense [17]. Therefore, if ex vivo antigen-specific B cells produce antibody classes/subclasses other than IgM, this shows that the memory cells have undergone immunoglobulin class switching in vivo [18], and the detection of a particular immunoglobulin class/subclass in this ELISPOT format establishes the quality of B cell/antibody memory.

Comprehensive immune monitoring, therefore, requires identifying the numbers and ratios of antigen-specific B cells producing antibodies of all classes and subclasses to a given antigen, i.e., IgM, IgG, IgA, and IgE, and the four subclasses of IgG: IgG_1, IgG_2, IgG_3, and IgG_4. To accomplish this goal, previously eight single color B cell ELISPOT assays would need to be run in parallel, each detecting one of the classes or subclasses. Here we report and communicate the protocol for combining these assays into a single seven color multiplex assay. Figure 1a shows a representative example of such a seven color assay. Of note, the assay was designed such that each analyte can be detected in a separate fluorescent channel or combination of channels without the leakage of signal (*see* **Note 2**). Panels b–g of Fig. 1 show the individual analyte planes for the seven color B cell assay described here. Analysis therefore can be done without the need for compensation, monochromatically for each of the analytes. In this chapter, we describe the seven color assay itself; additionally, we contributed other dedicated chapters on the experimental validation of multi-color analysis [19], as well as to the step by step process to its implementation [20].

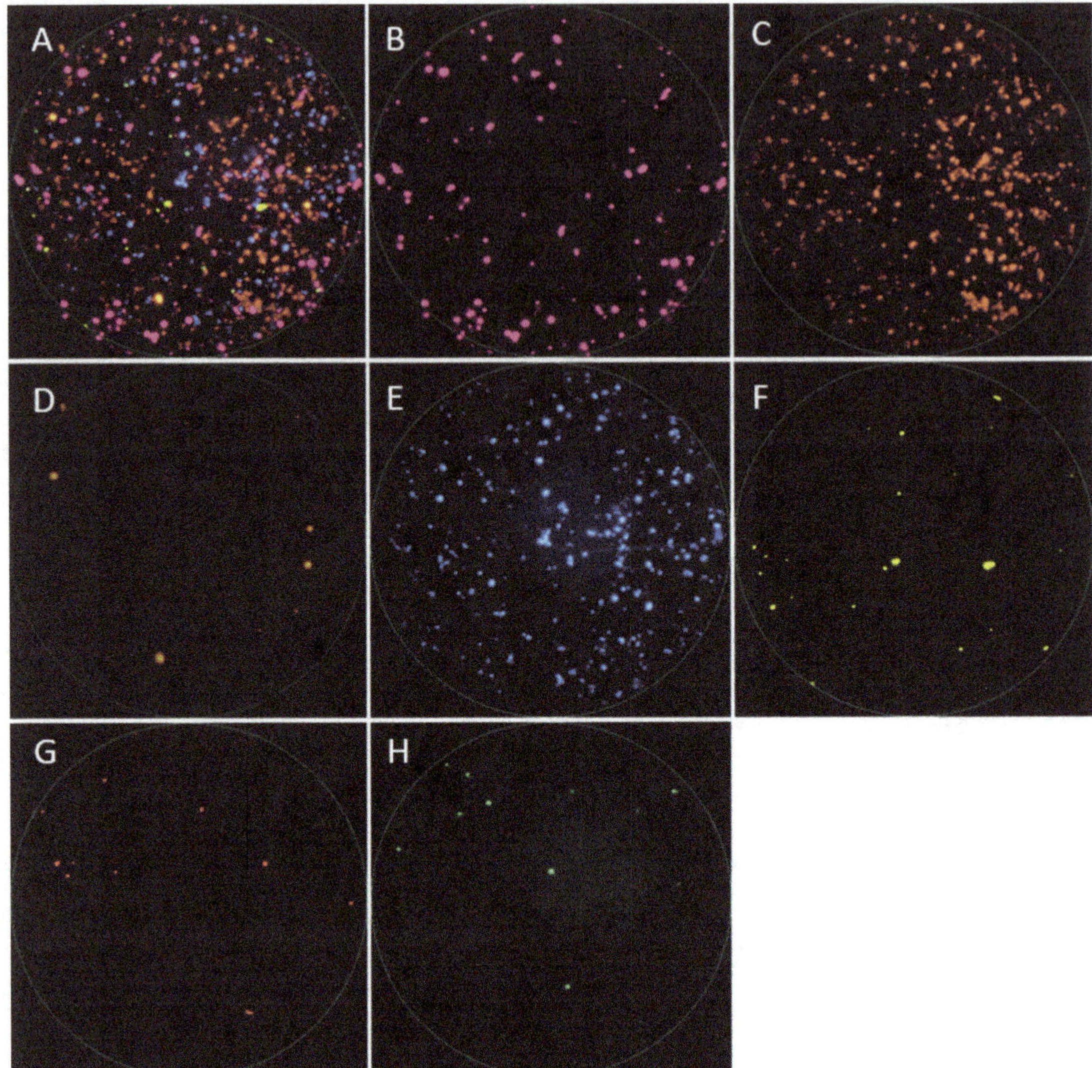

Fig. 1 Repereserative image of a seven color B cell ImmunoSpot® well. The assay was performed as described in this chapter. For analysis, each color is detected in a dedicated color plane (*see* **Note 2**). Each color plane is shown in one of the panels: IgA in Panel **b**, IgM in Panel **c**, IgE in Panel **d**, IgG$_1$ in Panel **e**, IgG$_2$ in Panel **f**, IgG$_3$ in Panel **g**, and IgG$_4$ in Panel **h**, respectively. Panel **a** shows the overlay of these images (*see* **Note 17**)

2   Materials

2.1   Isolation of PBMC from Whole Blood

1. Green vacutainer tubes with sodium heparin.

2. Ficoll-Paque™ Plus.

3. Ca^{2+}, Mg^{2+} free phosphate buffered saline (PBS) pH 7.2.

4. CTL-Wash™ Supplement 10× (Cellular Technology Ltd., CTL, Shaker Hts, OH, Cat# CTLW-010).

5. Centrifuge capable of spinning 50 mL conical tubes at 740 × *g*.

2.2 Thawing of Cryopreserved PBMC	1. Bead bath (set to 37 °C). 2. CTL-Test™ B Culture Medium (CTL, Cat# CTLTB-010), supplemented with 1% L-Glutamine. 3. Centrifuge capable of spinning 50 mL conical tubes at $330 \times g$.
2.3 Counting of PBMC	1. ImmunoSpot® Series 6 Ultimate Analyzer (CTL, Cat# S6UTM12), running LD Software for live/dead cell counting (CTL, Cat# LDA01). 2. CTL-LDC™ Live/Dead Cell Counting Kit (CTL, Cat# CTL-LDC-100-2).
2.4 Polyclonal Stimulation of Memory B Cells from PBMC	1. Cryopreserved or freshly isolated PBMC. 2. B-Poly-SE™ (CTL, Cat# hBPOLYSE-200). 3. Culture flask or plate. 4. Humidified CO_2 incubator set for 37 °C, 9% CO_2. 5. CTL-Test™ B supplemented with 1% L-Glutamine (CTL, Cat# CTLTB-010). 6. Centrifuge capable of spinning 50 mL conical tubes at $330 \times g$.
2.5 Elispot Assay	1. Commercially available, seven Color Fluorospot B Cell kit (CTL, Cat# hB7F) optimized to detect human IgM, IgA, IgE, IgG_1, IgG_2, IgG_3, and IgG_4 (*see* **Note 3**). 2. 0.05% Tween-PBS: 100 µL Tween-20 in 200 mL PBS (per plate). 3. PBS, sterile, 100 mL (per plate). 4. Distilled water, 100 mL (per plate). 5. 70% EtOH. 6. 0.1 µm syringe-driven filter. 7. Plate washer (CTL, Cat# 405LSR) (*see* **Note 4**). 8. Vacuum manifold (Millipore, USA). 9. ImmunoSpot® S6 Ultimate 5LED Analyzer (CTL, Cat# S6UTM12), running ImmunoSpot® 7.0 Software (CTL, Cat# IPS01).

---

3 Methods

3.1 Isolation of PBMC from Whole Blood	1. Obtain blood samples according to institution's IRB protocol. 2. Keeping donors' samples separate, pool each donor's blood into appropriately labeled 50 mL conical tubes. Rinse each vacutainer tube with PBS and add to blood. 3. Measure blood volume and dilute 1:1 with PBS.

4. Layer diluted blood slowly over Ficoll® taking care not to disrupt the interface (*see* **Note 5**).

5. Centrifuge balanced tubes at $740 \times g$ for 30 min with the centrifuge brake off.

6. Identify the cloudy interface between the Ficoll® and the plasma layer. Remove this interface with a serological pipette and transfer to a fresh 50 mL conical tube (*see* **Note 6**).

7. Dilute cells 1:2 with warm CTL-Wash™ Medium (for example, 15 mL cells + 30 mL medium) and spin at $330 \times g$ for 10 min with centrifuge brake on.

8. Decant supernatant and re-suspend cells in warm CTL-Wash™ Medium at approximately 1×10^6 cells/mL and take a sample for cell counting (*see* **Note 7**).

3.2 Thawing of Cryopreserved PBMC

1. Warm CTL-Test B™ Medium to 37 °C.

2. Place frozen cryovials (containing >1×10^7 cells per vial) in a 37 °C metal bead bath for 15 min.

3. Flip the cryovial twice 180° to re-suspend the cells.

4. Aspirate all liquid within cryovial using a serological pipette and transfer into a 50 mL conical tube.

5. Wash cryovial with 1 mL of fresh CTL-Test™ B Medium and add slowly to the rest of the cells.

6. Slowly add 8 mL of warm CTL-Test™ B Medium in the following manner: while swirling sample tube, add first 3 mL at the approximate rate of 1 mL/10 s, and the remaining 5 mL can be added progressively faster.

7. Centrifuge at $330 \times g$ for 10 min.

8. Re-suspend cells at approximately 1×10^6 cells/mL and take a sample for counting (*see* **Note 7**).

3.3 Counting of PBMC

1. For each sample to be counted, mix 50 µL CTL-LDC™ Reagent with 50 µL of the cell suspension, pipetting up and down three times.

2. Aspirate 10 µL of the stained cells and load into the hemocytometer chamber—the liquid will fill the chamber by capillary action and any excess will be collected in the overflow reservoir.

3. Count cells (*see* **Note 8**).

3.4 Polyclonal Stimulation of Memory B Cells from PBMC (See Note 9)

1. Use warm (37 °C) CTL-Test™ B Medium.

2. Adjust PBMC (freshly isolated from blood or thawed from cryopreserved PBMC) in CTL-Test™ B Medium to 4 million/mL.

3. Add B-Poly-SE™ reagent to PBMC in CTL-Test B™ 1:200 (e.g., 50 µL B-Poly-SE™ to 10 mL CTL-Test™ B).

4. Culture cells in a 37 °C humidified incubator at 9% CO_2 for 4–7 days (*see* **Notes 10** and **11**).

3.5 The seven Color ImmunoSpot® B Cell Assay

1. One day before plating cells, prepare 70% EtOH, Capture Antibody or Antigen working solutions.

2. Remove plate underdrain, pipette 15 μL of 70% ethanol into each well, and incubate for less than 1 min. Add 150 μL of PBS, decant, and wash with 150 μL of PBS two more times.

3. Replace underdrain and immediately (before plate dries) pipette 80 μL/well of the Capture Solution into the low-autofluorescence PVDF plate provided with the kit.

4. Seal plate with parafilm and incubate at 4 °C overnight.

5. The next day, count PBMC and centrifuge at 330 × *g* for 10 min, decant supernatant, then re-suspend cells to a concentration of 2×10^6 cells/mL.

6. Plate PBMC in serial dilution into the PVDF plate (*see* **Note 12**).

7. Incubate cells on plate overnight at 37 °C (*see* **Note 13**).

8. Prepare Detection Antibody working solution by following kit protocol.

9. After incubation, decant cells and wash plate two times with PBS and two times with 0.05% Tween-PBS, 200 μL/well each time (*see* **Notes 4** and **14**).

10. Decant wash buffer and add 80 μL/well of Detection Solution to plate, incubate 2 h at 4 °C.

11. Prepare a working Tertiary Solution containing the fluorescent tags by following kit protocol.

12. Wash plate three times with 0.05% Tween PBS, 200 μL/well.

13. Decant wash buffer and add 80 μL/well of Tertiary Solution to plate. Incubate at room temperature for 1 h.

14. Wash plate two times with distilled water, 200 μL/well each time.

15. Rinse membrane with tap water, decant, and repeat three times.

16. Remove protective underdrain, place plate face down on vacuum manifold and completely fill the backside of plate with water, then vacuum water through the membrane.

17. Let plate dry completely, protected from light (*see* **Note 15**).

18. Scan and count plate with compatible analyzer (*see* **Note 16**).

---

4 Notes

1. The affinity distribution of antigen-specific B cells can be readily studied using the ImmunoSpot® software: images of wells containing antigen-specific B cell ELISPOTs are converted

into FCS files, and these are plotted in a spot size vs. density diagram.

2. The detection of individual analytes using fluorochromes requires an analyzer configured to ensure that the signal from the dyes do not cross-bleed between the detection channels. In this way, each analyte is detected in a separate analyte plane. Each channel is defined by a narrow excitation wavelength in conjunction with a narrow emission filter and can be selected from an array of channels preinstalled on CTL fluorescent analyzers.

3. Kit is suited for detecting either antibody secreting cells that have been immunized/activated in vivo, or memory B cells that have been polyclonally stimulated in vitro to secrete antibody. Each kit contains capture and detection antibodies, fluorescent detection reagents, diluent buffers, serum-free B cell assay medium, low autofluorescence PVDF-membrane plates, and a polyclonal B cell activator.

4. Plate washes may also be performed manually, but for automated washing, the pin length and flow rate need to be customized so membranes and spots are not damaged, as has been done for the CTL 405LSR plate washer.

5. Alternately, the diluted blood can be added first, and the Ficoll® gently underlaid with a serological pipette.

6. While collecting the cells, be sure to aspirate as little Ficoll® as possible. At this point, interphase cells from two 50 mL tubes can be combined into one tube. If the proportion of Ficoll® is too high (>5 mL), a significant cell loss will occur.

7. As a point of reference, keep in mind that 1 mL of fresh blood should yield approximately 1×10^6 PBMC.

8. Live cells will fluoresce green (480/525) and dead cells will fluoresce red (570/620). Cells can be counted with either a fluorescence-capable microscope or using the LDA software of the ImmunoSpot® Analyzer.

9. Resting memory B cells do not secrete antibodies, and they can be detected in ELISPOT assays only after polyclonal stimulation. In contrast, the spontaneous production of antibodies by B cells in freshly isolated blood signifies recent and ongoing antigen stimulation in vivo.

10. For detection of all antibody classes except IgE, 4 day stimulation with CTL B-Poly-S™ is suitable. However IgE producing memory B cells occur in very low frequency. IgE class switching can be induced in vitro by culturing cells for 7 days with CD40L and IL-4.

11. If a 24-well plate is used, plate 1 mL of the cell suspension per well. For larger scale polyclonal stimulation cultures, traditional culture flasks can be used. Suggested conditions for culture

flasks are approximately 3 mL of 4 million/mL cell suspension per cm^2. For example, in a T-25 flask, we recommend 8 mL of total cell suspension, for a T-75 flask, 25 mL.

12. After in vitro stimulation, B cells secreting certain antibody classes and subclasses (such as IgA or IgG$_1$) can be rather high, whereas in vivo stimulated, spontaneously secreting B cells tend to occur in rather low frequencies. Therefore it is important to establish the frequency range for the test groups and antigens of interest, and then cover this range in serial dilutions. For the detection of low-frequency Ig-producing cells, we recommend plating cells at 1×10^6, 5×10^5, 2.5×10^5, and 1.25×10^5 cells per well. In the case of very rare Ig-secreting cells, magnetic bead-based enrichment of B cells is recommended. For high-frequency Ig-secreting cells, continue dilution of cells down to 15,000, 10,000, and 5000 cells per well. Keep the diluted PBMC in a CO_2 incubator with lid open until pipetting into the assay.

13. Do not stack plates in the incubator. Avoid disturbing incubator or plates during incubation so cells do not roll during the assay.

14. The membrane must not dry at any time during the analyte detection process.

15. To completely dry plate, place in running laminar flow hood for 2 h or on the bench top for 24 h at a 45° angle on paper towels. Do not dry the ELISPOT assay plates at temperatures exceeding 37 °C as this may cause the membrane to warp or crack. Spots may not be readily visible while the membrane is still wet and the background fluorescence may be elevated. Scan and count plates only after membranes have completely dried.

16. The multicolor analysis process is described, step by step, in a dedicated chapter of this book [19]. The experimental validation of multi-color analysis is described in another chapter of this book [20]. CTL has scanning and analysis services available, and offers a trial version of ImmunoSpot® Software with the purchase of a kit.

17. A comparison of the individual panels in Fig. 1b–h shows that spots present in one channel are not visible in any of the other channels, i.e., the individual colors are being selectively detected without cross-bleeding. Double positive spots, thus, are neither seen, nor expected to be seen, as B cells can produce only one class or subclass of immunoglobulin at each differentiation state.

References

1. Crotty S, Ahmed R (2004) Immunological memory in humans. Semin Immunol 16(3):197–203. https://doi.org/10.1016/j.smim.2004.02.008

2. Bottiger M, Gustavsson O, Svensson A (1998) Immunity to tetanus, diphtheria and poliomyelitis in the adult population of Sweden in 1991. Int J Epidemiol 27(5):916–925

3. Clerici M, Levin JM, Kessler HA, Harris A, Berzofsky JA, Landay AL, Shearer GM (1994) HIV-specific T-helper activity in seronegative health care workers exposed to contaminated blood. JAMA 271(1):42–46

4. De Maria A, Cirillo C, Moretta L (1994) Occurrence of human immunodeficiency virus type 1 (HIV-1)-specific cytolytic T cell activity in apparently uninfected children born to HIV-1-infected mothers. J Infect Dis 170(5):1296–1299

5. Rowland-Jones S, Sutton J, Ariyoshi K, Dong T, Gotch F, McAdam S, Whitby D, Sabally S, Gallimore A, Corrah T et al (1995) HIV-specific cytotoxic T-cells in HIV-exposed but uninfected Gambian women. Nat Med 1(1):59–64

6. Sester M, Gartner BC, Sester U, Girndt M, Mueller-Lantzsch N, Kohler H (2003) Is the cytomegalovirus serologic status always accurate? A comparative analysis of humoral and cellular immunity. Transplantation 76(8):1229–1230. https://doi.org/10.1097/01.TP.0000083894.61333.56

7. Zhu J, Shearer GM, Marincola FM, Norman JE, Rott D, Zou JP, Epstein SE (2001) Discordant cellular and humoral immune responses to cytomegalovirus infection in healthy blood donors: existence of a Th1-type dominant response. Int Immunol 13(6):785–790

8. Kuerten S, Pommerschein G, Barth SK, Hohmann C, Milles B, Sammer FW, Duffy CE, Wunsch M, Rovituso DM, Schroeter M, Addicks K, Kaiser CC, Lehmann PV (2014) Identification of a B cell-dependent subpopulation of multiple sclerosis by measurements of brain-reactive B cells in the blood. Clin Immunol 152(1–2):20–24. https://doi.org/10.1016/j.clim.2014.02.014

9. de la Hoz RE, Stephens G, Sherlock C (2002) Diagnosis and treatment approaches of CMV infections in adult patients. J Clin Virol 25(Suppl 2):S1–S12

10. Rawlinson WD (1999) Broadsheet. Number 50: diagnosis of human cytomegalovirus infection and disease. Pathology 31(2):109–115

11. Wrammert J, Ahmed R (2008) Maintenance of serological memory. Biol Chem 389(5):537–539

12. Bernasconi NL, Traggiai E, Lanzavecchia A (2002) Maintenance of serological memory by polyclonal activation of human memory B cells. Science 298(5601):2199–2202. https://doi.org/10.1126/science.1076071

13. Kurosaki T, Kometani K, Ise W (2015) Memory B cells. Nat Rev Immunol 15(3):149–159. https://doi.org/10.1038/nri3802

14. Altman JD, Paul AHM, Philip JRG, Barouch DH, McHeyzer-Williams MG, Bell JI, McMichael AJ, Davis MM (1996) Phenotypic analysis of antigen-specific T lymphocytes. Science 274(5284):94–96

15. Czerkinsky CC, Nilsson LA, Nygren H, Ouchterlony O, Tarkowski A (1983) A solid-phase enzyme-linked immunospot (ELISPOT) assay for enumeration of specific antibody-secreting cells. J Immunol Methods 65(1–2):109–121

16. Karulin AY, Lehmann PV (2012) How ELISPOT morphology reflects on the productivity and kinetics of cells' secretory activity. Methods Mol Biol 792:125–143. https://doi.org/10.1007/978-1-61779-325-7_11

17. Abbas AK, Lichtman AH, Pillai S (2014) Cellular and molecular immunology, 8th edn. Saunders, Philadelphia, PA

18. Harriman W, Volk H, Defranoux N, Wabl M (1993) Immunoglobulin class switch recombination. Annu Rev Immunol 11(1):361–384. https://doi.org/10.1146/annurev.iy.11.040193.002045

19. Karulin AY, Megyesi Z, Caspell R, Hanson J, Lehmann PV (2018) Multiplexing T- and B-Cell FLUOROSPOT Assays: Experimental Validation of the Multi-color ImmunoSpot® Software Based on Center of Mass Distance Algorithm. In: Kalyuzhny AE (ed.), Handbook of ELISPOT, Methods in Molecular Biology, 3rd ed. Springer, New York. pp 95–113

20. Megyesi Z, Lehmann PV, Karulin AY (2018) Multi-Color FLUOROSPOT Counting Using ImmunoSpot® Fluoro-X™ Suite. In: Kalyuzhny AE (ed) Handbook of ELISPOT, Methods in Molecular Biology, 3rd ed. Springer, New York. pp 115–131

Multiplexing T- and B-Cell FLUOROSPOT Assays: Experimental Validation of the Multi-Color ImmunoSpot® Software Based on Center of Mass Distance Algorithm

Alexey Y. Karulin, Zoltán Megyesi, Richard Caspell, Jodi Hanson, and Paul V. Lehmann

Abstract

Over the past decade, ELISPOT has become a highly implemented mainstream assay in immunological research, immune monitoring, and vaccine development. Unique single cell resolution along with high throughput potential sets ELISPOT apart from flow cytometry, ELISA, microarray- and bead-based multiplex assays. The necessity to unambiguously identify individual T and B cells that do, or do not co-express certain analytes, including polyfunctional cytokine producing T cells has stimulated the development of multi-color ELISPOT assays. The success of these assays has also been driven by limited sample/cell availability and resource constraints with reagents and labor. There are few commercially available test kits and instruments available at present for multi-color FLUOROSPOT. Beyond commercial descriptions of competing systems, little is known about their accuracy in experimental settings detecting individual cells that secrete multiple analytes vs. random overlays of spots. Here, we present a theoretical and experimental validation study for three and four color T- and B-cell FLUOROSPOT data analysis. The ImmunoSpot® Fluoro-X™ analysis system we used includes an automatic image acquisition unit that generates individual color images free of spectral overlaps and multi-color spot counting software based on the maximal allowed distance between centers of spots of different colors or Center of Mass Distance (COMD). Using four color B-cell FLUOROSPOT for IgM, IgA, IgG1, IgG3; and three/four color T-cell FLUOROSPOT for IL-2, IFN-γ, TNF-α, and GzB, in serial dilution experiments, we demonstrate the validity and accuracy of Fluoro-X™ multi-color spot counting algorithms. Statistical predictions based on the Poisson spatial distribution, coupled with scrambled image counting, permit objective correction of true multi-color spot counts to exclude randomly overlaid spots.

Key words ELISPOT, FLUOROSPOT, Polyfunctional, T cell, B cell, Immunoglobulin, Antibody, Cytokine, Center of mass, ImmunoSpot®, Fluoro-X™, Software, Fluorescence, Multi-color, Multiplex, Spot counting, Image analysis

1 Introduction

Dual-color ELISPOT assays based on traditional enzyme-tagged reagents and two to three color FLUOROSPOT assays based on fluorophore-tagged reagents have become increasingly popular in

Alexander E. Kalyuzhny (ed.), *Handbook of ELISPOT: Methods and Protocols*, Methods in Molecular Biology, vol. 1808, https://doi.org/10.1007/978-1-4939-8567-8_9, © Springer Science+Business Media, LLC, part of Springer Nature 2018

immunological research and immune monitoring. Recently, four color T-cell and seven color B-cell assays have also became commercially available. A number of commercial vendors now offer test kits and automated spot counters for simultaneous detection of various biological molecules secreted by activated T and B lymphocytes and other immune cells. There are two main reasons for multiplexing ELISPOT assays. First reason is purely pragmatic: detection of several analytes secreted by T or B cells in a single culture well reduces both the labor and the amount of cells/reagents required, and thus proportionally reduces the cost to perform the assay. Beyond cost, in clinical settings primary cells are frequently limited and quality controlled reagents also may be limited in the context of novel analytes. Secondly, it is increasingly clear that monitoring polyfunctional T-cell secreting multiple cytokines in various combinations at a time (like IL-2/IFN-γ or IL2/GzB/TNF-α) provides better assessment of protective immunity [1–13]. Although the procedural steps in performing multi-color cytokine (or antibody) FLUOROSPOT is not significantly different from a single-color ELISPOT, analyzing the results obtained, i.e., the spots with more than two colors, is a complex image analysis challenge. In case of FLUOROSPOT complex color recognition task can be reduced to a single-color analysis of separate single-color images generated for each individual analyte with subsequent detection of dual-/triple-/multi-color spots occupying the same location on the membrane. Such images can be readily generated using individual combinations of excitation/emission filters (fluorescent channel) optimized for each fluorochrome. The remaining issue is to develop an algorithm for accurately matching or "pairing" single-color spots from individual fluorescent channels to identify dual-, triple-, or multi-color spots. In the ImmunoSpot® Software v. 5.0 (September 2010 by CTL, Cleveland OH), we introduced a Center of Mass Distance algorithm based on the maximal allowed distance between centers of spots in individual color images. For bright fluorescence spots on a dark background, this "center of mass" corresponds to the center of light intensity inside the spot outline (often referred to in image analysis as "center of gray"). We found that due to several reasons discussed below, centers of gray (referred to as centers of mass from hereon) for individual colors never coincide precisely for true multi-color spots. To account for these color "shifts," we included a maximal allowed distance (in ImmunoSpot® Software, it is called Center of Mass Distance or COMD) parameter, which depends on the optical characteristics of a reader and specific fluorescent labels used. From the user perspective, any algorithm used for FLUOROSPOT multi-color image analysis is a "black box" and has to be validated. In this study, we propose an experimental validation approach based on two independent assays. One uses a four color B-cell FLUOROSPOT for human Ig classes and subclasses where no dual- or multi-color spots are possible due to allelic exclusion. The second assay is a three and four color T-cell FLUOROSPOT detecting analytes that T cells are known to co-express. Using statistical predictive approach and scrambled (distorted) spot positions, we are able to differentiate closely situated cells producing different cytokines, from a single cell producing multiple cytokines at a time.

2 Materials

1. Human cryopreserved PBMC of 2 HLA-A2-positive donors were obtained from our commercial ePBMC® library (CTL, Shaker Heights, OH). These PBMC had been previously HLA-typed at high resolution and characterized for T-cell reactivity to a variety of antigens previously (details are available at http://www.immunospot.com/ImmunoSpot-ePBMC).

2. Human IFN-γ/TNF-α/GzB (http://www.immunospot.com/immunospot-kits/human-interferon-gamma-tnf-a-granzyme-b-three-color-fluorospot) and IFN-γ/TNF-α/IL-2 (http://www.immunospot.com/immunospot-kits/human-interferon-gamma-tnf-a-il-2-three-color-fluorospot) FLUOROSPOT three color kits were obtained from CTL (Shaker Heights, OH).

3. Human four color B-cell FLUOROSPOT kit for simultaneous detection of total IgM, IgA, IgG1, and IgG3 producing cells (http://www.immunospot.com/immunospot-kits/human-igm-iga-igg1-igg3-four-color-fluorospot, CTL, Shaker Heights, OH).

4. FLUOROSPOT plates were scanned and analyzed using an ImmunoSpot® S6-Ultimate UV Reader (CTL, Shaker Heights, OH). Single-/dual-/multi-color spots were counted automatically by using the ImmunoSpot® v.7.0 Fluoro-X™ Software Suite (CTL, Shaker Heights, OH) as described in the Methods Subheadings 3.7 and 3.8.

3 Methods

3.1 Cell Preparation

Prior to testing, the PBMC cryo-vials, stored in the liquid N_2 vapor phase, were transferred to dry ice in styrofoam containers for transport to and short-term storage in the laboratory. Then the cells were thawed essentially following a protocol providing the optimal functionality and recovery for cryopreserved PBMC [14]. Specifically, cryo-vials were rapidly warmed up to 37 °C in the glass bead bath (CTL-BB-001, for 8 min at 37 °C). Warmed up cryo-vials were flipped twice to re-suspend the cells and the cell suspension (10 million cells in 1 mL) was gently transferred with a wide-bore 2-mL pipette into a 15-mL V-bottom Falcon tube. For complete cell recovery, the cryo-vials were rinsed with 1 mL warm (37 °C) CTL Anti-Aggregate-Wash™ medium (CTL-AA-005) containing benzonase. An additional 8 mL CTL Anti-Aggregate-Wash™ warm medium (37 °C) was added to the 15-mL tube at a rate of 2 mL per every 5 s. PBMCs were counted by fluorescence microscopy using Acridine Orange and Ethidium Bromide (AO/EB), then washed twice in 10 mL CTL-Test™ warm medium (CTLT-005) and re-suspended at a final concentration of 3×10^6/mL in the same medium. The freshly thawed PBMC (100 µL) were plated (within 1 h) into an ELISPOT 96 well plate (Msn HTS IP, Millipore, MA, USA).

3.2 T-Cell FLUOROSPOT

T-cell assays were performed following the manufacturer's protocols. Antigens EBV-dominant HLA-A2 restricted peptide LMP2A (426–434) and HCMV HLA-A2 restricted peptide pp65 (495–503) (EZ Biolab Inc., Carmel, IN, USA) were plated in 100 µL per well prior to cells into the capture antibody-coated assay plate. Final concentration of peptides was 1 µg/mL. The antigens were dissolved in CTL-Test™ medium (CTLT-005). Same test medium (without antigen) was used as negative control. The plates containing the antigens (or medium controls) were kept at 37 °C in a CO_2 incubator until the cells were ready to be plated. Final concentration of PBMC was 3×10^5/mL unless specified otherwise. In cell titration experiments, PBMC were diluted in CTL-test medium to the required concentrations and 100 µL/well. PBMC were always plated using wide-bore pipette tips, after which plates were gently tapped on each side to ensure even distribution of the cells. For the duration of the assay (24 h), plates were incubated at 37 °C in a CO_2 incubator.

3.3 B-Cell FLUOROSPOT

For multi-color B-cell FLUOROSPOT, human PBMC were prepared as described above. Prior to the assay, B cells were polyclonally pre-activated with R848 and human rIL-2 [15]. After pre-activation, cells were washed once in CTL-Test-B™ medium and counted as described above. PBMC were tested in 2× serial dilutions from 10,000 down to 78 cells per well. Plates with cells were incubated 24 h at 37 °C in a CO_2 incubator. B-cell FLUOROSPOT kit was used according to the manufacturer's protocols and recommendations. As capture reagents, mouse monoclonal antibodies against human Ig light κ/λ chains were used. Following protocol specified washing and developing steps, plates were air dried in a laminar hood.

3.4 Theoretical Calculations of Random Spot Overlays Based on Statistical Predictions

Assuming that cells in the ELISPOT plate well are distributed on the surface of the membrane according to the Uniform distribution law (any position has equal chance to be occupied by the spot) and each cell produces only single analyte at a time (such as in case of B-cell ELISPOT), we can postulate that the probability for spots of different color to overlay randomly (creating "false" multi-color spot) will follow Poisson Point Process [16].

Let Center of Mass Distances (COMD) be the maximum allowed distance between centers of masses of spots of different colors to form a multi-color spot, then $A_{\mathrm{thrs}} = \pi COMD^2$ will be the threshold area in the Poisson Point Process. Let N_i be the spot count/well of color i (for example, for blue $i = 1$, for red—2, red—3, and so on), A_{image} be the total well area, and $\lambda_i = N_i/A_{\mathrm{image}}$—the surface density of the color i spots. Let N_{ij} be the number of "false" dual-color spots containing colors i and j. According to the Poisson Point Processes, the probability that any well circular region A_{thrs} contains at least one spot of j color can be written as:

$$P_j \overset{\mathrm{def}}{=} e^{-\lambda_j A_{\mathrm{thrs}}} \tag{1}$$

Then the "false" dual-color count for spots containing colors i and j will be:

$$N_{ij} \overset{\mathrm{def}}{=} N_i P_j \tag{2}$$

In the general form, the number of "false" multi-color spots containing color i can be written as:

$$N_{i,j..n} \overset{\mathrm{def}}{=} N_i \prod_{k \in j..n} P_k \tag{3}$$

3.5 Monte Carlo Simulations

To prove our statistical predictions based on the Poisson Point Process, we used the Monte Carlo method [17]. Thousand artificial image sets were created with four colors in each. Random spots coordinates (center of mass positions) were generated using the uniform distribution independently for each of four colors. These artificial image sets were counted using standard Fluoro-X™ pairing algorithm (same way as real images are analyzed). Then the average numbers of dual-/multi-color spots were calculated among all sets. These simulations were repeated for different individual color spot numbers and different COMD.

3.6 Scrambled Image Counting

We also compare Poisson predictions with a method that can be applied on either artificial or real image sets. We refer to this method as "image scrambling." Relative orientations of individual color, real-well images (or artificially generated images) were randomly changed (scrambled), then standard spot pairing was performed to count multi-color spots. As in case of Monte Carlo simulation, counting was repeated for different spot numbers and different COMD.

Both of the abovementioned methods generate counting results for "false" positive multi-color spots formed by random overlays of the single-color spots.

3.7 Analysis of Individual Color Spots in Multi-color FLUOROSPOT

Analyzing of multi-color spots using a color image is not feasible owing to several reasons. Fluorescence intensity of individual fluorochromes are not equal due to their spectral properties (mainly extinction coefficient and quantum yield), and therefore are not directly comparable on a unitary scale. Therefore different exposures are needed to generate suitable spot images for each fluorochrome. The level of each cytokine secretion could be also radically different. When all fluorochromes are excited simultaneously, the overlap of the emission spectra will not permit reliable detection; particularly, when more than two colors are used. Also excitation spectrum of one fluorochrome may overlap with the emission spectrum of another, thus limiting the choice of labels for multi-color assay. Exciting one label at a time using computer-controlled, LED-based color illuminator and asynchronous excitation/emission filter selector completely eliminates the problem of spectral overlap and cross contamination of fluorescence between channels (*see* **Note 1**). In a well-designed optical system, no compensation is required between individual color channels (Fig. 1). The figure shows data for a B-cell IgG FLUOROSPOT assay where no dual-/multi-color spots are possible.

Basic principles of single-color FLUOROSPOT image analysis are similar to a single-color ELISPOT, including automatic sensitivity adjustment (SmartSpot™) and automatic spot size/intensity gating (AutoGate™) functions for the objective and reliable detection of true spots and eliminating background spots (not antigen induced) and artifacts (*see* **Note 2**). Details of single-color ELISPOT image analysis are published elsewhere in detail [18, 19], and are beyond the scope of this chapter. The main criterion for the accurate algorithm performance is linear relation between numbers of spots counted and numbers of cells plated per well [20, 21].

Results of the single-color spot counting for each cytokine in four color T-cell FLUOROSPOT are presented on Fig. 2a–c. For a visual control and publications multi-color images for any combinations of channels can be reconstructed by merging individual color images (shown with count overlays on Fig. 2d–f.

3.8 Center of Mass Distance Algorithm for Detection of Dual-, Triple-, and Multi-color Spots

For each detected single-color spot, X–Y coordinates of the center of masses are calculated and recorded. These center of mass coordinates are then compared between all channels, and spots whose Center of Mass Distances (COMD) are less than maximum COMD are paired (considered to be generated by the same cell) (*see* **Note 3**). To speed up the process, such comparisons are performed in a certain vicinity of the spots and performed in parallel. The algorithm "qualifying"

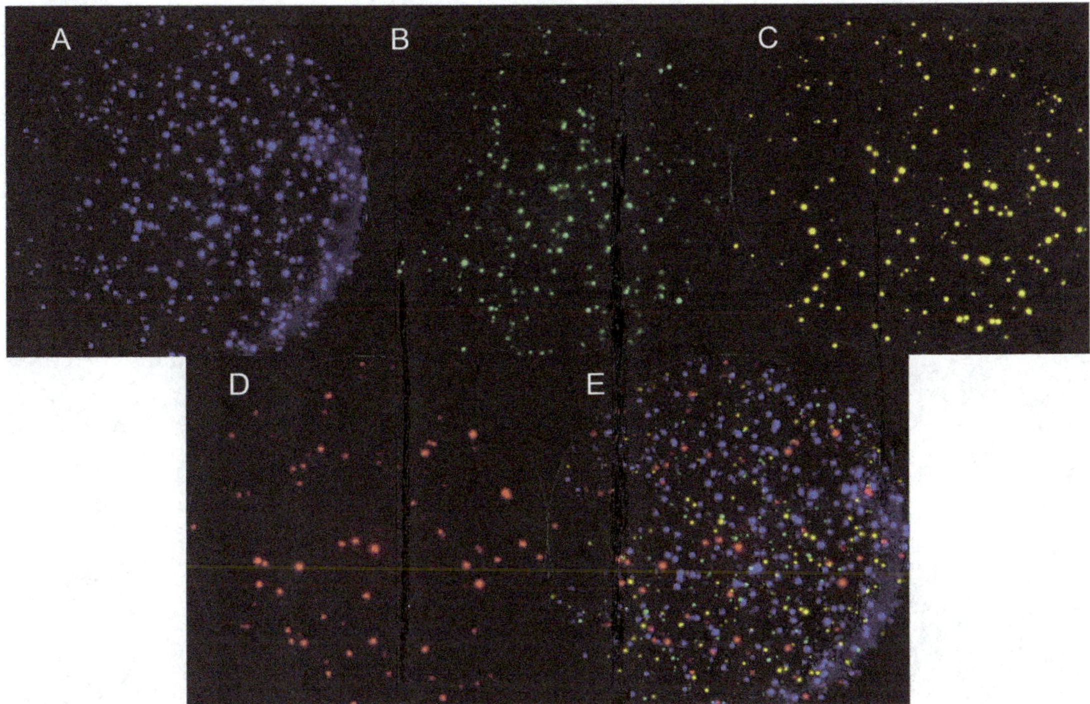

Fig. 1 Capturing of individual color spots in four color human IgG3 (**a**), IgG1 (**b**), IgA (**c**), IgM (**d**) B-cell FLUOROSPOT assay using individually selectable combinations of the excitation/emission bands (channels). Merged from individual channels four color image is shown in panel **e** (not used for counting). No cross contamination of fluorescent signals was observed at optimal image capture conditions

spots as dual-/triple-/multi-color is similar to a computer neural network (Fig. 3).

The relations between individual color objects are analyzed based on the maximum COMD parameter and the set of pairing rules. For example, to qualify for a triple-color spot, all distances in the cluster should be inside the COMD (Fig. 4d). To avoid ambiguities in situations when spot of one color (green for example) has the same distance to two different spots of another color (for example, red), the cluster with higher dimension (if a blue spot is also close enough to a green spot) is favored in this case (Fig. 4f). If partially overlapping spots (red on Fig. 4c) were not separated by Spot Separation function, Fluoro-X™ Software calculates "virtual" centers of masses and pairs them to centers of masses of other color spots (green on Fig. 4c) (*see* **Note 4**). There are other rules for processing unseparated clusters of closely situated spots; together, they guarantee accurate dual-/multi-color spot detection even in crowded wells.

After individual color spots are counted in all channels and paired where appropriate, the single-, dual-, triple-, and multi-color events are generated by the algorithm and all parameters

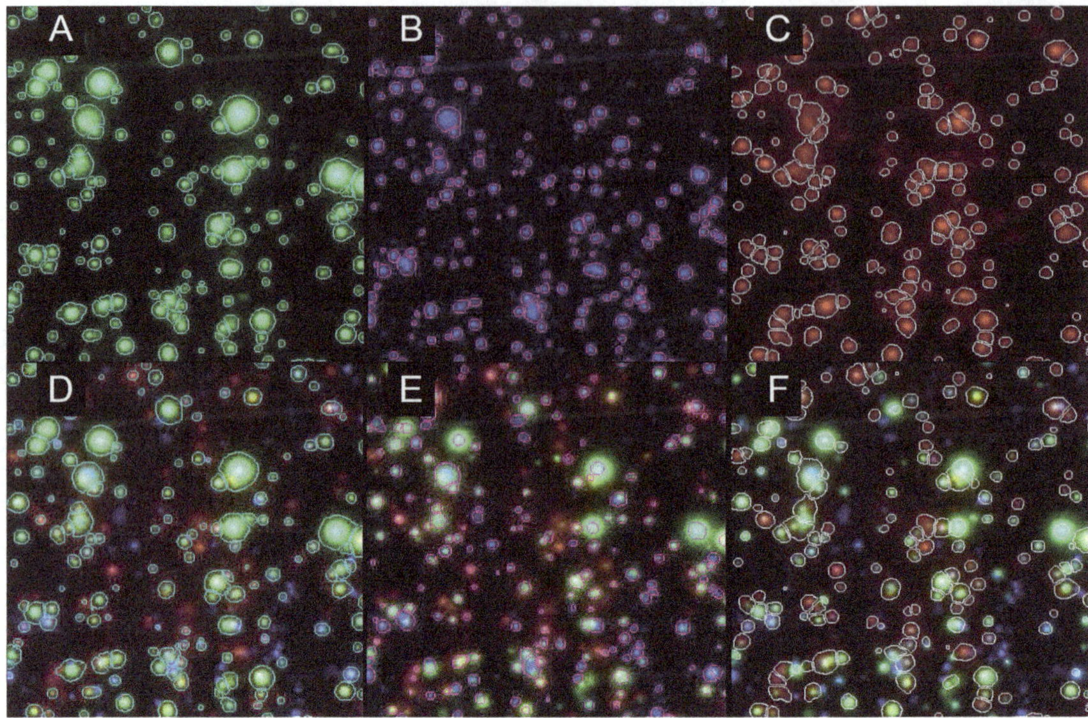

Fig. 2 Counting of individual color spots in the triple-color human IFN-γ (green), TNF-α (blue), and IL-2 (red) T-cell FLUOROSPOT assay. Magnified regions of the well scanned and counted using individual color detection is shown on top panels **a**, **b**, and **c**. Single-color spots count overlays are also shown on the merged triple-color images (bottom panels **d**, **e**, and **f**). Partially overlapping spots were separated by spot separation function of ImmunoSpot® Software

associated with each event are recorded (size, color density, time, etc.). These data can be retrieved (as Flow Cytometry Standard .fcs file) for a *post-hoc* detailed high-content analysis using either Fluoro-X™ Data Management module or any commercial flow cytometry software. The detailed workflow for the multi-color counting using ImmunoSpot® 7.0 Software is presented in [22].

3.9 Validation of Counting Algorithms Using Four Color B-Cell FLUOROSPOT

For the multi-color counting validation, we used four color B-cell FLUOROSPOT assays of human Ig classes/subclasses (IgM, IgA, IgG1, IgG3). Polyclonally pre-activated PBMC [15] were tested in linear titrations using anti-κ/λ chain monoclonal antibodies as a capture reagent and anti-Ig class/subclass detection antibodies. Because individual B cells, due to the allelic exclusion, can only express a single type of Ig molecule, this model is optimally suited for validating multi-color algorithms and for determining frequencies of false positive multi-color spots.

Figure 5 depicts four color FLUOROSPOT for human IgA, IgM, IgG1, and IgG3. The number of individual color spots (for each subtype) closely follows linear relationship to the number of

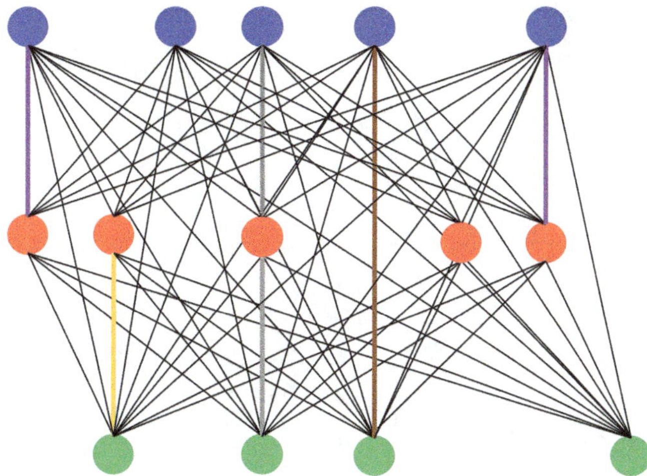

Fig. 3 Spot pairing algorithm for multi-color events generation. Center of mass X–Y coordinates for individual spots of one color (blue for example) are compared to those of other colors (red and green) in certain neighborhood (shown in a single dimension). Every pairwise comparison between individual spots coordinates in blue, red, and green images (or layers) is shown as connecting black line. If the distance between centers of masses of spots in different layer is smaller than COMD, these two spots are paired to form a two color event. Such pairing is shown as violet lines (for blue/red spots), yellow (red/green spots) and brown line (blue/green spots). Gray lines indicate blue/red/green triple-color event

PBMCs plated (panel a), validating the accuracy of the single-color counting algorithm [20, 21]. Slight deviation from the linearity at highest used cell numbers (overcrowded wells with over 1000 spots) results from the large percentage of partially overlapping spot separated by counting algorithm.

Even when no true dual-/multi-color spots were produced (as is the case in Fig. 5), certain number of random overlays of individual color spots giving an appearance of multi-color spots was always observed. In contrast to the genuine spots, the counts of random overlay spot numbers drop in geometrical progression with cell numbers and numbers of colors (Fig. 5b, c). For example for the dual-color situation at highest cell concentration (10,000/ well), 1200 green spots and 1400 blue spots resulted in 145 random overlays (about 6%). For half of the cells plated (5000/well) random overlays counts dropped down to 20 (about 2%) and so on. Random triple-color spots overlays are much rarer events: at highest cell numbers used, 1200 green, 1400 blue, and 500 red spots resulted in only 0.2% of triple-color random overlays. Quadruple random overlays were not detectable even at highest cell numbers used. Similar results were obtained among 12 donor

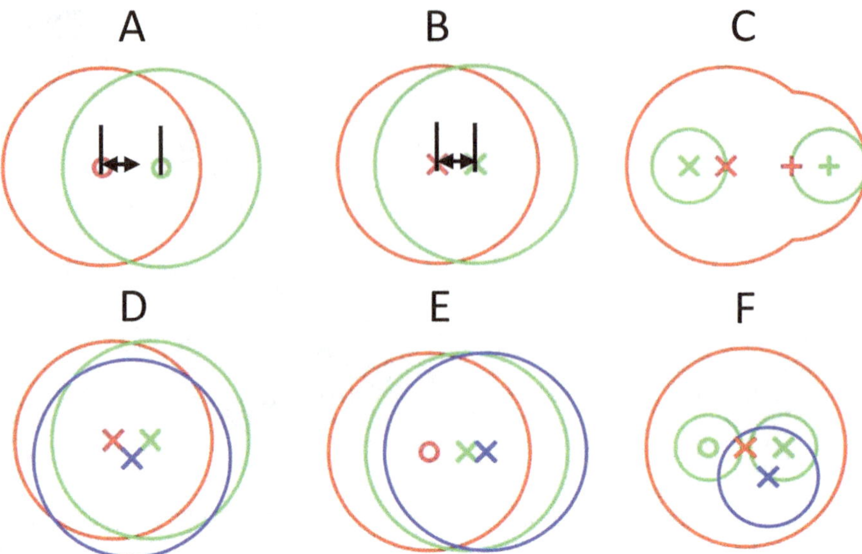

Fig. 4 Spot pairing rules for multi-color events generation are based on the minimal centers of mass distance (COMD). Counting overlays for individual color spots are shown as red, green, and blue circles, and their centers of masses are indicated by "x" (if spots are paired) or "o" if they are not paired. In Panel **a**, the distance between red and green centers is greater than minimal allowed value (shown by double point arrow) and spots are not paired, whereas in **b** it is smaller than/equal to COMD and a two color event (spot) is generated. In **c**—when two overlapping spots (red) are not resolved by spot separation function, "virtual" centers of masses (red crosses) are calculated and two dual-color events are generated. In panel **d**, a triple-color spot is shown with all distances between centers of masses smaller than COMD. In panel **e**, pairing resulted in one green/ blue dual-color spot (as indicated by green and blue "x") and one single-color spot (red "o"). In panel **f**, right green spot (green "x" center) was paired to the blue spot (blue "x"). In this example, red spot center (red "x") is equidistant from the right green (green "x")- and the left green (green "o") spots. In such an instance of equal distances, the algorithm favors higher order events (spots with more colors) resulting in one triple red/ green/blue and one single-color green spot. The less favorable alternative would be two dual-color spots (red with left green and blue with right green spot). COMD distances are shown larger in magnitude in the diagram for better visual representation

PBMC samples tested in both three color (Ig class) and four color IgG class/subclass assays (data not shown).

3.10 Statistical Predictions and Scrambled Image Analysis Permit Correction of Random Overlays of Spots

If counting algorithm works properly, the number of "false" dual-/ multi-color spots detected in B-cell assays should match theoretical (statistical) predictions for random spot overlays. We used statistical calculations based on the Poisson Point Process to evaluate the effect of such random overlays on the counting results.

Statistical calculations were performed by using both Poisson formula (3) and Monte Carlo simulations (*see* Subheadings 3.4 and 3.5). The results of Monte Carlo simulations closely matched Poisson formula, thus validating the use of latter method for the prediction of "false" positive multi-color spot frequencies (data not shown).

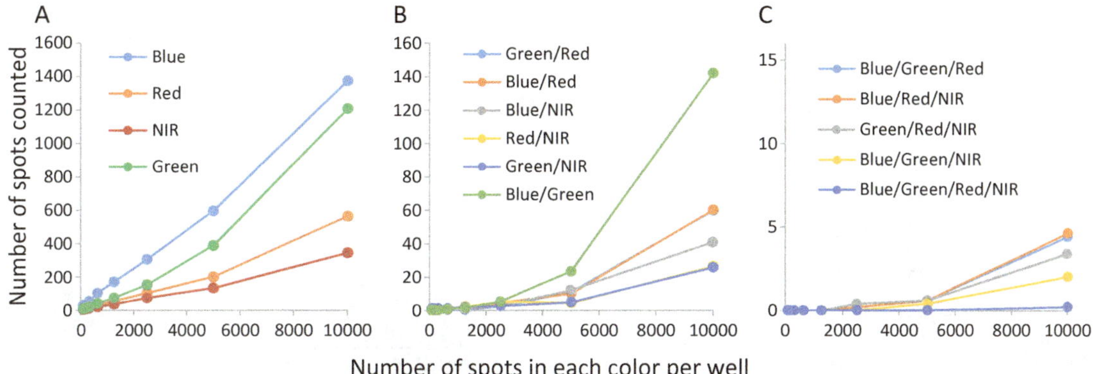

Fig. 5 Frequencies of the random spot overlays in four color B-cell FLUOROSPOT vs. numbers of pre-activated PBMCs plated per well. Panel **a** shows linear relationship between numbers of PBMC plated (*X*-axis) and the numbers of counted spots (*Y*-axis) in individual single-color images (labelled: IgG3 as blue, IgA—red, IgG1—green and IgM—near infrared (NIR)). Panel **b** shows numbers of detected random overlay (false positive dual-color spots) for all dual-color combinations plotted vs. numbers of PBMC/well. Panel **c** similarly shows data for three and four color spots. Maximum 145 of false positive two color spots were counted for 1400 blue spots and 1200 green spots (about 6% at COMD = 0.5%). Maximum number of random triple-color spots did not exceed 0.2%. In contrast to the linear function for single-color spots, dual-/triple-color spot numbers dropped in geometrical progression with decreasing cell concentrations plated. False positive four color spots were not detectable even at highest cell numbers

Two independent methods of generating random spot overlays (theoretical Poisson model and scrambled image counts described in Subheading 3.6) (*see* **Note 5**) exactly matched results of B-cell FLUOROSPOT (Fig. 6), validating the multi-color spot counting algorithm used (*see* **Note 6**). The monotonicity of the graphs in Fig. 6 (where results for all 6 two color combination are plotted together) proves that frequencies of "false" dual-color spots (actually counted or simulated) do not depend on which two colors are used.

Statistical prediction shows that the number of random overlays grows with the increase of COMD (compare Fig. 6a, b). In the ImmunoSpot® Software, COMD is expressed as percentage of an image vertical size. It makes COMD independent of image pixel size. In case of two colors (shown in Fig. 6) with total 1000 spots of both color per well, COMD equal to 0.5 results in the 19–20 random overlays (about 2%), whereas at COMD equal to 0.75 there will be about 50 random overlays (5%). In practice, the COMD parameter depends mainly on the chromatic aberrations of the optical system (*see* **Note 7**). Automatic correction for the random overlays implemented in the ImmunoSpot® Software makes precise settings of COMD unnecessary. Minimal value must guarantee detection of all true dual-/multi-color spots (see below) and

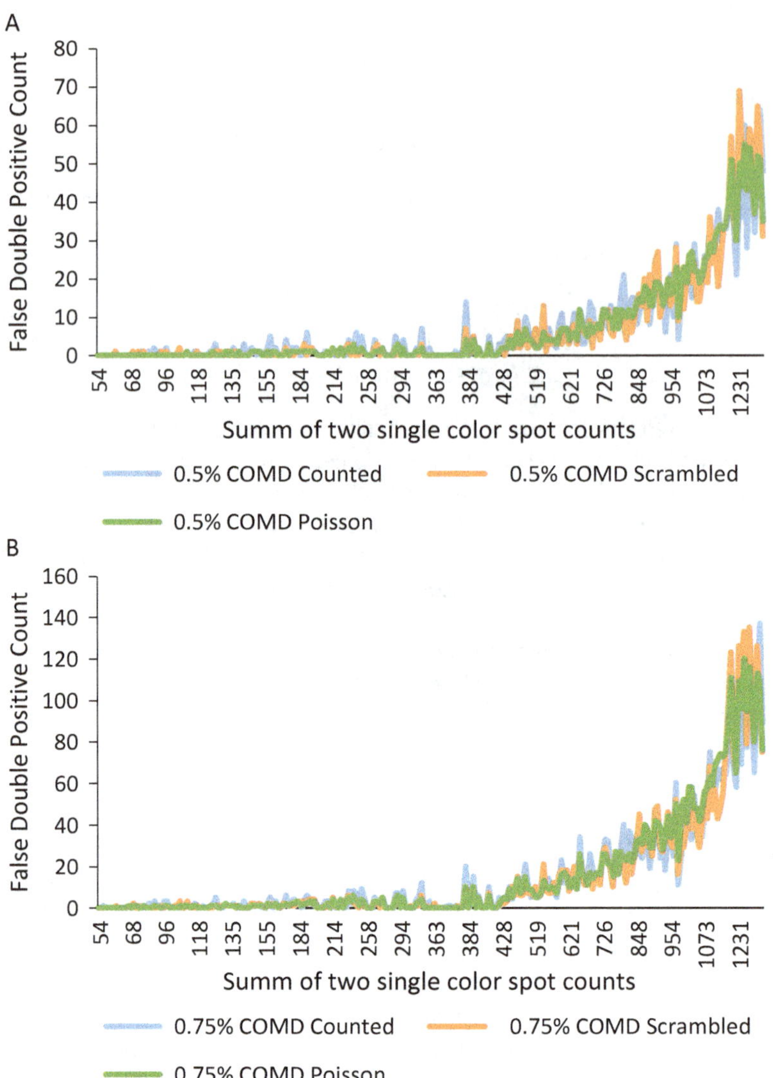

Fig. 6 Statistically predicted and experimentally counted numbers of "false" dual-color spots in four color B-cell FLUOROSPOT (*see* legend to Fig. 5 for additional details). Two COMD values equal to 0.5% (panel **a**) and to 0.75% (panel **b**) were used for both counting and simulations. Numbers of false positive dual-color spots (*Y*-axis) are plotted vs. total number of spots in every possible two color combination (*X*-axis). For example, with COMD 0.5, about 20 "false" dual-color spots resulted from 600 blue and 400 green spots (total 1000 on *X*-axis) and about 9 "false" dual-color spots resulted from 600 blue and 200 red spots (total 800 on *X*-axis). With COMD 0.75, the same two combinations resulted in about 50 and 20 "false" dual-color spot counts, respectively. The same PBMC sample shown in Fig. 5 at the same dilutions was used for the experimental counts. The proportion of the individual color spots in every dual-color combinations can be found in Fig. 5a. The blue line reflects results of the experimentally counted dual-color spots, green corresponds to the probabilistic predictions based on Poisson model, and orange line shows results for counting of image with scrambled spot coordinates

maximal value should not result in the numbers of random overlays significantly higher than the numbers of true multi-color spots. Typical values lay between 0.5 and 0.8% of the image size (Fig. 6). For 1000 × 1000 pixels image, the COMD is in the range of 5–8 pixels. Sometimes cells are moving during the secretion period which may require higher COMD settings.

3.11   Linear Cell Titrations in Four Color FLUOROSPOT Prove Accurate Detection of Polyfunctional T Cell

The use of overlaid multi-color images (shown with counted spots outlines in Fig. 7) enables visual control of multi-color counting for each possible color combination. However the most reliable way to validate true frequencies of dual- or multi-color spots produced by cytokine secreting T cells is to perform serial dilutions of cells. Dual and triple concentric overlays (shown in different color on Fig. 7) indicate dual- and triple-positive spots, respectively.

As demonstrated in the previous section, the frequencies of random spot overlays diminish in the geometrical progression when cells are linearly diluted. The relative frequencies (percentage) of real multi-color spots should stay the same (linearly decreasing with cell dilution). Representative data from such validation study is shown in Fig. 8 utilizing the human IFN-γ/TNF-α/GzB triple-color FLUOROSPOT kit. When counting parameter are set correctly, counted numbers of dual- and triple-color spots perfectly follow linear function validating the accuracy of multi-color counting algorithm. A CD8 cell response of a single A2 restricted donor to CMV peptide pp65 (495–503) is shown in Fig. 8 for all possible color combinations. Experiments were repeated for over 50 donor/antigen combinations using both MHC Class 1 restricted peptides (CD8 responses) and full protein antigens (CD4 responses). For all responses studied, the relationship between number of dual-/multi-color spots and cell concentrations were uniformly linear (data not shown).

A scientifically validated, accurate, single-color spot counting algorithm is an absolute prerequisite for the accurate multi-color spot recognition in T- and B-cell FLUOROSPOT assay. The use of SmartCount™ and AutoGate™ functions makes single-color spot count objective and user independent (*see* **Note 2**). ImmunoSpot® single-color counting software has been validated in multiple reported studies including "blind" multi-laboratory studies [23, 24].

The multi-color spot recognition method implemented in ImmunoSpot® Fluoro-X™ Suite is based on the individual single band fluorescent images and Center of Mass Distance pairing algorithm. The ability to create optimal for a given set of fluorescent tags combination of excitation/emission bands maximizes the number of colors which can be analyzed simultaneously and allows for the detection of polyfunctional cytokine producing cells, where

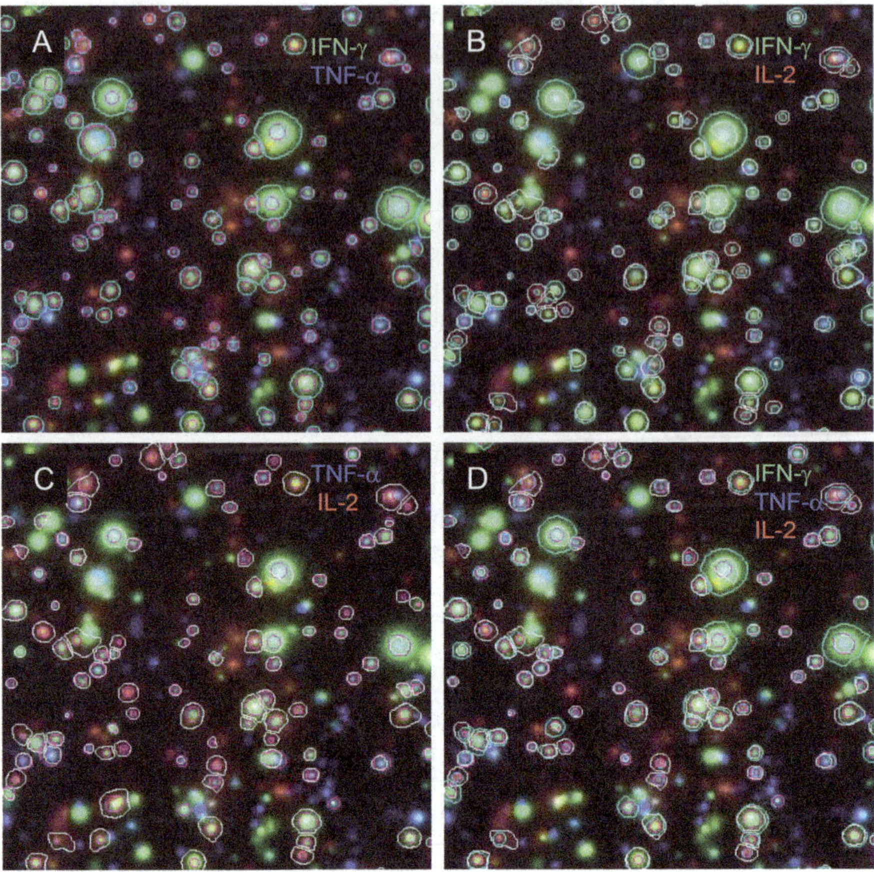

Fig. 7 Counting of dual- and triple-color spots in the human IFN-γ (green), TNF-α (blue), and IL-2 (red) T-cell FLUOROSPOT assay (magnified region of the well is shown). All combinations of two color spot overlays (panels **a**, **b**, and **c**) and triple-color spot overlays (panel **d**) are shown superimposed over the merged triple-color image

the individual cytokine levels produced may be quantitatively different (*see* **Note 1**). Even significant (hundreds and thousands of times) excess of one analyte will not obstruct the detection of the other/s. Another important advantage of this approach is the selective excitation of one label at a time. This approach eliminates potential bleeding of fluorescent signals emitted by fluorochromes into each other's channels when their emission spectra partially overlap. There is no need for highly selective narrow band filters for close emission spectra resolution, and wide band emission filters can be used for maximizing detection sensitivity. CTL Series 7 Ultimate ImmunoSpot® analyzer is capable of resolving up to twelve color fluorescence using commercially available organic fluorochromes in visual spectrum range (400–900 nm) with maximum possible sensitivity.

When pairing spots from individual color images (channels), we allow for certain small distances between their centers of masses

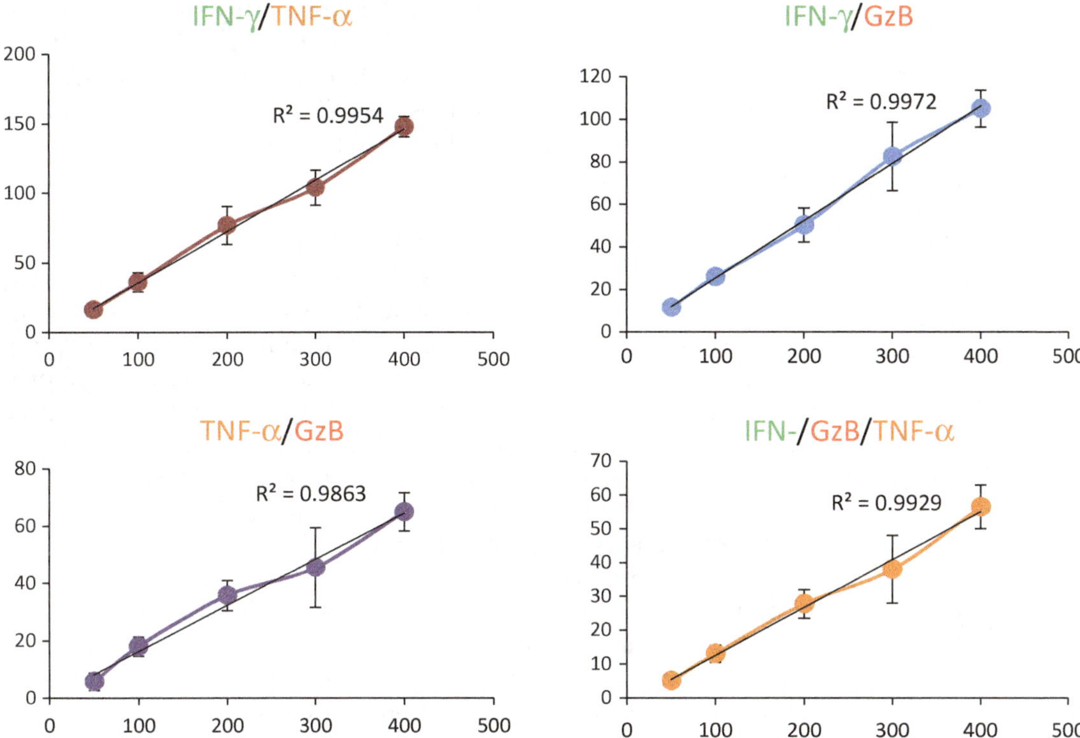

Fig. 8 Validation of the multi-color counting in the triple-color human IFN-γ/TNF-α/GzB assay (*see* Subheadings 2 and 3). Numbers of dual-/triple-color spots counted in ImmunoSpot® Fluoro-X™ Software (*Y*-axis) are plotted vs. the numbers of PBMCs plated (shown in thousands on *X*-axis). Single-color spot counts were performed using SmartSpot™ and AutoGate™ functions with pairing algorithm minimal COMD set to 0.5%. Vertical error bars represent ±1 SD calculated from four repetitive wells. The linear regression coefficient, R^2, for all color combinations was close to one reflecting direct linear relationship between the numbers of dual-/triple-color spots and the number of cells plated per well (decreasing cell numbers lead to the proportional reduction of dual-/triple-color spot counts)

(COMD). There are few reasons why centers of spots of different color do not coincide precisely. First is the accuracy of center of mass detection: it is never precise at the microscopic pixel level, particularly with small spots. Second is the chromatic aberration of the optical system: though modern lenses are corrected for chromatic aberrations, there is still some shift in the relative position of spots of different colors. Such minute shift is consistent across all spots in the image for any given scan and can thus be corrected with high confidence. Third reason is cell movement: activated T and B cells can move on the membrane during the secretion period (*see* **Note 3**). The probability of movement increases proportionally with the assay incubation time which for IL-17 can be as long as 72 h [25]. If two cytokines are produced by the same cell with different kinetics (like IFN-γ and GzB [26, 27], or IFN-γ and IL-17 [25, 28]), corresponding color spots will be shifted as a result of such cellular movement. First two factors are constant for a given instrument and color combination, default factory settings for COMD are usually the best. If cell movement is affecting counting results, some increase of COMD could be needed. However, even in this case the COMD settings are constant for a specific analyte combination and do not need to be adjusted each time (*see* **Note 7**).

Ex vivo frequencies of polyfunctional T cells expressing two and more cytokines could be as low as just a few percent [1–13] which is in the same range as the frequencies of random dual-color spot overlays theoretically predicted for high count wells (starting at about 200–300 individual color spots and geometrically progressing after that). This entails correction for random overlays a mandatory part of any multi-color spot counting algorithm (*see* **Note 5**). We used two methods to calculate random spot overlays. First is statistical prediction: if cells are randomly distributed over the membrane surface, their positions (X–Y coordinates) have to be distributed according to the Poisson spatial distribution function [16]. Using actual numbers of individual color spots counted per well, ImmunoSpot® Fluoro-X™ Software calculates probabilities for centers of masses of the spots of different colors to be at or closer than COMD using Poisson model. In a second approach, the software counts dual-/triple-/multi-color spots using scrambled images where original relative positions of spots of different colors were randomly modified (*see* Subheading 3.6). Though either method provides practically identical results, both of them are implemented in the ImmunoSpot® Software (*see* **Note 5**).

Automatic correction for the frequencies of random spot overlays permits pairing algorithm parameters (primarily COMD) vary in wide range without affecting the accuracy of true multi-color spot counts. In principle, once the fluorescent reader, testing reagents, and protocols are tested and optimal counting parameters are established for a given combination of cytokines, validation by serial dilution of cells is not required anymore. We still recommend performing cell titrations for unknown samples/antigen combinations to identify optimal cell concentrations for a given assay.

Another important factor that affects multi-color counting is the partially overlaying of spots. Even in uncrowded wells (50–100 spots), there are certain numbers of doublets, triplets, or rarely, multiples detected (Figs. 1, 2, and 7). If two (or more) partially overlaid spots (of the same color) are detected as a single object, the resultant center of mass will not be correct for either of these spots. If, for example, one of these overlaid spots was of dual-color, the pairing will fail and a dual-positive event will not be generated. Also, a large number of false positive multi-color events may be generated if one single-color cluster is mistakenly paired to another color cluster. Similar to the random overlays, the frequencies of partially overlapping single-color spots will rise in geometrical progression with the numbers of spots extant per well. ImmunoSpot® Software implements powerful algorithms to separate touching/overlapping spots. In addition, the Fluoro-X™ pairing algorithm is able to calculate "virtual" centers of masses for partially overlapping spots (Fig. 4c) insuring accurate counting even in the crowded wells (*see* **Note 4**).

Each manufacturer of FLUOROSPOT instruments could present multiple arguments in favor of their hardware and/or software. However, the only way for the user to objectively assess system performance is to conduct a validation study. As discussed earlier, major problems/errors in multi-color counting are spot number dependent. Hence, the best proof of accurate analysis is the direct linear relationship between the numbers of cell plated (single-color spot counts) and the numbers of single-/dual-/multi-color spots detected. Such validation data are presented on Fig. 8 (*see* **Note 8**). As we demonstrate, the frequency of false positive spots drops in a geometrical progression, while true multi-color spots show a direct linear relationship to the number of cells plated. In this study, using objective corrections for the random spot overlays and intelligent pairing algorithms, we achieve accurate counts (linear spot/cells titrations), even in crowded wells with over a thousand spots for each individual analyte for multi-color T- and B-cell FLUOROSPOT assays (*see* **Note 9**).

4 Notes

1. Using individual monochromatic images (channels) instead of analyzing multiband color images eliminates the necessity for sophisticated color recognition algorithms and allows using optimal for each fluorochrome combinations of the excitation/emission wavelengths (bands).

2. The use of SmartCount™ and AutoGate™ functions makes single-color spot count objective and user independent. ImmunoSpot® single-color counting Software has been validated in multiple studies.

3. CTL Fluoro-X™ multi-color analysis Suite utilizes individual color spots pairing algorithm based on the maximal allowed Center of Mass Distances between spot centers (COMD) correcting for chromatic aberrations and possible cells movement.

4. The COMD-based algorithm is capable of accurate pairing of partially overlapping spots (spot clusters which were not fully separated) from the single-color images.

5. Correction for the "false" multi-color spots resulting from the random overlay of individual color spots is a mandatory component of the multi-color counting software. Fluoro-X™

Software Suite provides two independent methods for the "random" spots overlay correction based on the statistical probabilities and on the analysis of scrambled experimental images.

6. Analysis of four color B-cell FLUOROSPOT using serial dilutions proves accuracy of random spot overlays correction methods used.

7. The COMD settings are constant for a specific optics and fluorochrome combination and do not need to be adjusted for each assay.

8. Multi-color T- and B-cell FLUOROSPOT analysis using serial cell dilutions is the only way to validate multi-color data analysis system.

9. Direct linear relationship between cell numbers and the numbers of dual-, triple- and quadruple-spots in the four color T-cell FLUOROSPOT fully validates the COMD-based multi-color spot analysis system.

References

1. Zimmerli SC, Harari A, Cellerai C, Vallelian F, Bart PA, Pantaleo G (2005) HIV-1-specific IFN-gamma/IL-2-secreting CD8 T cells support CD4-independent proliferation of HIV-1-specific CD8 T cells. Proc Natl Acad Sci U S A 102(20):7239–7244

2. Betts MR, Nason MC, West SM, De Rosa SC, Migueles SA, Abraham J, Lederman MM, Benito JM, Goepfert PA, Connors M, Roederer M, Koup RA (2006) HIV nonprogressors preferentially maintain highly functional HIV-specific CD8+ T cells. Blood 107(12):4781–4789

3. Almeida JR, Price DA, Papagno L, Arkoub ZA, Sauce D, Bornstein E, Asher TE, Samri A, Schnuriger A, Theodorou I, Costagliola D, Rouzioux C, Agut H, Marcelin AG, Douek D, Autran B, Appay V (2007) Superior control of HIV-1 replication by CD8+ T cells is reflected by their avidity, polyfunctionality, and clonal turnover. J Exp Med 204(10):2473–2485

4. Papagno L, Almeida JR, Nemes E, Autran B, Appay V (2007) Cell permeabilization for the assessment of T lymphocyte polyfunctional capacity. J Immunol Methods 328(1–2):182–188

5. Day CL, Mkhwanazi N, Reddy S, Mncube Z, van der Stok M, Klenerman P, Walker BD (2008) Detection of polyfunctional Mycobacterium tuberculosis-specific T cells and association with viral load in HIV-1-infected persons. J Infect Dis 197(7):990–999

6. Duvall MG, Precopio ML, Ambrozak DA, Jaye A, McMichael AJ, Whittle HC, Roederer M, Rowland-Jones SL, Koup RA (2008) Polyfunctional T cell responses are a hallmark of HIV-2 infection. Eur J Immunol 38(2):350–363

7. Hutnick NA, Carnathan D, Demers K, Makedonas G, Ertl HC, Betts MR (2010) Adenovirus-specific human T cells are pervasive, polyfunctional, and cross-reactive. Vaccine 28(8):1932–1941

8. Owen RE, Heitman JW, Hirschkorn DF, Lanteri MC, Biswas HH, Martin JN, Krone MR, Deeks SG, Norris PJ, NIAID Center for HIV/AIDS Vaccine Immunology (2010) HIV+ elite controllers have low HIV-specific T-cell activation yet maintain strong, polyfunctional T-cell responses. AIDS 24(8):1095–1105

9. Akinsiku OT, Bansal A, Sabbaj S, Heath SL, Goepfert PA (2011) Interleukin-2 production by polyfunctional HIV-1-specific CD8 T cells is associated with enhanced viral suppression. J Acquir Immune Defic Syndr 58(2):132–140

10. El Fenniri L, Toossi Z, Aung H, El Iraki G, Bourkkadi J, Benamor J, Laskri A, Berrada N, Benjouad A, Mayanja-Kizza H, Betts MR, El Aouad R, Canaday DH (2011) Polyfunctional Mycobacterium tuberculosis-specific effector memory CD4+ T cells at sites of pleural TB. Tuberculosis 91(3):224–230

11. Han Q, Bagheri N, Bradshaw EM, Hafler DA, Lauffenburger DA, Love JC (2012)

Polyfunctional responses by human T cells result from sequential release of cytokines. Proc Natl Acad Sci U S A 109(5):1607–1612

12. Samri A, Bacchus-Souffan C, Hocqueloux L, Avettand-Fenoel V, Descours B, Theodorou I, Larsen M, Saez-Cirion A, Rouzioux C, Autran B, ANRS VISCONTI study group (2016) Polyfunctional HIV-specific T cells in post-treatment controllers. AIDS 30(15):2299–2302

13. Smith SG, Zelmer A, Blitz R, Fletcher HA, Dockrell HM (2016) Polyfunctional CD4 T-cells correlate with in vitro mycobacterial growth inhibition following Mycobacterium bovis BCG-vaccination of infants. Vaccine 34(44):5298–5305

14. Kuerten S, Batoulis H, Recks MS, Karacsony E, Zhang W, Subbramanian RA, Lehmann PV (2012) Resting of cryopreserved PBMC does not generally benefit the performance of antigen-specific T cell ELISPOT assays. Cell 1(3):409–427

15. Pinna D, Corti D, Jarrossay D, Sallusto F, Lanzavecchia A (2009) Clonal dissection of the human memory B-cell repertoire following infection and vaccination. Eur J Immunol 39(5):1260–1270

16. Kingman JFC (1993) Poisson processes, Oxford studies in probability, vol 3. Clarendon Press, New York

17. Kroese DP, Taimre T, Botev ZI (2011) Handbook of Monte Carlo methods. Wiley, New York

18. Lehmann PV (2005) Image analysis and data management of ELISPOT assay results. Methods Mol Biol 302:117–132

19. Zhang W, Lehmann PV (2012) Objective, user-independent ELISPOT data analysis based on scientifically validated principles. Methods Mol Biol 792:155–171

20. Karulin AY, Caspell R, Dittrich M, Lehmann PV (2015) Normal distribution of CD8+ T-cell-derived ELISPOT counts within replicates justifies the reliance on parametric statistics for identifying positive responses. Cell 4(1):96–111

21. Karulin AY, Karacsony K, Zhang W, Targoni OS, Moldovan I, Dittrich M, Sundararaman S, Lehmann PV (2015) ELISPOTs produced by CD8 and CD4 cells follow log normal size distribution permitting objective counting. Cell 4(1):56–70

22. Megyesi Z, Lehmann PV, Karulin AY (2018) Multi-color FLUOROSPOT counting using ImmunoSpot® Fluoro-X™ suite. In: Kalyuzhny AE (ed) Handbook of ELISPOT, Methods in molecular biology, 3rd edn. Springer, New York

23. Zhang W, Caspell R, Karulin AY, Ahmad M, Haicheur N, Abdelsalam A, Johannesen K, Vignard V, Dudzik P, Georgakopoulou K, Mihaylova A, Silina K, Aptsiauri N, Adams V, Lehmann PV, McArdle S (2009) ELISPOT assays provide reproducible results among different laboratories for T-cell immune monitoring--even in hands of ELISPOT-inexperienced investigators. J Immunotoxicol 6(4):227–234

24. Sundararaman S, Karulin AY, Ansari T, BenHamouda N, Gottwein J, Laxmanan S, Levine SM, Loffredo JT, McArdle S, Neudoerfl C, Roen D, Silina K, Welch M, Lehmann PV (2015) High reproducibility of ELISPOT counts from nine different laboratories. Cell 4(1):21–39

25. Wunsch M, Zhang W, Hanson J, Caspell R, Karulin AY, Recks MS, Kuerten S, Sundararaman S, Lehmann PV (2015) Characterization of the HCMV-specific CD4 T cell responses that are associated with protective immunity. Virus 7(8):4414–4437

26. Nowacki TM, Kuerten S, Zhang W, Shive CL, Kreher CR, Boehm BO, Lehmann PV, Tary-Lehmann M (2007) Granzyme B production distinguishes recently activated CD8(+) memory cells from resting memory cells. Cell Immunol 247(1):36–48

27. Kuerten S, Nowacki TM, Kleen TO, Asaad RJ, Lehmann PV, Tary-Lehmann M (2008) Dissociated production of perforin, granzyme B, and IFN-gamma by HIV-specific CD8(+) cells in HIV infection. AIDS Res Hum Retrovir 24(1):62–71

28. Duechting A, Przybyla A, Kuerten S, Lehmann PV (2017) Delayed activation kinetics of Th2- and Th17 cells compared to Th1 cells. Cell 6(3)

Chapter 10

Multi-Color FLUOROSPOT Counting Using ImmunoSpot® Fluoro-X™ Suite

Zoltán Megyesi, Paul V. Lehmann, and Alexey Y. Karulin

Abstract

Multi-color FLUOROSPOT assays for simultaneous detection of several T-cell cytokines and/or classes/sub-classes of immunoglobulins secreted by B cells have recently become a major new avenue of development of ELISPOT technology. Advances in assay techniques and the availability of commercial test kits stimulated development of multi-color FLUOROSPOT data analysis platforms. The ImmunoSpot® Fluoro-X™ Software Suite was developed by CTL as an integrated data acquisition, analysis, and management solution for automated high-throughput processing of multi-color T- and B-cell FLUOROSPOT assay plates. The Fluoro-X™ software counting module is based on SmartSpot™/AutoGate™ technologies and utilizes CTL's Center of Mass Distance algorithm for the detection of multi-color spots. The Fluoro-X™ software provides an objective, user error-free means for analyzing multi-color FLUOROSPOT data. An integrated quality control module, with optional GLP and CFR Part 11 compliant package and role-based security, enables data validation, review, and approval with complete audit trails. The extensive multi-format data output and presentation capabilities of the Fluoro-X™ software allow further analysis of FLUOROSPOT data using any commercial flow cytometry software and facilitate the generation of professional reports and presentation. In this article, we present a detailed step-by-step workflow for the analysis of a human four-color IFN-γ, IL-2, TNF-α, and GzB antigen-specific T-cell assay using the Fluoro-X Software Suite.

Key words T cell, B Cell, Cytokines, Immunoglobulins, Antibodies, ELISPOT, FLUOROSPOT, Multiplex, Multi-Color, Spot counting, Objective, Center of mass, AutoGate™, SmartSpot™, SmartCount™ Quality Control, Software, Fluoro-X™, Fluorescence, Label

1 Introduction

Over past decade, ELISPOT has become the gold standard for monitoring T- and B-cell immunity in clinical trials. This is primarily to its capacity for single cell resolution, high throughput, and ability to detect antigen-specific responses directly ex-vivo. Recent advances in multi-color fluorescent spot detection made FLUOROSPOT a fast-developing method for simultaneous measurements of up to seven analytes at a time [1]. Whereas the main criteria for objective, user independent single color ELISPOT counting are well established [2, 3], and commercial analysis

Alexander E. Kalyuzhny (ed.), *Handbook of ELISPOT: Methods and Protocols*, Methods in Molecular Biology, vol. 1808, https://doi.org/10.1007/978-1-4939-8567-8_10, © Springer Science+Business Media, LLC, part of Springer Nature 2018

software has been available for a number of years, a multi-color FLUOROSPOT analysis software is new to the majority of the ELISPOT users. Here we present the main principles as well as a step-by-step workflow for four-color T-cell FLUOROSPOT data analysis. CTL's Fluoro-X™ multi-color assay platform utilizes individual monochromatic images taken at the excitation/emission conditions (fluorescent channels) optimized for each fluorochrome used. This approach, as opposed to the analysis of a single multi-color image, allows for the detection of cells secreting highly variable amounts of individual cytokines (or other analytes). Further, this eliminates both the necessity of employing complex color recognition algorithms and the possibility of spectral cross-bleeding from different fluorochromes.

At the first step of the analysis, individual monochromatic images for each fluorescent channel are collected and counted in exactly the same manner as has been established for single color ELISPOT analysis. Objective user-independent single-color analysis is facilitated by two main features of the ImmunoSpot® Software—SmartSpot™ and AutoGate™ [2, 3].

At the second step, spots from the monochromatic images for each individual channel are "paired" to identify double-, triple-, quadruple-analyte producing cells using the experimentally validated Center of Mass Distance (COMD) algorithm [4]. Different color spots (scanned trough individual fluorescent channels) form a multi-color event if each of their "centers of mass" is less than the maximal allowed COMD apart. These multi-color events are recorded the same way as in flow cytometry data analysis. Multiple measurements are extracted from each single or multi-color event, including spot sizes, max/average/total intensities, peak intensity values, XY coordinates, and more. In addition to the proprietary ImmunoSpot® data format, Fluoro-X™ software saves Flow Cytometry Standard (FCS) files, which can be further analyzed using the Fluoro-X™ Manage Data module, or with any commercial flow cytometry software to establish detailed statistical analysis of different analyte-producing/co-producing cell populations. In this chapter, we provide an overview of multi-color counting, quality control, and the advanced data management/presentation features of the ImmunoSpot® Fluoro-X™ Suite.

2   Materials

- Software: ImmunoSpot® Fluoro-X™ Software Suite Version 7.0 by CTL (Shaker Heights, OH).

- Hardware: ImmunoSpot® S6 ULTIMATE analyzer by CTL.

- Four-color FLUOROSPOT kit for human IFN-γ/IL-2/TNF-α/ Granzyme B by CTL (http://www.immunospot.com/

immunospot-kits/human-interferon-gamma-il-2-tnf-a-granzyme-b-four-color-fluorospot).

- Human cryopreserved PBMC sample of HLA-A2-positive donor was obtained from CTL's commercial ePBMC® library. These PBMC had been previously HLA-typed at high resolution and characterized for T-cell reactivity to a variety of antigens (details are available at http://www.immunospot.com/ImmunoSpot-ePBMC).

- FLUOROSPOT assay shown was performed on a single HLA-A2 positive donor PBMC sample stimulated with HCMV HLA-A2 restricted peptide pp65 (495–503) (EZ Biolab Inc., Carmel, IN, USA) according to the test kit instructions.

- Throughout the article, *"single color spots"* refers to those spots that appear only on a single fluorescent channel, and *"multi-color spots"* to those appearing in multiple channels. When evaluating the results, it is important to distinguish objects that appear *exclusively* on a specific channel or combination of channels (*exclusive* results), from objects that are visible in other channels (or combinations of channels) as well (*inclusive* results).

---

3   Methods

3.1   Main Fluoro-X™ Switchboard

The main switchboard of the Fluoro-X™ Software Suite (Fig. 1) is designed to activate key software functions, including scanning multi-color fluorescence plates, counting multi-color T- and B-cell spots, quality control and data management of the counted results (*see* **Note 1**).

3.2   Scanning and Loading FLUOROSPOT Plates for Counting

As in conventional single-color ELISPOT analysis, FLUOROSPOT plates are first scanned on the ImmunoSpot® analyzer (*see* Subheading 2). For high-throughput assays, 384-well plates can be used in place of standard 96-well plates [5]. After loading a scanned plate (or multiple plates), the first step is to fine-tune parameters, including setting the spot-size gates for all analytes/channels before autocounting of the whole plate/plates. When scanning multi-color FLUOROSPOT plates, individual channels are organized as single-color plates. Once the counting parameters and spot size gates have been set for all channels, the autocount feature can be enabled to count all wells in multi-color mode. After the count is complete, it is possible to verify, quality control, visualize, and export the multi-count data. These steps are discussed and illustrated next.

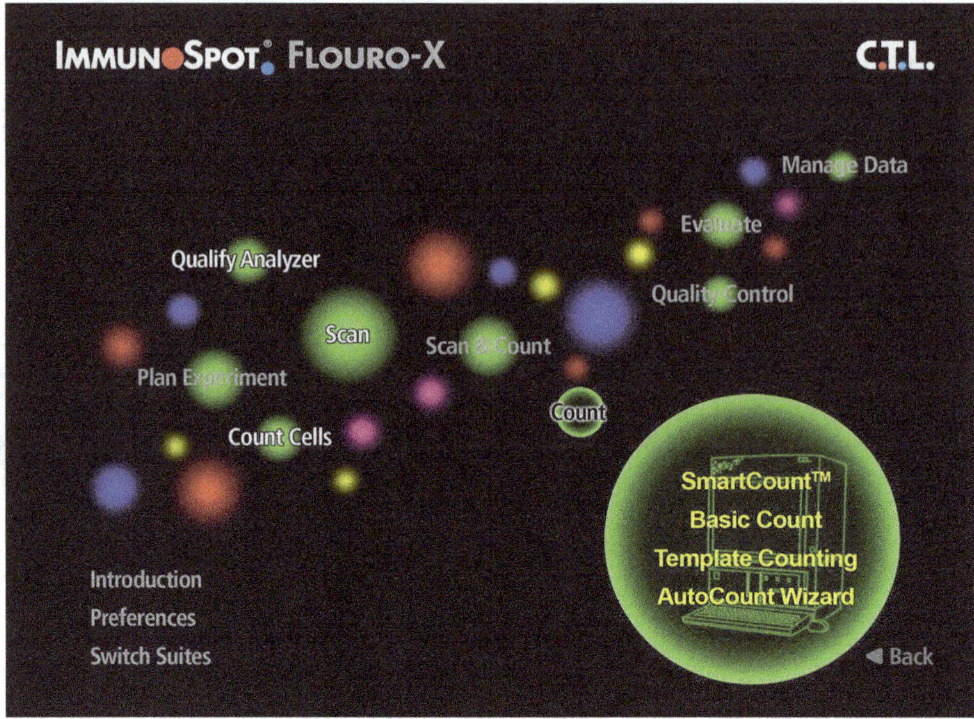

Fig. 1 ImmunoSpot® Fluoro-X™ Suite switchboard

3.2.1 Setting up Counting Parameters for all Channels Using SmartSpot™

Multi-color analysis starts with single-color (for each separate channel) counting, based on the established and validated ELISPOT counting algorithms implemented in the ImmunoSpot® Software. The input is a set of monochromatic images captured under conditions optimized for each individual fluorochrome/channel. This set of images records objects that may or may not appear in multiple channels, and the task is to identify and count objects of each individual fluorescent channel and all possible combinations of these.

To optimize parameters for the entire plate (or set of plates), it is recommended to set the counting parameters on a selection of typical wells representative of the type(s) of response(s) seen in the plate(s) (including both negative control and positive wells). It is also recommended to test the parameters on both sparsely and densely populated wells. Individual wells can be selected using the well navigation/selection interface (*see* red dot-marked well selection on Fig. 2) by clicking on the well of interest.

Since the scanned plates contain images for multiple channels, it is important to have single color counting fine-tuned for all channels. The channels for a currently selected well can be switched through the channel selection interface (*see* highlighted selection on Fig. 3).

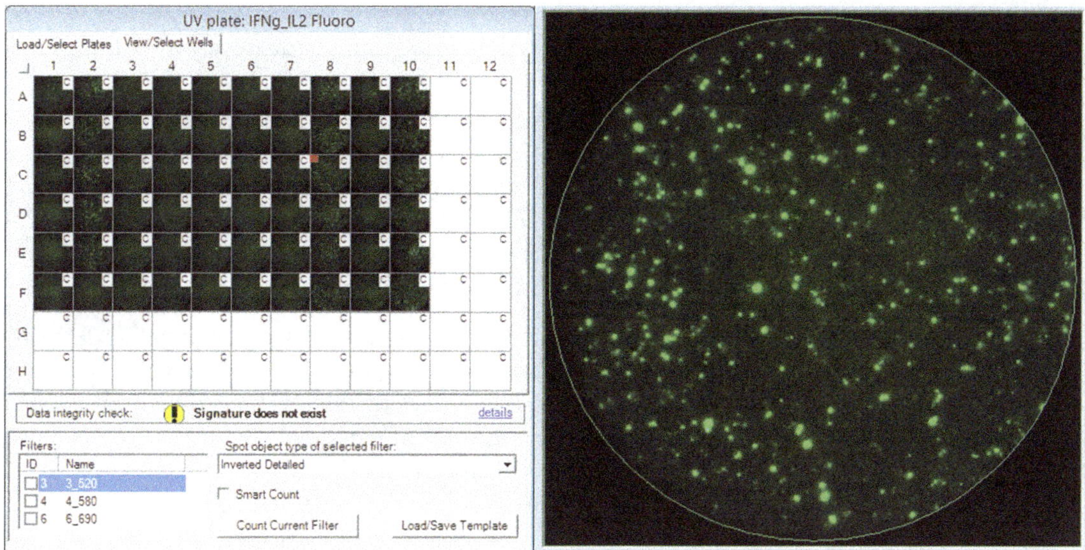

Fig. 2 Plate navigation and well selection interface

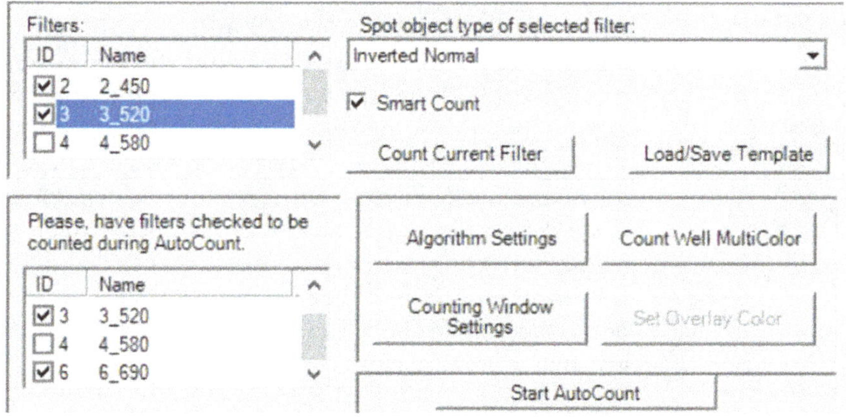

Fig. 3 Fluorescence channel selection window with all major function call buttons. In the upper-left "Filters" panel, the highlighted channel indicates the image to be displayed during a single well test count, checkboxes select which spot outlines will be shown on this image after it is counted during the setup. In the example shown, a 520 nm (green) channel image will be shown after counting with 520 nm (green) and 450 nm (blue) spot outlines. In the bottom left "Autocount" panel, checkboxes select channels to be included in the batch autocount

ImmunoSpot® software allows for the optimization of multiple counting parameters for ensuring accurate results (*see* below for list); however, the only parameter which may need to be adjusted in the majority of assays is the minimal spot intensity or "Sensitivity." ImmunoSpot® Software implements SmartCount™ mode for automatic recognition of spots of different morphologies on various backgrounds. SmartCount™ mode is based on the SmartSpot™ object/background recognition algorithm, and provides an objective user-independent means for analyzing spot data (*see* **Note 2**). The accuracy, reliability, and reproducibility of SmartCount™ mode were confirmed during multiple studies including a multi-laboratory ELISPOT validation study [6, 7].

Additionally, spot morphology may vary depending on the affinity of the capture antibodies and the kinetics of the analyte secretion by different cells [8]. To account for such morphological differences, ImmunoSpot® Software includes additional parameters chief among these being the following (*see* Fig. 4):

- Diffuseness (Diffuse Processing): This parameter handles differences in spot morphology and mainly reflects the relationship between spot sizes and densities. If the plate contains tight intense spots, it is best set at "normal" level. For large faint ("diffuse") spots, Diffuse Processing should be set to "Large" or "Largest," whereas for bright small spots the "Detailed" is the best choice.

- Background Balance: ELISPOT and FLUOROSPOT wells sometimes show uneven background staining. Among other possible reasons, "ELISA effect" (where an abundance of cytokine or other analyte is released into the culture medium during the assay incubation period, and then binds uniformly to capture antibody on the well surface) and leaking wells (if the assay is not performed in the optimal way) may create such strong uneven membrane coloration. This can be compensated for by the Background Balance feature, which detects unevenness of the background and normalizes (balances) it. This parameter is proportional to the size of the background area. It is important to note that setting this parameter too high may not sufficiently balance the background, whereas setting it too low may eliminate large spots of interest.

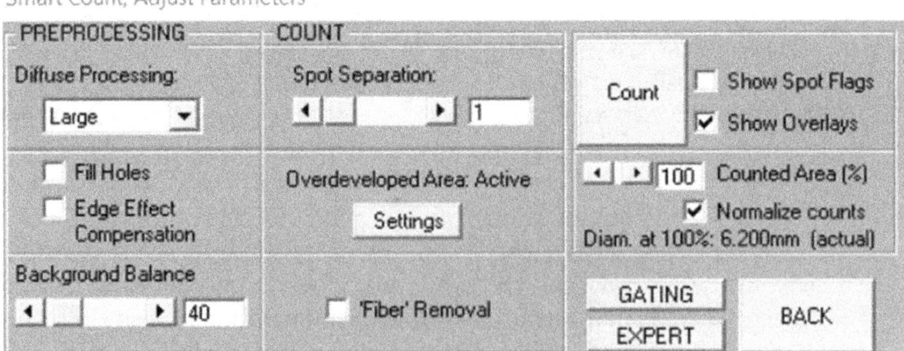

Fig. 4 SmartCount™ parameters window of ImmunoSpot® Fluoro-X™ suite

- Spot Separation: Closely situated or partially overlapping spots can potentially be mistakenly counted as a single object. To separate such touching or overlapping objects, ImmunoSpot® software implements intelligent spot separation function. The algorithm is based on detailed analysis of the spot-intensity profiles, and has proven to be robust even when separating large spot clusters in overcrowded wells. The parameter is proportional to the sizes of the spots to be separated, i.e., the smaller the spots, the lower this parameter should be set.

It must be noted that spot intensities and morphologies, along with differences in background staining, can be different for different analytes. Therefore, in multi-color analysis, counting parameters must be optimized for each fluorescent channel individually. However, as we emphasized earlier, in the majority of cases, the pre-set default settings for these parameters will be close to optimal and will not need adjustment. Additionally, ImmunoSpot® Fluoro-X™ Suite contains a standard set of counting templates (sets of parameters) optimized for each CTL multi-color B- and T-cell kit. For using pre-set, standard, or user-modified templates, the Load/Save Template function can be activated from the main channel/well selection interface (Fig. 3).

3.2.2 Setting Spot Size Gates for all Fluorescent Channels Using the AutoGate™ Function

As demonstrated previously, the range of spot sizes produced by antigen-stimulated T-cells uniformly (for different cytokines, cell donors and antigens) follows a Log Normal distribution [9]. Knowing the expected spot size statistics allowed the implementation of the AutoGate™ function (*see* **Note 2**). This facilitates the automatic discrimination between the relevant spots produced by stimulated cells, and irrelevant spots produced by bystander cells, which may be present either in both negative and positive wells (background production) or in positive wells only (bystander activation), such as when there is antigen-induced IFN-γ, IL-10, or IL-4 production by T cells, as well as background/bystander secretion of these cytokines by NK cells, monocytes, and basophils, respectively [3, 10, 11].

Background and bystander spots are usually smaller than antigen-induced spots and can be excluded from the final counts using automatic size gating. Gating options can be accessed from the counting parameters interface (Fig. 4) by pressing GATING button. The autogating interface (Fig. 5) prompts users to select first a few typical (for the specific cytokine/analyte) positive wells, containing stimulated and potentially bystander cell, then if applicable, select a few typical negative wells (background spots only).

After the selected wells are counted, and spot size statistics are calculated from these cumulative counts for both induced and background spots, the auto-adjust function can be executed to automatically set minimum and maximum size gates (Fig. 6).

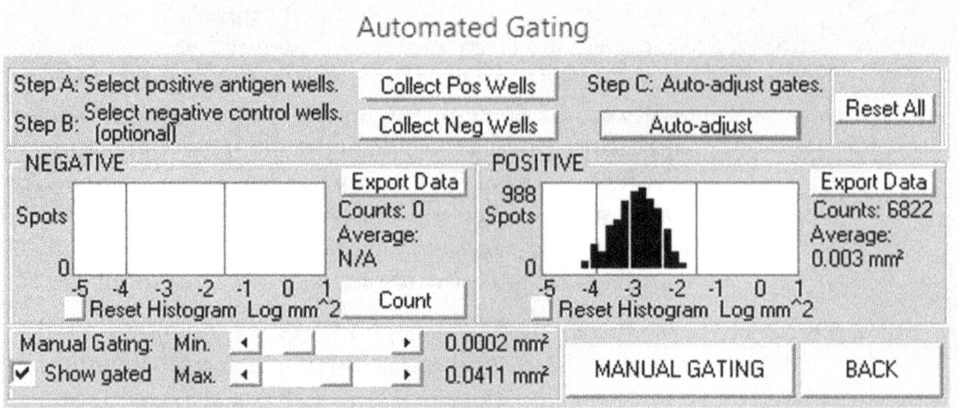

Fig. 5 AutoGate™ window. Main functions inlude selection of positive and negative (background) wells for autogating, execute autogating (Auto-adjust) button, and link to the manual gating window. In the example shown, autogating was done on positive wells only using Log Normal model

If negative wells are not available, or collectively do not have enough spots for statistical calculations, gates can be automatically set using positive wells only, using a Log Normal spot size distribution model (Fig. 5). It should also be mentioned that wells for autogating can be selected from different plates loaded for batch counting.

The result of the AutoGate™ function can be seen in Fig. 6. Vertical blue lines show Min/Max gate positions on negative (top) and positive (bottom) spot size histograms for the corresponding selected wells (labeled on the well navigation interface with letters "N" and "P," respectively). Note the reduced count and white outlines marking undersized spots after gating was applied (Fig. 7).

ImmunoSpot® Software also allows the user to set minimum and maximum spot size gates manually by moving Min/Max sliders or by sampling the smallest and largest spots to be counted (Fig. 5). Manual gating can be used when there is not a sufficient amount of spots available for statistically significant results, or when a subpopulation of cells with a different cytokine productivity is to be evaluated separately. Spot-size statistics and gate settings can be reviewed/modified using the Verify Gates window of the Quality Control module (Fig. 6).

Because spot size distributions differ between cytokines/analytes, it is important to set spot size gates for all fluorescents channels individually. Well selections can be different between channels.

3.2.3 Setting Up Parameters for Multi-Color Spot Recognition

Once spot counting has been completed for all individual fluorescent channels, the next step is to establish the relationship between spots from the different channels using a pairing algorithm, which is based on spot coordinates within the well image. Spots of different colors occupying the same (or highly proximate) positions on

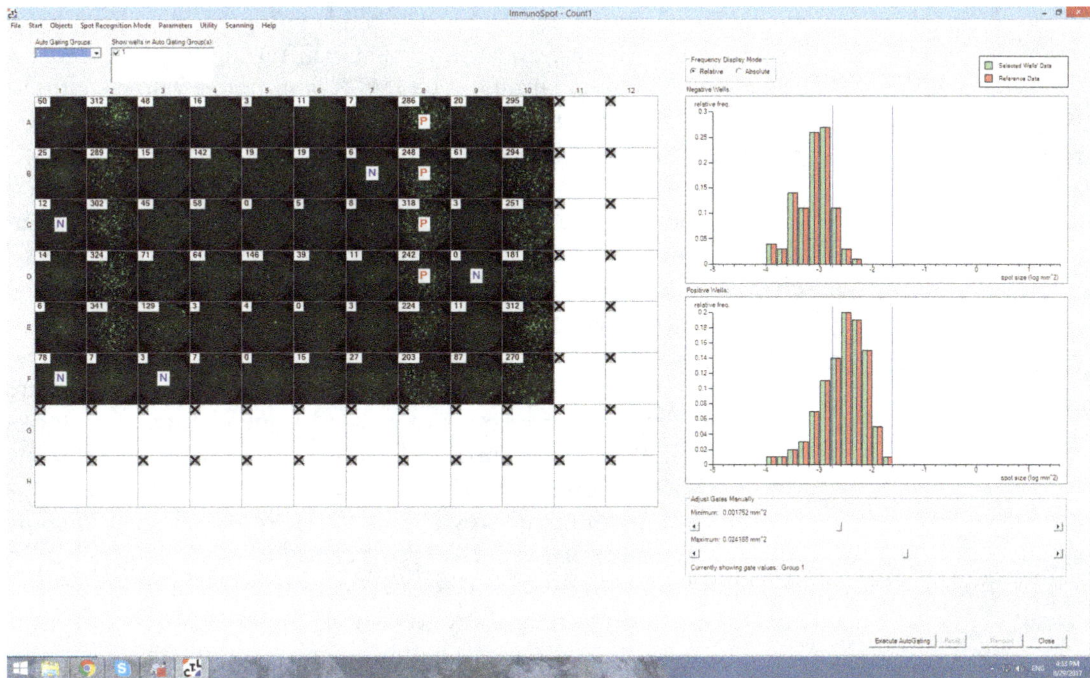

Fig. 6 Verify Gates window. On the left, wells selected for positive (P) and negative background (N) wells are shown in the plate navigation control. On the right, negative background (top) and positive (bottom) spot histograms calculated from the selected wells are shown with the auto-adjusted gates (blue vertical lines). Red histograms are calculated for reference (selected for autogating) wells. Green histograms are calculated for any other positive and negative wells chosen specifically for this gate verification process. In the example shown, no additional wells for gate verification are selected and both red and green histograms are the same

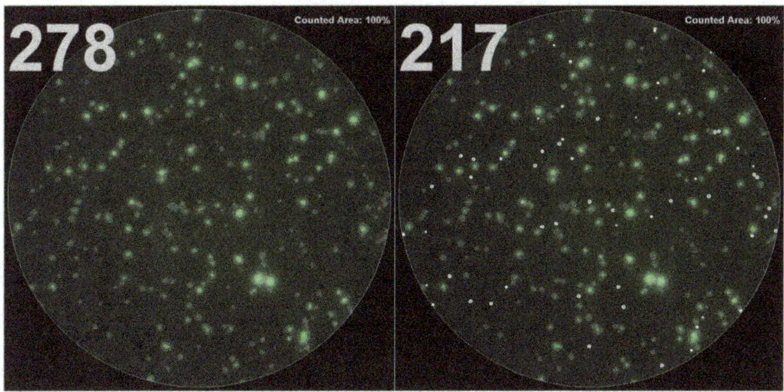

Fig. 7 Results of autogating on the spot counts in the 520 nm (green) fluorescence channel. Image on the left shows counting prior size gating, and image on the right shows counting with AutoGate™ enabled. Spots inside size gates are marked with purple outlines, and undersized background spots are shown with white outlines (these are excluded from the final count)

the well membrane are counted as multi-color. We tested multiple different algorithms, and found that pairing algorithm based on the Center of Mass Distance (COMD) is the most reliable among all of these to accurately determine co-localization of spots between different channels (*see* **Note 3**).

The Center of Mass Distance is defined as a maximal allowed distance between centers of masses (in image analysis, it is often referred to as centers of gray) of two spots of different colors/channels. Extensions of this algorithm include resolving partial overlaps of spots in the same channel and processing of spot clusters.

The algorithm basically determines the precise coordinate location of the center of mass of a spot in one channel, and looks for spots in all other channels whose center(s) of mass are below the maximum allowed COMD. The spot and its multi-color pairs are removed from further tests. This step is repeated until all spots on all filters are processed. If a spot's center of mass appears within the COMD on multiple filters, it is considered a multi-color spot (or "event" using the analogy to flow cytometry).

The result of the multi-color pairing is two-/three-/multi-color spots (events) indicated on the counted images with double, triple, etc. concentric spot outlines of different colors (colors of outlines are selectable, Fig. 8). The pairing algorithm also returns inclusive and exclusive numbers of double-, triple-, multi-color spots for every possible filter combination. In the case of our four-color T-cell FLUOROSPOT, there are 11 combinations of multi-color spots: six double color, four three-color and one four-color. Inclusive double color results list all spots of two certain colors including three- and four-color spots; in contrast, exclusive results list only double color counts.

The COMD parameter depends primarily on the optics of an analyzer and is practically constant for each model of analyzer. However, if new fluorescent channels or different optical zoom factors are used, or if cells are moving during the incubation period (in case of asynchronous cytokine secretion by the same cell), it is recommended to fine-tune the COMD parameter using the Algorithm Setting option (Figs. 3 and 9). The unit for this tolerance parameter is defined as a percentage of the well bottom diameter. So, the zoom factor, or image scaling, will not affect this value (e.g., 1% of a 6 mm well would mean 0.06 mm tolerance regardless of zooming, *see* Fig. 9). With an image vertical resolution of 1000 pixels per well, the COMD equal to 1 is equivalent to 10 pixels. Integrated correction for "false" positive multi-color spots (by statistically determining the expected number of random co-localization events for a given number of spots in each channel) ensures that the final counts are accurate, even when the COMD is set higher then optimal [4].

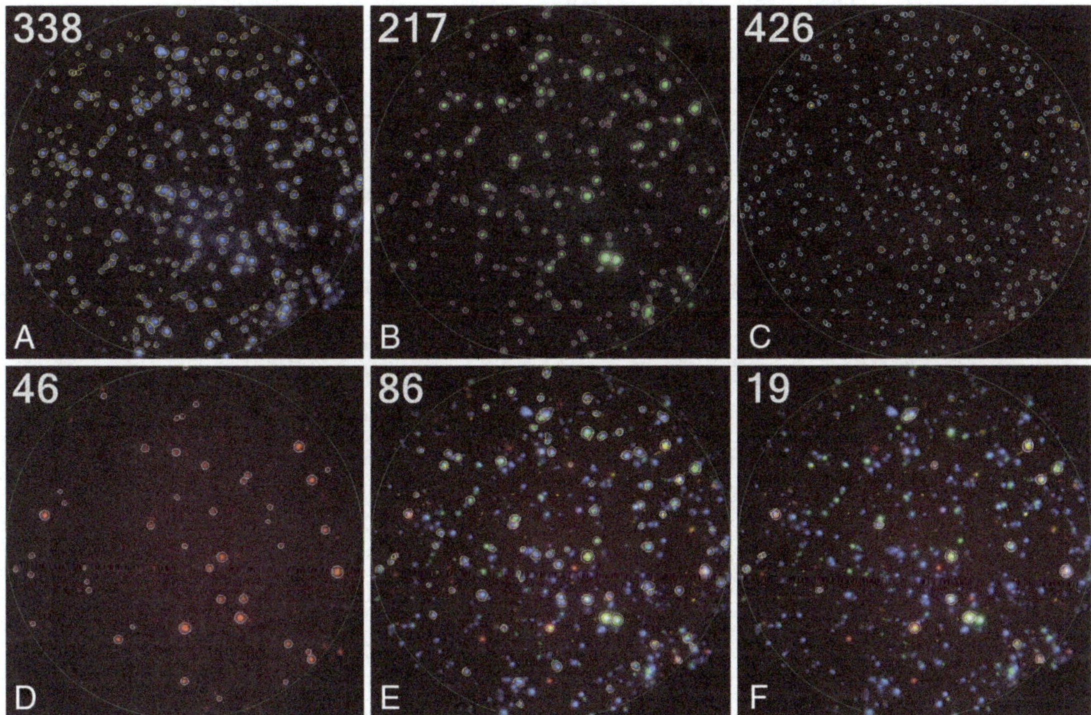

Fig. 8 Multi-color counting results: single-color spot outlines are shown for the individual fluorescence channels: GzB—450 nm blue (**a**), IFN-γ—520 nm green (**b**), TNF-α—580 nm yellow (**c**), and IL-2—690 nm red (**d**). Triple-color and four-color outlines are shown for GzB/IFN-γ/TNF-α triple-positive (**e**) and GzB/IFN-γ/TNF-α/IL-2 qudrouple-positive spots on the four-color merged image (**f**)

Fig. 9 Pairing parameters setup dialog for fine-tuning Center of Mass Distance

The object pairing algorithm can be tested on a well by well basis by pressing "Count Well Multicolor" (Fig. 3). Pairing results for each possible color combination can be easily visualized and verified by enabling/disabling corresponding channel selection checkboxes (top left on Fig. 3) (*see* **Note 4**). An example of a triple-color pairing can be seen in Fig. 8. In this illustration, single-color spot outlines are shown on the individual channel images (A, B, and C) and triple-color spot outlines (objects that are present on all three filters) are shown on a merged multi-color image (D).

After all counting parameters, including min/max spot size gates and pairing parameters, are optimized, the Start Autocount command can be executed (Fig. 3). All wells for all pre-loaded plates will be counted, and the results will be written to Excel, XML, and Flow Cytometry Standard (FCS) files once the multi-color counting is completed.

3.3 Quality Control

The next step is to quality control and evaluate the results. The quality control (QC) module of ImmunoSpot® software is designed to provide maximal visual feedback on the levels of full plate overview as well as on the individual wells basis. The quality control process allows the user to verify or change counting parameters and gates (manually or automatically), remove artifacts and/or overdeveloped areas, and recount individual wells or batches of wells. It is also possible to adjust the COMD for the multi-color spot pairing. When the GLP (Good Laboratory Practice) Compliance Package is used, the software keeps a complete audit trail of all changes done to the original counts during QC using secure Code for Federal Regulations (CFR) Part 11 compliant database (*see* **Note 5**). The GLP Compliance Package also provides a role-based security feature, allowing pre-defined users and groups to perform certain individual tasks, like plate scanning, plate counting with locked parameters, changing counting parameters, or performing quality control, depending on the roles (permissions) set in the ImmunoSpot® Software.

3.4 Multi-Color Data Management

The evaluation of multi-color counting results is a complex task. The multi-dimensional nature of the counted data (multiple individual channel images plus multiple spot outlines for each possible color combination) makes it difficult to see the connections between the results. To this end, ImmunoSpot® Fluoro-X™ QC and Manage Data modules implement a Multi-Color View function which can be activated for each selected well (Fig. 10). The Multi-Color View function provides a tool that can combine (or merge) together and recolor any combination of the individual channel images and spot outlines into a single image, allowing visual cross-checking of the spot images and outlines.

The channel recolor tool is particularly helpful when fluorescent channels (600, 630, and 690 nm, for example) will generate similar red RGB images, which would be difficult to visually distinguish otherwise. All spot count outlines can be enabled, disabled, and recolored for better visual evaluation. The Multi-Color View tool also provides controls for automatic or manual image enhancement, and for weight/intensity control of individual selected col-

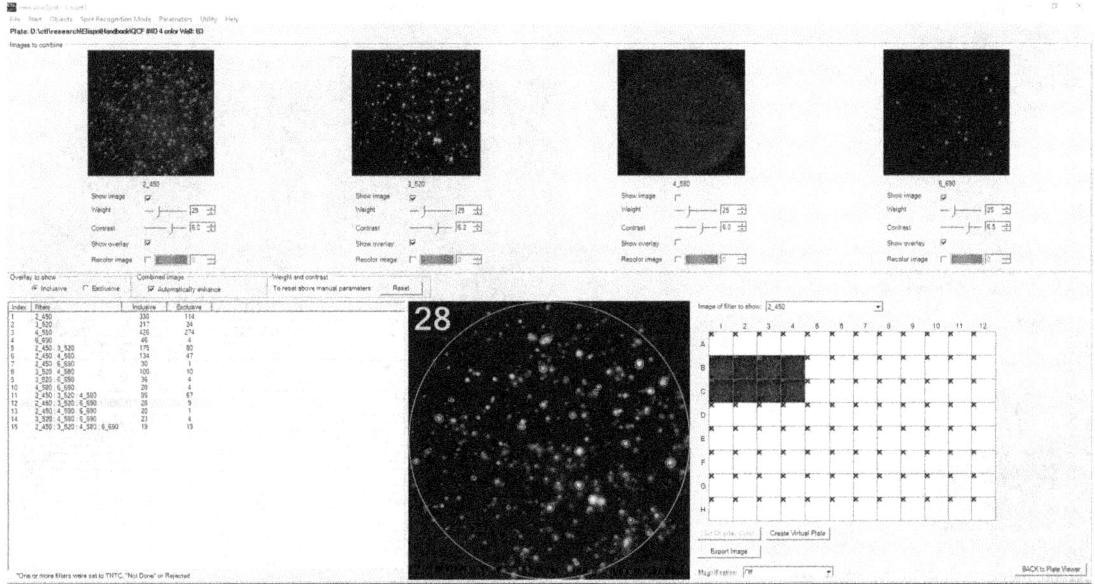

Fig. 10 Fluoro-X™ Multi-Color View window for Manage Data and Quality Control modules. Any combination of individual channel images and spot outlines can be created for any well (plate navigation is to the right of the well image) . Specific spot outline combinations can be generated for exclusive and inclusive counts using the selection list (bottom left panel)

ors in the resulting merged image. In the example shown in Fig. 10, three original well images (450, 520, and 690 nm channels) from well B3 are shown in the merged image, together with the triple color (exclusive) spot outlines for these three channels.

Both QC and Manage Data modules share the same well browsing interface for exporting well images from scanned/ counted/quality controlled plates. The images may be arbitrarily arranged, and any individual filter or any combination of the filters can be exported (using image merging). In the example shown on Fig. 11 counted wells B2, B3, B4, C2, C3, and C4 are selected for the Well Survey using two rows by three columns format for the combination (merged image) of 450, 520, 580 and 690 nm fluorescent channels with exclusive quadruple color spots outlines. After evaluating the results, these Well Surveys can be exported as Power Point slides.

The Multi-Color View interface also allows the user to create a virtual plate (for presentation purposes) containing both original scanned well images merged from selected filters, and selected combinations of spot outlines (Create Virtual Plate button on Fig. 10).

The Data Management tool can open any saved data file format created by the counting and QC modules. The counted data are exported to different formats including Excel workbook, XML, and Flow Cytometry Standard format (FCS). The Excel and XML outputs also contain estimations for the probability of random sin-

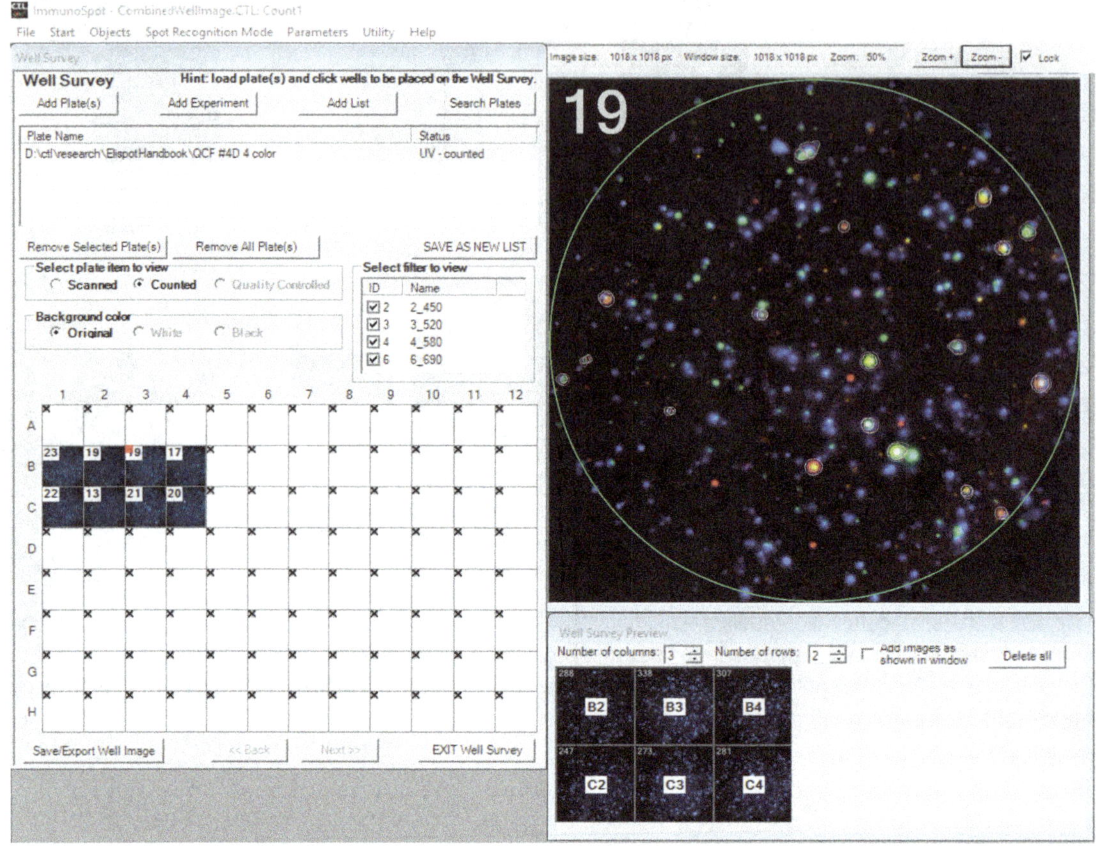

Fig. 11 Fluoro-X™ Well Survey window for exporting of individual images and arranged groups of images to a PPT presentation. In the example shown, a three by two image survey is created for wells marked in the plate navigator window

	Inclusive Spot Counts					Probabilistic Inclusive Spot Counts			
	2_450: 3_520	2_450: 6_690	3_520: 6_690	2_450: 3_520: 6_690		2_450: 3_520	2_450: 6_690	3_520: 6_690	2_450: 3_520: 6_690
B1	167	25	34	24	B1	25	5	4	0
B2	156	34	46	28	B2	23	7	5	1
B3	175	30	36	28	B3	28	6	4	1
B4	170	27	35	27	B4	24	5	4	0

Fig. 12 A fragment of Excel workbook sections displaying numbers of double- and triple-spots for 450 nm (blue), 520 nm (green), and 590 nm (red) channels counted in wells B1, B2, B3, B4 (on the left) and numbers of calculated "false" positive random spots overlays (on the right)

gle-color spots overlays using statistically validated tools (Fig. 12 shows a sample of Excel output).

The Excel workbook stores results in separate sheets. The first two sheets store inclusive and exclusive multi-count results with filters in separate charts, while the next two sheets combine these results into a single chart (well ID versus filter combination). Additional sheets store probabilistic counts of random single-color

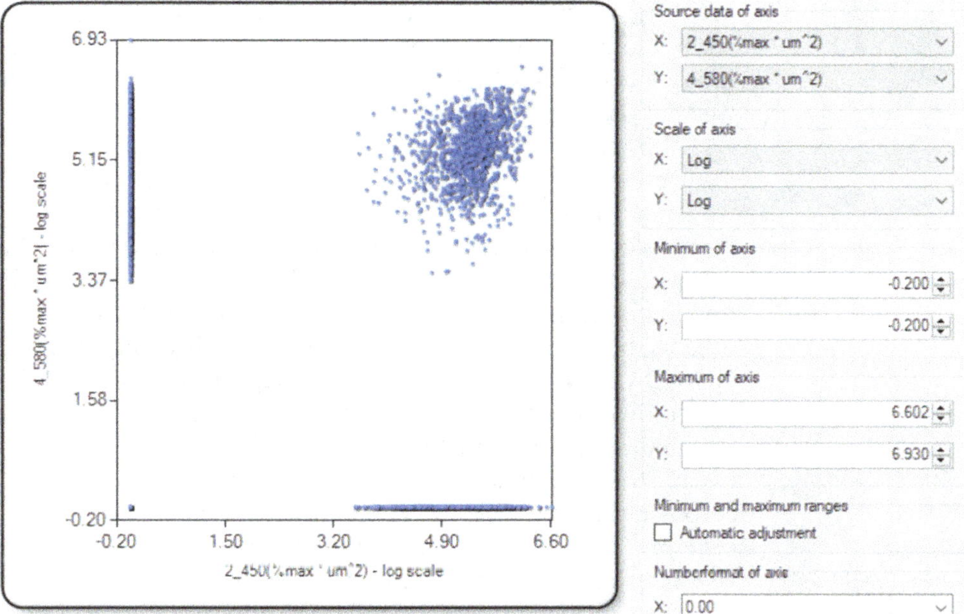

Fig. 13 A Flow Cytometry Standard (FCS) file opened using Fluoro-X™ Data Management module. A standard dot-plot graph is shown as total spot fluorescence for TNF-α 580 nm (yellow) and GzB 450 nm (blue) spots in Log scale. Single-color GzB and TNF-α spots are aligned along X and Y axis, respectively, and double color spots form a cluster in the upper-right quadrant of the plot. Average total intensities of these two cytokines in single color spots are practically the same as in double color spots

spots overlays using different methods. The last sheet stores all parameters used for counting.

The XML format provides a bridge between the ImmunoSpot® Software and customer databases using Common Laboratory System.

For more detailed analysis of sub-populations of T cells producing different combinations of cytokines, and High Content analysis of T- and B-cell produced spots based on the spot morphologies [8] ImmunoSpot®, Fluoro-X™ Suite generates Flow Cytometry Standard (FCS) files (*see* **Note 6**). The individual fluorescence channel data that is exported to the FSC file include maximal, mean and total spot fluorescence, spot size, circularity, and image-based XY center of mass. FCS files can be opened by either Fluoro-X™ Manage Data module as a standard dot-plot (Fig. 13) or in any commercial Flow Software. In Fig. 13, the total spot intensities in 450 nm (GzB) and 580 nm (TNF-α) fluorescent channels are shown as a dot-plot in Log scale. Single color TNF-α and GzB spots are aligned along the X and Y axis (no compensation required), with the double positive population in the upperright quadrant. For more detailed analysis including gating on different populations, 2D and 3D dot-plot statistics, histogram statistics, and cluster analysis, any commercial Flow Cytometry analysis software can be used. In most cases, the number of spots in a single well may not be sufficient for building a good quality high-resolution dot-plot or histogram. Fluoro-X™ Manage Data module provides a function to merge multiple similar (repetitive) well data to a single FCS file.

Although Fluoro-X™ software contains multiple functions and features, the user interface is intuitive and easy to use (*see* **Note 1**). As we reported earlier, single-color algorithms used for individual color spots recognitions are robust, user error-free and guarantee objective counts over a wide range of spot numbers per well (*see* **Note 2**). The multi-color spot detection algorithm is based on the maximal allowed distance between spot centers and contains only a single parameter—COMD (*see* **Note 3**). This parameter depends primarily on the configuration of the optics of the analyzer used, and does not need to be adjusted between assays if the same fluorescent channels are used. To maximize the accuracy of multi-color counting, Fluoro-X™ software automatically calculates numbers of false positive multi-color spots resulting from random overlays of single color spots of different channels for each well (*see* **Note 7**). An integrated quality control system provides data security and validation by authorized QC-users (*see* **Note 5**). Extended data output includes Excel workbooks, Power Point graphical output, Common Laboratory System compatible XML files, and Flow Cytometry Standard files for detailed analysis of different sub-populations and High Content analysis (*see* **Note 6**). Built-in image and data export features help to prepare publications, reports, and Power Point presentations (*see* **Note 8**).

Although we demonstrated the Fluoro-X™ Suite using a four-color T-cell FLUOROSPOT, the same principles and procedures are applicable to any numbers of the fluorescent channels. The current ImmunoSpot® 7.0 platform supports scanning and counting of up to twelve different analytes in both T- and B-cell modes.

4   Notes

1. ImmunoSpot® Fluoro-X™ Suite is an integrated data acquisition, analysis, and management solution for high-throughput processing of multi-color T- and B-cell FLUOROSPOT plates.

2. ImmunoSpot® Software utilizes SmartCount™ mode, which is based on the SmartSpot™ automatic object recognition algorithm and statistically validated AutoGate™ function for objective user-independent data analysis.

3. Fluoro-X™ multi-color spot detection algorithm is based on the maximal allowed distance between centers of masses of spots, the Center Of Mass Distance (COMD), in individual fluorescent channels.

4. The Software provides options for setting parameters for the major steps of multi-color counting (counting, size-gating, and

multi-color spot detection) and has a built-in validation tool for evaluation and visualization of multi-color counting results.

5. The integrated quality control (QC) module with an Optional GLP and CFR Part 11 compliance package enables multi-color counting data review, validation, and approval with complete audit trail and data security.

6. Multiple counted data output formats include Flow Cytometry Standard (FCS) files for extended High Content spot morphology analysis and XML files for Laboratory Information Management System (LIMS) compatibility.

7. For maximal accuracy of true multi-color spots counting, the Fluoro-X™ Software calculates frequencies of "false" positive multi-color spots (random spots overlays) using two independent statistical methods.

8. Built-in data and image exporting tools assist in composing high quality data presentations and reports.

References

1. Caspell R, Lehmann PV (2018) Detecting all immunoglobulin classes and subclasses in Multiplex 7 Color ImmunoSpot® assays. In: Methods in molecular biology, 3rd edn. Springer Verlag GmbH, New York

2. Lehmann PV (2005) Image analysis and data management of ELISPOT assay results. Methods Mol Biol 302:117–132

3. Zhang W, Lehmann PV (2012) Objective, user-independent ELISPOT data analysis based on scientifically validated principles. Methods Mol Biol 792:155–171

4. Karulin AY, Megyesi Z, Caspell R, Hanson J, Lehmann PV (2018) Multiplexing T- and B-cell FLUOROSPOT assays: experimental validation of the Multi-Color ImmunoSpot® software based on center of mass distance algorithm. In: Methods in molecular biology, 3rd edn. Springer Verlag GmbH, New York

5. Hanson J, Sundararaman S, Caspell R, Karacsony E, Karulin AY, Lehmann PV (2015) ELISPOT assays in 384-well format: up to 30 data points with one million cells. Cells 4(1):71–83

6. Zhang W, Caspell R, Karulin AY, Ahmad M, Haicheur N, Abdelsalam A, Johannesen K, Vignard V, Dudzik P, Georgakopoulou K, Mihaylova A, Silina K, Aptsiauri N, Adams V, Lehmann PV, McArdle S (2009) ELISPOT assays provide reproducible results among different laboratories for T-cell immune monitoring—even in hands of ELISPOT-inexperienced investigators. J Immunotoxicol 6(4):227–234

7. Sundararaman S, Karulin AY, Ansari T, BenHamouda N, Gottwein J, Laxmanan S, Levine SM, Loffredo JT, McArdle S, Neudoerfl C, Roen D, Silina K, Welch M, Lehmann PV (2015) High reproducibility of ELISPOT counts from nine different laboratories. Cell 4(1):21–39

8. Karulin AY, Lehmann PV (2012) How ELISPOT morphology reflects on the productivity and kinetics of cells' secretory activity. Methods Mol Biol 792:125–143

9. Karulin AY, Karacsony K, Zhang W, Targoni OS, Moldovan I, Dittrich M, Sundararaman S, Lehmann PV (2015) ELISPOTs produced by CD8 and CD4 cells follow log normal size distribution permitting objective counting. Cell 4(1):56–70

10. Karulin AY, Hesse MD, Yip HC, Lehmann PV (2002) Indirect IL-4 pathway in type 1 immunity. J Immunol 168(2):545–553

11. Guerkov RE, Targoni OS, Kreher CR, Boehm BO, Herrera MT, Tary-Lehmann M, Lehmann PV, Schwander SK (2003) Detection of low-frequency antigen-specific IL-10-producing CD4(+) T cells via ELISPOT in PBMC: cognate vs. nonspecific production of the cytokine. J Immunol Methods 279(1–2):111–121

B-Cell ELISpot Assay to Quantify Antigen-Specific Antibody-Secreting Cells in Human Peripheral Blood Mononuclear Cells

Haw Hwai, Yi-Ying Chen, and Shiang-Jong Tzeng

Abstract

Peripheral blood is commonly used to assess the cellular and humoral immune responses in clinical studies. It is a convenient sample to collect for immunological research as compared to the surgically excised and biopsied lymphoid specimens. To determine the functional status of immune system from peripheral blood, the enzyme-linked immunospot (ELISpot) assay is a popular method of choice owing to its high sensitivity, great accuracy, and easy performance. The ELISpot allows detection and quantification of cellular functionality at the single-cell level. Therefore, ELISpot assay is commonly applied to detect cytokines and cytotoxic granules released from T cells as well as to measure antibodies secreted from B cells. Because the ELISpot assay has been increasingly used for evaluation of the vaccine efficacy in clinical trials, standardization and reproducibility are crucial to minimize assay variability amongst samples from different sources. Here we introduce methods to isolate human peripheral blood mononuclear cells (PBMCs) for quantification of the antigen-specific antibody-secreting cells using the ELISpot assay.

Key words Enzyme-linked immunospot (ELISpot), B cells, Antibody-secreting cells (ASCs), Peripheral blood mononuclear cells (PBMCs), Vaccine

1 Introduction

The ELISpot assay was originally developed by Dr. Cecil Czerkinsky in 1983 for the purpose to detect antigen (Ag)-specific antibody (Ab)-secreting cells (ASCs) [1]. Over the years, the ELISpot has become an important method for the detection and quantification of ASCs in vaccine research. The technology of ELISpot assay is a combination of enzyme-linked immunoabsorbance assay (ELISA) and western blotting to enable quantification of a specific cell population based on their secretory molecules with superior sensitivity to detect a single positive cell [2]. Therefore, ELISpot assay has been increasingly adopted for the identification and enumeration of cytokine-producing T cells as well as Ag-specific ASCs [2–4]. Although the conventional ELISA and flow cytometry-based

Alexander E. Kalyuzhny (ed.), *Handbook of ELISPOT: Methods and Protocols*, Methods in Molecular Biology, vol. 1808, https://doi.org/10.1007/978-1-4939-8567-8_11, © Springer Science+Business Media, LLC, part of Springer Nature 2018

cytokine bead arrays and intracellular staining can provide extremely useful information of the cells, they have less sensitivity and accuracy than ELISpot in the quantification of rare Ag-specific cells [5, 6]. These advantages make the ELISpot assay frequently applied to directly monitor Ag-specific B-cell response in PBMCs.

In an ELISpot assay for detecting Ag-specific ASCs, the polyvinylidene difluoride (PVDF) membranes in a 96-well microtiter plate require pre-coating with the Ag to be assayed. After blocking and washing steps, purified PBMCs are serially diluted to seed into wells of the ELISpot plate for incubation. The Ag-specific ASCs secrete Abs, which are captured directly on the membrane surface by the immobilized Ag to prevent diffusion into culture medium. Subsequent detection steps utilize a detection Ab, typically conjugated with horseradish peroxidase (HRP) or alkaline phosphatase (AP) enzyme, in order to visualize the secretory fingerprint of individual ASCs [7]. Because ELISpot is capable of detecting a single Ag-specific cell, direct ex vivo measurement of Ag-specific ASCs from PBMCs is frequently adopted in vaccine trials [8, 9]. In vitro differentiation of memory B cells from PBMCs into ASCs is an option for long-term assessments of vaccine-induced humoral response [10–12]. Because the processing of blood samples is amenable to scale up, ELISpot assay is suitable for investigating Ag-specific Ab response in a large-scale and multicenter vaccine trial.

The protocols described include isolation of PBMCs (~1 h) and detection of total and Ag-specific IgG ASCs (~4 h) in small amounts of blood (~10 mL). Other than culturing cells overnight, the hands-on steps normally take less than 6 h. The whole procedures can be performed in a resource-poor setting.

2   Materials

2.1 Isolation of Human PBMCs

1. Autoclaved double distilled water (ddH_2O).

2. Sterile 0.5 M ethylenediaminetetraacetic acid (EDTA) solution (9.3 g of EDTA disodium and 1.12 g of NaOH dissolved in 50 mL ddH_2O).

3. Blood sample drawing equipment: tourniquet, rubber gloves, disinfection swabs, 3M micropore tape, adhesive dressing, and needle disposal box.

4. 10 mL syringe with 20G or 22G needle.

5. Sterile 15 and 50 mL conical tubes.

6. Red blood cells (RBC) lysis buffer: 155 mM NH_4Cl, 10 mM $NaHCO_3$, 0.1 mM EDTA.

7. Autoclaved phosphate-buffered saline (PBS, NaCl 137 mM, KCl 2.7 mM, Na_2HPO_4 10 mM, KH_2PO_4 2 mM, pH 7.4) and PBS-T (PBS with 0.1% Tween 20).

8. RPMI 1640 culture medium supplemented with 10% fetal calf serum (FCS), 10 mM penicillin/streptomycin, and 10 mM L-glutamine (*see* **Notes 1** and **2**).

9. Centrifuge machine that allows spinning 10 and 50 mL conical tubes at $500 \times g$.

10. Trypan blue solution (0.5%).

11. Hemocytometer (Hausser Scientific, Horsham, PA, USA) to count PBMCs under the microscope.

12. Upright microscope equipped with bright-field illumination and phase contrast condenser.

13. A protocol approved by the Internal Review Board (IRB) of investigators' institutions for the use of human blood to perform ELISpot assays. Note: the protocol (no. 201307019RINB) to use human peripheral blood was approved by the IRB of National Taiwan University Hospital for this study.

2.2 ELISpot Assays

1. PVDF membrane-bottomed 96-well filter plates, 0.45 µm pore size (Merck Millipore, Billerica, MA, USA).

2. Tetanus toxin.

3. Goat anti-human IgG conjugated with alkaline phosphatase (AP) (Fcγ fragment specific).

4. Bromochloroindolyl phosphate-nitro blue tetrazolium (BCIP/NBT) substrate solution (Sigma-Aldrich, St. Louis, MO, USA).

5. C.T.L. ImmunoSpot analyzer (Cellular Technology Limited, Cleveland, OH, USA).

3 Methods

3.1 Isolation of Human PBMCs

1. Collect 10 mL of venous blood from a donor with a tube containing 20 µL of 0.5 M EDTA (final concentration: 5 mM) (*see* **Notes 3** and **4**).

2. Transfer blood into a 50 mL conical tube.

3. Fill tube to 50 mL with RBC lysis buffer and incubate at room temperature (RT) for 5 min (*see* **Notes 5** and **6**).

4. Spin down cells at $500 \times g$ (or 1500 rpm) at RT for 5 min.

5. Decant supernatant carefully.

6. Resuspend PBMCs with 10 mL of sterile PBS.

7. Centrifuge at $500 \times g$ for 5 min.

8. Decant supernatant carefully.

9. Resuspend PBMCs gently with 1 mL of culture medium.

10. Take 10 µL, transfer into an Eppendorf tube, and add 90 µL culture medium (10× dilution).

11. Mix cells 1:1 with trypan blue dye and incubate 1–2 min at RT.

12. Pipette 20 µL from the mixture into a V-shaped well of one side of hemocytometer under a coverslip.

13. Count cells under the phase contrast microscope using 20× lens (*see* **Note 7**).

14. Aliquot desired numbers of cells into separate Eppendorf tubes.

15. Cells are ready for seeding into the ELISpot plate (Fig. 1).

3.2 ELISpot Assays

1. Pre-wet the membranes with 30 µL of 35% ethanol per well in ELISpot plates for 30 s. Avoid touching the membrane in wells at all times during pipetting (*see* **Note 8**).

2. Decant ethanol.

3. Add 150 µL of sterile ddH_2O into each well and incubate at RT for 5 min.

4. Decant ddH_2O.

5. Add 200 µL of sterile PBS into each well and incubate at RT for 3 min.

6. Decant PBS.

7. Pre-coat the plate with 50 µL per well of 10 µg/mL of Ag (e.g., tetanus toxin) (*see* **Note 9**).

8. Incubate overnight at 4 °C (preferred) or alternatively at 37 °C for 2 h.

9. Empty the wells and wash with 200 µL of PBS per well for three times.

10. Decant PBS thoroughly.

11. Add 200 µL of culture medium per well for blocking at RT for 2 h.

12. Decant culture medium and briefly wash wells with 200 µL of PBS.

13. Seed 5×10^5, 2.5×10^5, 1.25×10^5 PBMCs per donor's sample into wells, respectively. Bring up volume to 100 µL in wells with culture medium (*see* **Note 10**).

14. Incubate the plate in a 37 °C incubator with 5% CO_2 overnight. Do not shake or move the plate (*see* **Note 11**).

15. Decant cells and culture medium.

16. Wash the plate with 200 µL per well of PBS-T at RT for 3 min for five times (*see* **Note 12**).

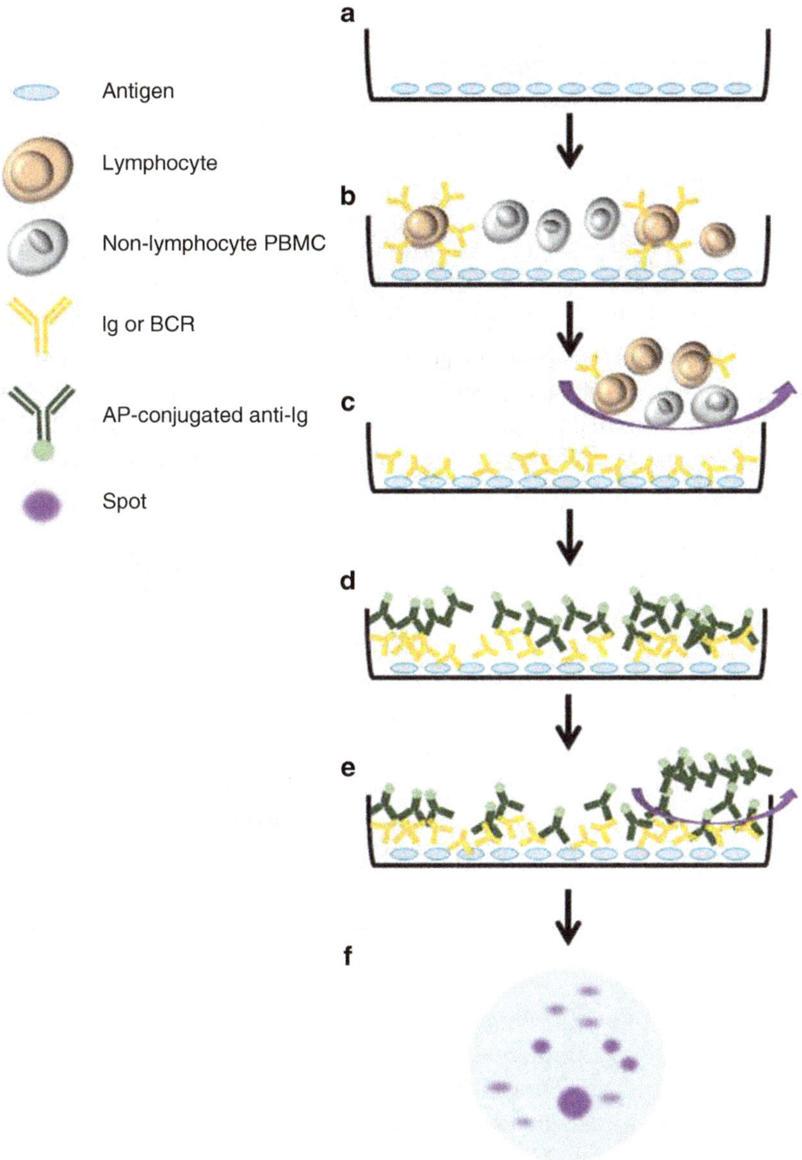

Fig. 1 A schematic flowchart of ELISpot assay to detect Ag-specific ASCs. (A) Pre-coat the wells of the ELISpot plate with an Ag, e.g., tetanus toxin. (B) Seed serial diluted PBMCs into wells of the plate, respectively. Culture overnight (minimum: 8 h). (C) Wash off cells with PBS-T. (D) Add AP-conjugated detection Abs specific to IgM, IgG, or IgA. (E) Wash off unbound Abs. (F) Develop the spots with BCIP/NBT substrate solution

17. Add goat anti-human IgG-AP (Fcγ-specific, 1:5000 in PBS with 1% BSA) into wells and incubate at RT for 2 h in the dark.

18. Wash the plate three times with 200 μL of PBS-T.

19. Add 50 μL of BCIP/NBT substrate solution and incubate at RT. Purple-colored spots normally appear in 10–30 min (*see* **Note 13**).

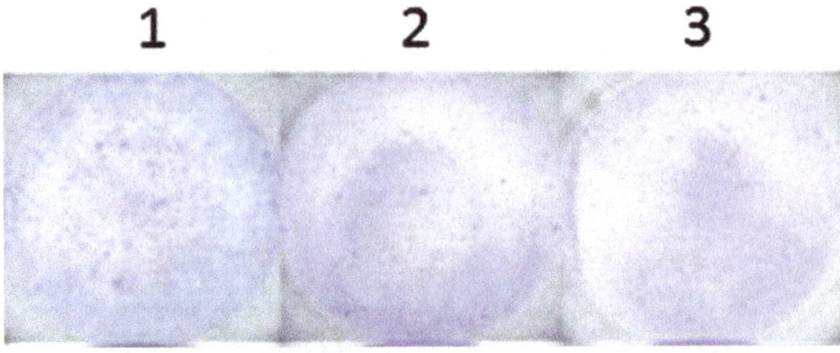

Fig. 2 Representative ELISpot images of tetanus toxin-specific IgG ASCs detected from PBMCs. PBMCs were isolated from a healthy donor 2 weeks after receiving a booster of tetanus toxin. ELISpot plate was pre-coated with 50 μL/well of tetanus toxin (10 μg/mL in PBS). Aliquots of 5×10^5, 2.5×10^5, and 1.25×10^5 PBMCs (#1, #2 and #3) were seeded into wells of the ELISpot plate, respectively. Tetanus toxin-specific IgG ASCs were detected and illustrated

20. Stop enzymatic reaction by adding 100 μL ddH$_2$O into each well to prevent over-development of spots.

21. Take the underdrain off the plates and wash both sides of the membrane with tap water (*see* **Note 14**).

22. Allow plates completely air dried and store plates in the dark before scanning (*see* **Note 15**).

23. Count the spots on membrane surface (Fig. 2) using a C.T.L analyzer or an automated plate reader equipped with an image acquisition and analysis unit (*see* **Note 16**).

4   Notes

1. Complements in FCS may inhibit or destroy cells, e.g., via complement-dependent cytotoxicity, or affect the results of immunoassays, e.g., via binding to the Fc portion of Abs. If this is a concern, inactivate the serum at 56 °C for 30 min. Filtrate serum with a 0.2 μm sterile filter if precipitates occur after cooling.

2. If human serum is necessary to replace FCS in culture medium, pre-test the serum in different batches to avoid nonspecific activation to cultured cells, which may cause background spot formation. Heat inactivation of human serum before use is recommended.

3. Vacutainer blood collection tubes, which contain 1–2% of spray-dried K$_2$EDTA, are often adopted in vaccine trials. K$_2$EDTA is recommended by the CLSI (Clinical & Laboratory Standards Institute) and the ICSH (International Council for Standardization in Hematology). It is important to mix the sample immediately after collection to ensure no blood clot formation.

4. If sodium citrate is used as the anticoagulant, add 1 part sodium citrate (3.2% or 0.109 M) to 9 parts blood. Incubate at RT for 5 min [13].

5. Ficoll gradient is also commonly used to prepare PBMCs from fresh blood [7, 14]. Make sure no mixing of blood with Ficoll to gain good separation of buffy coat and high yield of PBMCs. In our experience, the purity and the yield of PBMCs isolated from either direct RBC lysis or Ficoll gradient methods are comparable.

6. Purified PMBCs can be cryopreserved until use. Typically, PBMCs can be frozen and stored at $1–2 \times 10^6$ cells/mL in cold cryoprotective medium containing 90% FCS and 10% dimethyl sulfoxide (v/v).

7. The hemocytometer is generally divided into nine major squares of 1 mm^2 area in the middle square part. Add ~20 μL of cell suspension between hemocytometer and cover glass. The goal is to distribute roughly 50–100 cells/square. Count five squares—typically four corner and the center squares. Take the average of cellular counts per square, multiply it by the dilution factor (multiply by 1 if not diluted) and then multiply by 10^4 = the number of cells/mL. Alternatively, an automated cell counter is quick and convenient and highly suitable for processing multiple samples at a time.

8. Pre-wetting of the PVDF membrane with 35–70% ethanol or methanol improves hydrophobicity and greatly increases protein binding. By contrast, the nitrocellulose membrane-bottomed filter plates require no pre-treatment and they are not compatible with ethanol or methanol.

9. To detect all ASCs in PBMCs, the plate can be pre-coated with a single Ab, the F(ab')$_2$ fragment of anti-human (IgM + IgG + IgA). Use F(ab')$_2$ fragment of Ig rather than the whole Ig to reduce background signals resulting from potential cross-reactivity of Fc fragment with the detection Abs [7].

10. Seeding of serial diluted PBMCs is necessary to obtain a quantifiable number of spots for counting. The practical limit of spot detection generally depends on the number of cells seeded to form a tight monolayer on the membrane surface. Typically, $2–3 \times 10^5$ PBMCs in a well is recommended. The goal is to get ~50–200 spots. Although up to a maximum of 10^6 cells is acceptable for detection of rare events, it should be noted that over-seeding of cells may lead to piling up of cells and compromise the linearity between cell input and spot frequency.

11. Disturbing cultured cells in the plate may cause the development of weakly stained and fuzzy spots and the formation of "snail trail" or "comet tail" spots. Do not stack plates to prevent the edge effect—few or no spots at the outer wells of the plate.

12. Squirt bottle is preferred over multichannel pipettes for manual wash to prevent damaging of the membrane. When a microplate washer is used, make sure the protruding prongs are properly adjusted to avoid puncturing the membrane. An automatic plate washer is highly convenient and effective. After completing the wash, tap the plates on a dry paper towel to remove residual liquid contents to prevent increasing background signals. Repeat tapping motion when necessary.

13. BCIP/NBT reaction produces an insoluble NBT diformazan end product that is blue to purple in color. Alternatively, use AEC (9-ethylcarbazol-3-amine) substrate solution for HRP-conjugated Abs. If using biotinylated detection Abs, incubate with streptavidin-AP or -HRP proteins before adding respective substrate solutions.

14. For enzymatic reaction steps, removing the base of the plate before addition of substrates can further reduce background signals as reagents can leak through the membrane into the bottom underdrain of the plate.

15. It is necessary to allow the ELISpot plate completely air dried in the dark before analysis in that wet membranes appear dark and obscure the detection of weak and small spots.

16. Spot counting can be performed manually via a dissecting microscope.

Acknowledgments

This study was supported by a research grant from the Ministry of Science and Technology of the Executive Yuan of Taiwan (NSC99-2320-B-002-011).

References

1. Czerkinsky CC, Nilsson LA, Nygren H et al (1983) A solid-phase enzyme-linked immunospot (ELISPOT) assay for enumeration of specific antibody-secreting cells. J Immunol Methods 65:109–121

2. Saletti G, Çuburu N, Yang JS et al (2013) Enzyme-linked immunospot assays for direct ex vivo measurement of vaccine-induced human humoral immune responses in blood. Nat Protoc 8:1073–1087. https://doi.org/10.1038/nprot.2013.058

3. Wulf M, Hoehn P, Trinder P (2009) Identification and validation of T-cell epitopes using the IFN-γ ELISPOT assay. Methods Mol Biol 524:439–446. https://doi.org/10.1007/978-1-59745-450-6_32

4. Sedegah M (2015) The ex vivo IFN-γ enzyme-linked immunospot (ELISpot) assay. Methods Mol Biol 1325:197–205. https://doi.org/10.1007/978-1-4939-2815-6_16

5. Hagen J, Zimmerman R, Goetz C et al (2015) Comparative multi-donor study of IFNγ secretion and expression by human PBMCs using ELISPOT side-by-side with ELISA and flow cytometry assays. Cell 4:84–95. https://doi.org/10.3390/cells4010084

6. Pike KA, Hui C, Krawczyk CM (2016) Detecting secreted analytes from immune cells: an overview of technologies. Methods Mol Biol 1458:111–124. https://doi.org/10.1007/978-1-4939-3801-8_9

7. Tzeng SJ (2016) The isolation, differentiation, and quantification of human antibody-secreting B cells from blood: ELISpot as a functional readout of humoral immunity. J Vis Exp. https://doi.org/10.3791/54582

8. Ahlén G, Frelin L (2016) Methods to evaluate novel hepatitis C virus vaccines. Methods Mol Biol 1403:221–244. https://doi.org/10.1007/978-1-4939-3387-7_11

9. Fiore-Gartland A, Manso BA, Friedrich DP et al (2016) Pooled-peptide epitope mapping strategies are efficient and highly sensitive: an evaluation of methods for identifying human T cell epitope specificities in large-scale HIV vaccine efficacy trials. PLoS One 11:e0147812. https://doi.org/10.1371/journal.pone.0147812

10. Crotty S, Aubert RD, Glidewell J et al (2004) Tracking human antigen-specific memory B cells: a sensitive and generalized ELISPOT system. J Immunol Methods 286:111–122

11. Weiss GE, Ndungu FM, McKittrick N et al (2012) High efficiency human memory B cell assay and its application to studying *Plasmodium falciparum*-specific memory B cells in natural infections. J Immunol Methods 375(1–2):68–74. https://doi.org/10.1016/j.jim.2011.09.006

12. Tzeng SJ, Li WY, Wang HY (2015) FcγRIIB mediates antigen-independent inhibition on human B lymphocytes through Btk and p38 MAPK. J Biomed Sci 22:87–98. https://doi.org/10.1186/s12929-015-0200-9

13. Wiese J, Didwania A, Kerzner R et al (1997) Use of different anticoagulants in test tubes for analysis of blood lactate concentrations: Part 2. Implications for the proper handling of blood specimens obtained from critically ill patients. Crit Care Med 25:1847–1850

14. Heine G, Sims GP, Worm M et al. (2011) Isolation of human B cell populations. Curr Protoc Immunol Chapter 7, Unit 7.5. doi:https://doi.org/10.1002/0471142735.im0705s94

Identification of Novel Mycobacterial Targets for Murine CD4⁺ T-Cells by IFNγ ELISPOT

Alison J. Johnson, Steven C. Kennedy, Tony W. Ng, and Steven A. Porcelli

Abstract

Enzyme-linked immunospot (ELISPOT) is an assay used to detect secretion of cytokines from immune cells. The resolution and sensitivity of ELISPOT allow for the detection of rare T cell specificities and small quantities of molecules produced by individual cells. In this chapter, we describe an epitope screening method that uses CD4⁺ T cell ELISPOT assays to identify specific novel mycobacterial antigens as potential vaccine candidates. In order to screen a large number of candidate epitopes simultaneously, pools of predicted MHC class II peptides were used to identify mycobacterial specific CD4⁺ T cells. Using this method, we identified novel mycobacterial antigens as vaccine candidates.

Key words ELISPOT, CD4⁺ T cell, Epitope, Mycobacteria, Cytokine

1 Introduction

The concept of the enzyme-linked immunospot (ELISPOT) assay is based on the sandwich variant of the enzyme-linked immunosorbent assay (ELISA) that uses antibody pairs to detect the molecule of interest. Unlike ELISA, ELISPOT contains modifications that allow for the detection of cytokine secretions from individual cells [1]. In the T cell ELISPOT assay, the antibody pairs consist of a capture antibody that recognizes cytokines secreted by T cells and a detection antibody that binds to a different epitope on the cytokine from where the capture antibody binds [2]. CD4⁺ T cells are rested on the surface of a cellulose based micro titer plate precoated with the capture antibody. Activation of the CD4⁺ T cells through the presentation of their cognate antigens by antigen presenting cells leads to the secretion of cytokine by the activated immune cells [3]. The released cytokine is captured by the precoated capture antibody, and in subsequent steps bound by detection antibody, thus forming a sandwich configuration similar to ELISA. The detection antibody used in ELISPOT is biotinylated so that an avidin-linked enzyme can be used to cleave a substrate

Alexander E. Kalyuzhny (ed.), *Handbook of ELISPOT: Methods and Protocols*, Methods in Molecular Biology, vol. 1808,
https://doi.org/10.1007/978-1-4939-8567-8_12, © Springer Science+Business Media, LLC, part of Springer Nature 2018

when added [4]. Cleavage of the substrate produces a colorimetric change that leaves a spot on the cellulose membrane corresponding to the secretion of cytokine by an individual CD4+ T cell.

Identification of novel antigens by methods such as T cell hybridoma reactivity screening [5, 6] or analysis of eluates directly from the MHCII binding groove [7] is costly, time-consuming, and has variable sensitivity. The relative speed, incredible sensitivity, and cost-effective setup of ELISPOT allow for large-scale screening of putative antigens [3]. Thus, using a large peptide library and consecutive CD4+ T cell ELISPOT assay, we efficiently identified novel subdominant mycobacterial antigens that are usually difficult to detect within the vast mycobacterial proteome. Purified CD4+ T cell populations from mycobacteria-immunized mice were re-stimulated with peptide library pools covering 880 predicted mycobacterial CD4+ T cell epitopes and assayed by IFNγ ELISPOT [5]. Pools that yielded IFNγ responses in the initial ELISPOT assay were then deconvoluted. CD4+ T cell responses to the individual peptides within the positive pools were evaluated in an additional round of ELISPOT assay to identify the specific mycobacterial CD4+ T cell epitope. This method of consecutive ELISPOT assays allowed for screening of an otherwise intractable antigen library quickly and with exceptional sensitivity.

2   Materials

2.1   ELISPOT Plates, Buffers, and Media

1. ELISPOT Plates: 96-well plates with mixed cellulose esters filter membrane (0.45 μm).

2. Phosphate Buffered Saline (PBS).

3. Blocking Buffer: 1% bovine serum albumin (BSA) in PBS.

4. Substrate Buffer: ultrapure water (deionized water, purified to 18 MΩ-cm at 25 °C).

5. Wash Buffer: 0.05% Tween-20 in PBS.

6. Complete Medium: RPMI-1640 with additives for T cell culture (0.1% 2-ME, 1% HEPES, 1% nonessential amino acid mixture, and 1% Pen/Strep) plus 10% fetal calf serum (FCS) (*see* **Note 1**).

2.2   Antibodies and Detection Reagents

1. Coating Antibody: purified anti-mouse IFNγ monoclonal antibody: dilute to a final concentration of 10 μg/mL in sterile PBS.

2. Detecting Antibody: biotin conjugated anti-mouse IFNγ monoclonal antibody: dilute to a final concentration of 1 μg/mL in PBS.

3. Streptavidin-Alkaline phosphatase (SA-AP): dilute per manufacturer's direction in Blocking Buffer (*see* **Note 2**).

4.Substrate: 5-bromo-4-chloro-3-indolyl-phosphate   (BCIP), nitroblue tetrazolium chloride (NBT) tablets: dissolve one tablet in 10 mL Substrate Buffer.

2.3 Cells

1. CD4$^+$ T cell magnetic isolation kit.

2. CD4$^+$ T cells: isolated from immunized or infected mice.

3. Antigen presenting cells (APCs): T cell-depleted splenocytes from naïve syngeneic mice (*see* **Note 3**).

2.4 Antigens

The design of peptide libraries and Class II MHC binding prediction by the consensus method are previously described [5, 8]. Briefly, 15-mer peptides based on the protein sequences of the mycobacterium under investigation are ranked by predicted binding affinity for the appropriate MHC Class II allele using the consensus method [8]. To limit the number of peptides to be screened, peptides with significant overlap are removed. To screen a large library, peptides can first be screened as pools of up to 20 peptides. Peptides from the pools that generate a positive response from the CD4$^+$ T cells are then examined separately.

All antigens are prepared at 4× final concentration in Culture Media.

1. Peptide pools are generally screened at a final concentration of 2.5 μg/mL for each peptide. Individual peptides are generally used at a final concentration of 10 μg/mL. Titration of new antigens is recommended.

2. Positive control: Concanavalin A (ConA).

3. Negative control: same media used to reconstitute lyophilized peptide.

3 Methods

A flowchart of the ELISPOT protocol is provided in Fig. 1.
Day 0

1. Calculate the number of wells/plates needed for the experiment, figuring three replicates per condition.

2. Coat plate with Coating Antibody diluted in sterile PBS to a final concentration of 10 μg/mL, and adding 50 μL/well. Gently tap plate to ensure antibody has completely covered the membranes (*see* **Note 4**).

3. Wrap plate in plastic wrap and incubate at 4 °C overnight (*see* **Note 5**).

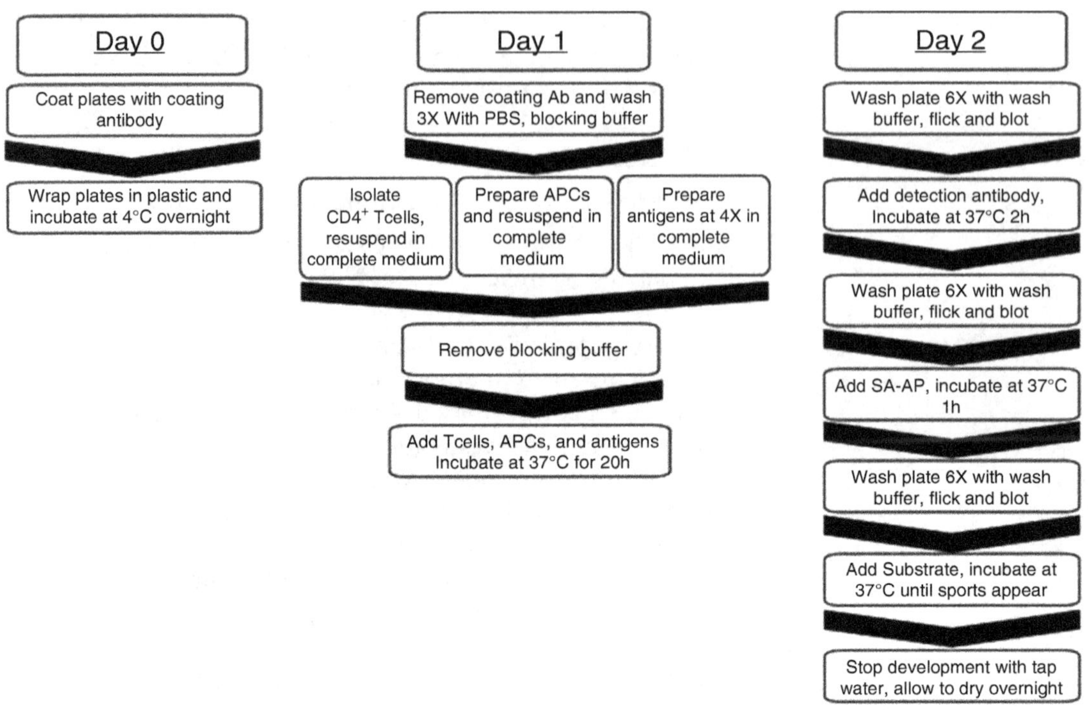

Fig. 1 Flowchart detailing the ELISPOT protocol at a glance

Day 1

4. Remove Coating Antibody from plate by flicking.

5. Wash plate with 200 μL/well *sterile* PBS.

6. Flick the plate and repeat washing step twice, for a total of three PBS washes.

7. Flick the plate and add Blocking Buffer (200 μL/well *sterile* 1% BSA in PBS). Incubate at least 2 h at ambient temperature (while cells and other reagents are prepared).

8. Isolate CD4$^+$ T cells using magnetic isolation kits per manufacturer's directions (*see* **Note 6**).

9. Resuspend isolated CD4$^+$ T cells at 8×10^6 per mL in Complete Medium. When 25 μL are added to each well of the plate, this will yield 2×10^5 CD4$^+$ T cells per well (*see* **Note 7**).

10. Prepare APCs and resuspend at 10^7 per mL in Complete Medium. When 50 μL are added to each well of the plate, this will yield 5×10^5 APCs per well.

11. Prepare antigens in Complete Medium at 4× final desired concentration.

12. Remove Blocking Buffer by flicking plate.

13. Add 25 μL/well CD4$^+$ T cells, 50 μL/well APCs, and 25 μL/well antigen. Total volume = 100 μL/well, with 2×10^5 CD4$^+$ T cells, 5×10^5 APCs, and antigen at desired final concentration.

14. Incubate at 37 °C in 5% CO_2 incubator for 20 h (*see* **Note 8**).

    Day 2

15. Wash plate 6× with Wash Buffer (200 μL/well), with 5 s of agitation between washes (can use an automated plate washer, as sterility is no longer required).

16. Flick the plate to remove the last wash, and blot plate on paper towels.

17. Add prepared Detection Antibody, 50 μL/well.

18. Cover plate with foil and incubate 2 h at 37 °C (*see* **Note 9**).

19. Wash plate 6× as above.

20. Flick the plate to remove the last wash, and add the prepared SA-AP, 50 μL/well.

21. Cover plate with foil and incubate 1 h at 37 °C.

22. Wash plate 6× as above.

23. Flick the plate to remove the last wash, and add 50 μL/well of prepared substrate.

24. Cover plate with foil and incubate ~10 min at 37 °C. *Important: examine the plate every few minutes to assess development of spots and background.*

25. Stop development when dark, distinct spots appear. Stop development before background gets too dark (though some of the background will fade when the plates are fully dried).

26. Stop development by washing plate under running tap water.

27. Remove the plastic scaffolding from the back of the plate. Wash the plate thoroughly again under running tap water.

28. Dry the plate at ambient temperature overnight before analysis (*see* **Note 10**).

29. Count spots with the aid of computer-assisted image analysis (ELISPOT plate reader), or manually by light microscopy. Images of developed too numerous to count (TNTC), positive, and negative wells are provided for reference in Fig. 2. Express the net number of IFNγ-producing CD4$^+$ T cells per 10^6 CD4$^+$ T cells, determined as ([number of spots against relevant peptide/antigen] − [number of spots against irrelevant control]) × 5.

4 Notes

1. It is important to screen FCS lots. Ensure the FCS yields high foreground but low background in the ELISPOT assay. FCS lots can vary considerably.

2. When using SA-AP as described here, the substrate is BCIP/NBT, yielding dark purple or blue-black spots.

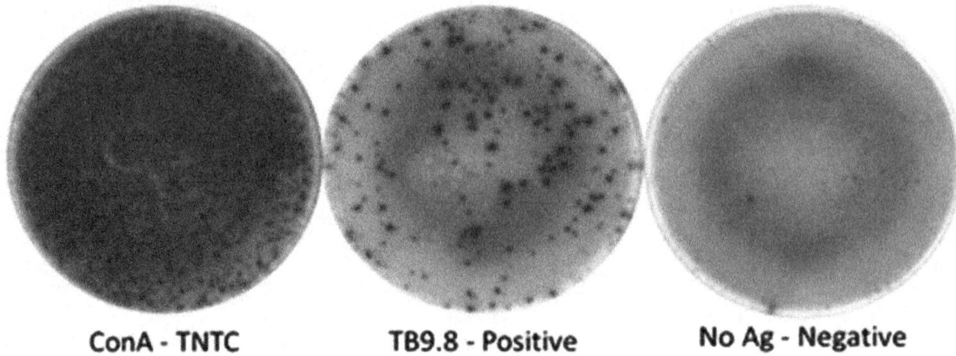

Fig. 2 Examples of TNTC, positive, and negative ELISPOT wells. After development and drying, ELISPOT wells were imaged using an ELISPOT plate reader. The first well is an example of a well that is too numerous to count, or TNTC. The second well is a positive well with distinct and easily separated spots. The third well is a negative well containing only cell debris and no spots

Streptavidin-horseradish peroxidase (HRP) could also be used, in combination with the substrate 3-amino-9-ethylcarbazole (AEC, yielding red spots) or 3,3′,5,5′-tetramethylbenzidine (TMB, yielding blue spots).

3. Other sources of APCs that have been used successfully in ELISPOT for mycobacterial antigens include: lipopolysaccharide (LPS) blasts [5, 9, 10], bone marrow-derived cells [11], and peripheral blood mononuclear cells (PBMCs) [12, 13].

4. In our hands, 10 μg/mL Coating Antibody and 1 μg/mL Detection Antibody were found to yield strong results in IFNγ ELISPOT. When assessing other cytokines by ELISPOT, the concentration of Coating and Detection Antibodies may vary. Therefore, it is important to titrate the antibody pairs prior to use to ensure appropriate detection and development.

5. Alternatively, plate can be coated the same day (Day 1) as cells are to be added to the plate for culture. Coat plate as above, incubate at 37 °C for 2 h, and then proceed with washing and blocking as in **steps 4–7**.

6. Considering experiments in which the immunized mice may have antigen in the tissue at the time of sacrifice for ELISPOT, it is important to isolate CD4$^+$ T cells. For example, BCG will persist for many weeks, resulting in very high background in the ELISPOT assay unless the BCG-infected macrophages and dendritic cells are removed. When mice have been immunized with non-persisting bacteria or antigens, T cell purification is not required, and whole splenocytes can be used instead of the combination of purified T cells plus naïve APCs described here.

7. The number of CD4$^+$ T cells added to each well is somewhat flexible. If limited CD4$^+$ T cells are available, it may be possi-

ble to add fewer cells per well and still achieve adequate data. The number of CD4$^+$ T cells required for each well is also dependent on the frequency of the antigen-specific-CD4$^+$ T cell within the tissue/mouse. Therefore, the number of CD4$^+$ T cells added to each well may need to be adjusted to obtain a response adequate for detection and analysis.

8. In our hands, 20 h incubation is sufficient to obtain adequate data. However, if the response is weak or undetectable, incubation time can be increased to 48 h. Incubation times longer than 48 h will likely require the addition of survival factors like IL-2 to the culture.

9. Alternatively, after addition of the Detection Antibody, plate can be wrapped in plastic and stored at 4 °C for up to 7 days before finishing development, continuing forward from **step 19**.

10. For BSL-3 experiments, all steps through **step 26** above are performed in BSL-3 lab. After **step 26**, submerge the plate in a 1% solution of Vesphene IIse disinfectant. Remove the plastic scaffolding from the back of the plate and discard. Return the plate to the Vesphene solution and soak for an additional 5 min. The plate can then be removed from the BSL-3 facility. Wash the plate thoroughly under running tap water and dry the plate overnight before proceeding with analysis (**steps 28** and **29**).

References

1. Kalyuzhny AE (2005) Chemistry and biology of the ELISPOT assay. Methods Mol Biol 302:15–31

2. Czerkinsky CC, Nilsson LA, Nygren H et al (1983) A solid-phase enzyme-linked immunospot (ELISPOT) assay for enumeration of specific antibody-secreting cells. J Immunol Methods 65:109–121

3. Kouwenhoven M, Ozenci V, Teleshova N et al (2001) Enzyme-linked immunospot assays provide a sensitive tool for detection of cytokine secretion by monocytes. Clin Diagn Lab Immunol 8:1248–1257

4. Navarrete MA, Bertinetti-Lapatki C, Michelfelder I et al (2013) Usage of standardized antigen-presenting cells improves ELISpot performance for complex protein antigens. J Immunol Methods 391:146–153

5. Johnson AJ, Kennedy SC, Lindestam Arlehamn CS et al (2017) Identification of mycobacterial RplJ/L10 and RpsA/S1 proteins as novel targets for CD4$^+$ T cells. Infect Immun 85:e01023–e01016. https://doi.org/10.1128/IAI.01023-16

6. Fonteneau J-F, Larsson M, Somersan S et al (2001) Generation of high quantities of viral and tumor-specific human CD4+ and CD8+ T-cell clones using peptide pulsed mature dendritic cells. J Immunol Methods 258:111–126

7. Bozzacco L, Yu H (2013) Identification and quantitation of MHC class II-bound peptides from mouse spleen dendritic cells by immunoprecipitation and mass spectrometry analysis. Methods Mol Biol 1061:231–243

8. Wang P, Sidney J, Kim Y et al (2010) Peptide binding prediction for HLA DR, DP and DQ molecules. BMC Bioinformatics 11:568. https://doi.org/10.1186/1471-2105-11-568

9. Krieger JI, Grammer SF, Grey HM et al (1985) Antigen presentation by splenic B cells: resting B cells are ineffective, whereas activated B cells are effective accessory cells for T cell responses. J Immunol 135:2937–2945

10. Pasquetto V, Bui H-H, Giannino R et al (2005) HLA-A*0201, HLA-A*1101, and HLA-B*0702 transgenic mice recognize numerous poxvirus determinants from a wide

variety of viral gene products. J Immunol 175:5504–5515

11. Beamer GL, Flaherty DK, Vesosky B (2008) Peripheral blood gamma interferon release assays predict lung responses and *Mycobacterium tuberculosis* disease outcome in mice. Clin Vaccine Immunol 15:474–483

12. Lindestam Arlehamn CS, McKinney DM, Carpenter C et al (2016) A quantitative analysis of complexity of human pathogen-specific CD4 T cell responses in healthy *M. tuberculosis* infected South Africans. PLoS Pathog 12:e1005760. https://doi.org/10.1371/journal.ppat.1005760

13. Mothé BR, Lindestam Arlehamn CS, Dow C et al (2015) The TB-specific CD4[+] T cell immune repertoire in both cynomolgus and rhesus macaques largely overlap humans. Tuberculosis 95:722–735

Chapter 13

ELISPOT-Based "Multi-Color FluoroSpot" to Study Type-Specific and Cross-Reactive Responses in Memory B Cells after Dengue and Zika Virus Infections

Paulina Andrade, Josefina Coloma, and Eva Harris

Abstract

Co-circulation and re-emergence of antigenically related viruses such as dengue (DENV), Zika (ZIKV), and yellow fever (YF) in the Americas has brought a sense of urgency in the field to further define the genesis and to more fully describe the immune response. The recent explosive epidemics of Zika in the Americas and the co-circulation of ZIKV with the phylogenetically similar DENV has raised important questions and concerns regarding the role of cross-reactive immunity in protection and potential enhancement of severity of subsequent ZIKV or DENV infections in pre-immune individuals and the safety of vaccines against both viruses in endemic populations. Antibodies are a critical part of the immune response for clearing flavivirus infections, but the role of pre-existing antibodies in protection or enhancement of subsequent infection and disease with closely related viral species and strains is still not fully understood. We have developed a novel Multi-Color FluoroSpot (MCF) assay based on our ELISPOT-derived assay, previously designated the Quad-color FluoroSpot (QCF), in order to study the development of type-specific versus cross-reactive responses within the B cell pool of Zika virus (ZIKV)- and/or dengue virus (DENV)-infected patients. The QCF is based on a panel of four fluorescent Qdots, each conjugated to a monoclonal antibody specific to one of the four DENV serotypes; now we have included a fifth color (Qdot) for ZIKV to enable analysis of the specificity versus cross-reactivity of B cell populations at a single-cell level for all four DENV serotypes and ZIKV. This novel assay allows us to analyze unique human samples from long-term studies of dengue and Zika in Nicaragua to investigate the nature of B cell/antibody responses and their role in pathogenesis and/or protection in secondary flavivirus infections and could have important implications for vaccine development for Zika and dengue.

Key words Multi-color FluoroSpot, Peripheral blood mononuclear cells, Human memory B cells, Qdots, Type-specific versus cross-reactive responses, Dengue, Zika

---

1 Introduction

Flaviviruses are medically important arthropod-borne enveloped viruses with a ~11 kb positive-stranded RNA genome consisting of three structural (capsid (C), pre-membrane/membrane (prM/M), and envelope (E)) and seven nonstructural proteins. Dengue and Zika are important examples of flaviviral diseases affecting populations

Alexander E. Kalyuzhny (ed.), *Handbook of ELISPOT: Methods and Protocols*, Methods in Molecular Biology, vol. 1808, https://doi.org/10.1007/978-1-4939-8567-8_13, © Springer Science+Business Media, LLC, part of Springer Nature 2018

worldwide. The incidence of dengue has increased dramatically over the last 50 years; an estimated 3.9 billion people in 128 countries are at risk of infection and up to ~390 million infections occur annually, causing up to 100 million dengue cases [1]. Since 2015, ZIKV has also spread rapidly to many countries in the Americas affecting millions of susceptible individuals. According to the WHO, 84 countries have reported ZIKV infections to date, including 48 countries in the Americas, many of which reported a concurrent increase in ZIKV-associated congenital birth defects, including microcephaly, and Guillain Barré Syndrome [2–4].

Antibodies are a critical part of the immune response for clearing flavivirus infections, but the role of pre-existing antibodies in protection from subsequent infection and disease with closely related viral species and strains is still not fully understood. Co-circulation and re-emergence of antigenically related flaviviruses such as dengue (DENV), Zika (ZIKV), and yellow fever (YFV) in the Americas has brought a sense of urgency in the field to further define the genesis and to more fully describe the protective immune response.

Following a primary (1°) infection, most of the antigen-specific B cells differentiate as plasma cells that transiently secrete a first wave of antibodies, but a portion persist as memory B cells (MBCs), surviving long term after highly selective germinal center differentiation [5]. B cell-mediated memory immune responses generate two distinct subsets of cells, MBCs and long-lived plasma cells (LLPCs). MBCs maintain the antigen-specific immunoglobulin in a membrane-bound form as the B cell receptor (BCR). In contrast, LLPCs are terminally differentiated cells that no longer express a BCR but continuously secrete antibody without antigenic stimulation. Protection from a secondary (2°) infection depends in part on the quality and quantity of pre-existing serum antibodies secreted by LLPCs as a first line of defense and MBCs that are rapidly reactivated to produce antibodies as a second line of defense [6].

Secondary infections with pathogens that possess antigenic similarity to the primary infection can result in ineffective 2° immune responses that in some circumstances can contribute to pathogenesis or severity, as seen in certain viral diseases such as dengue. DENV includes four serotypes (DENV1–4) that share 60–75% identity at the amino acid level [7] and cause a spectrum of illness ranging from asymptomatic infection to fatal Dengue Shock Syndrome. Cross-reactive antibodies are produced after a 1° infection but provide only transient protection against the other three serotypes, and progression to severe dengue is often associated with a 2° infection with a different (heterotypic) DENV serotype [8, 9].

Since the recent explosive epidemic of Zika in the American continent, ZIKV co-circulates in the same areas where other flaviviruses are prevalent, including DENV and YFV, as well as YF vaccination. DENV and ZIKV share 54–59% identity in amino acid sequence in the E protein [10]. The phylogenetic similarity of ZIKV and DENV has raised important concerns regarding the role of cross-reactive immunity in protection and potential enhancement of severity in subsequent ZIKV or DENV infections in previously exposed individuals and the safety of vaccines against both viruses in endemic populations.

In order to study the development of type-specific versus cross-reactive responses within the B cell pool of ZIKV- and/or DENV-infected patients, we have developed a novel Multi-Color FluoroSpot (MCF) assay based on our ELISPOT-derived assay previously designated the Quad-color FluoroSpot (QCF) [11]. The Multi-Color FluoroSpot differs from the conventional ELISPOT in that its configuration has been flipped from the traditional format consisting of an antigen-coated surface of each well that captures antibodies secreted by the B cells of interest, followed by detection of these specific antibodies in independent wells. In the FluoroSpot, the wells are instead coated with anti-human IgG or IgM, such that the antibodies secreted by B cells from peripheral blood mononuclear cells (PBMC) samples are captured, followed by incubation with multiple purified viruses and visualization with a panel of type-specific monoclonal antibodies (mAbs) conjugated to unique fluorophores (Qdots)—thus allowing detection of multiple antigen specificity in a single well (Fig. 1). The QCF is based on a panel of four Qdots, with specific light emission/color, each conjugated to a mAb specific to one of the four DENV serotypes; now we have included a fifth color for ZIKV to enable analysis of the specificity versus cross-reactivity of B cell populations for all four DENV serotypes plus ZIKV. Overall, this format enables the determination of serotype specificity on a single-cell basis, rather than only at the cell-population level [11], and it can be used to study plasmablasts directly ex vivo or MBCs after in vitro stimulation [11].

Our results show that we can characterize the MBC population from in vitro-stimulated PBMCs from ZIKV-infected pediatric patients in a dengue-endemic region. We were able to capture and quantify the ZIKV-specific MBC response and to differentiate it from DENV cross-reactive responses in ZIKV-infected DENV-naïve and DENV-immune patients during early and late convalescence. To obtain these results, we adapted our initial QCF assay using a multi-step approach. The initial step involved obtaining and testing a mAb specific to ZIKV, with no cross-reactivity against DENV. In parallel, a ZIKV strain isolated from a patient from the recent epidemic in Nicaragua was propagated and purified using Optiprep® centrifugation to be used as antigen. The assay requires concentrated, high-quality and pure mAb and antigen, as determined by ELISA, SDS-PAGE, and RT-PCR. Purified ZIKV-specific mAbs were then labeled with a Qdot fluorophore following

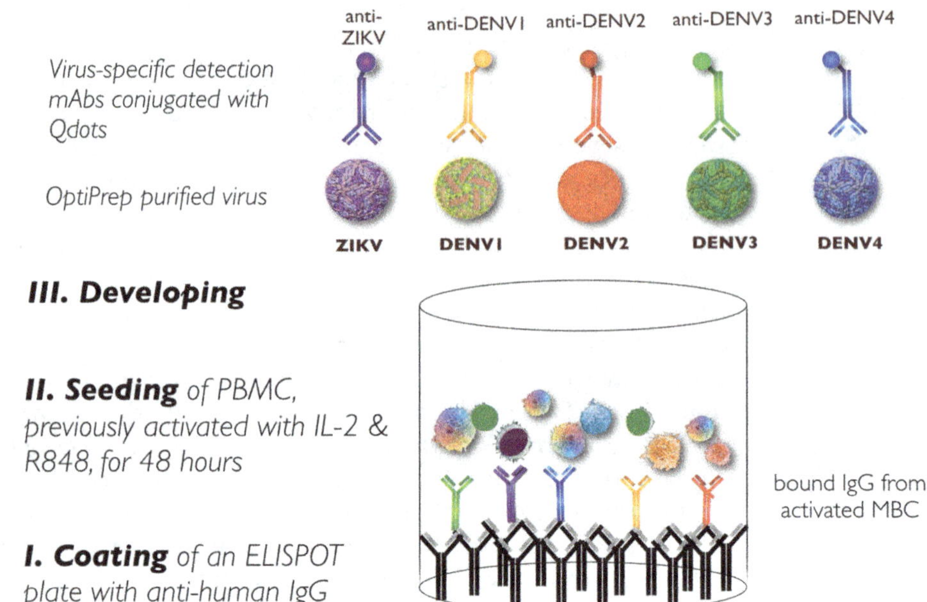

Fig. 1 Schematic diagram of the MCF

the recommended protocol. These ZIKV-specific reagents were then combined with purified antigen and purified mAbs labeled with different Qdots for each of the four DENV serotypes and included in the MCF assay. Finally, the CTL Analyzer was adjusted in two ways: (1) to prevent bleed-through of fluorescence emission between the different Qdots, filters with narrow light emission spectra were used (Table 1) and (2) the ImmunoSpot software was fine-tuned to allow accurate quantification of cross-reactive and type-specific responses to all five antigens simultaneously.

The B cells that react with an antigen are visualized with the CTL Analyzer as spots representing single cells. Each antigen corresponds to one filter and each filter corresponds to one Qdot-labeled mAb (Table 1). The CTL Analyzer generates images from each filter; thus, five different images are created per well and when merging these images, the ImmunoSpot software is able to distinguish type-specific responses from cross-reactive ones. In our analysis, we identified type-specific responses against ZIKV, which are seen as purple spots, as well as cross-reactive responses against DENV represented by different colors due to the merging of different Qdot colors, depending on the specificity of the B cell (Fig. 2). The ImmunoSpot software creates an excel document that details the number of spots found in each filter and indicates whether they are specific for one filter (type-specific responses) or for multiple filters (cross-reactive responses).

The MCF assay represents a unique and powerful tool to study MBC responses at a single-cell level in longitudinal samples and

Table 1
Characteristics of laser excitation and emission filters used in the CTL Analyzer for the MCF

Qdot	Excitation laser	Emission filter
525	405	525/40
565	405	580/23
625	405	625/30
700	405	690/50
800	405	845/55

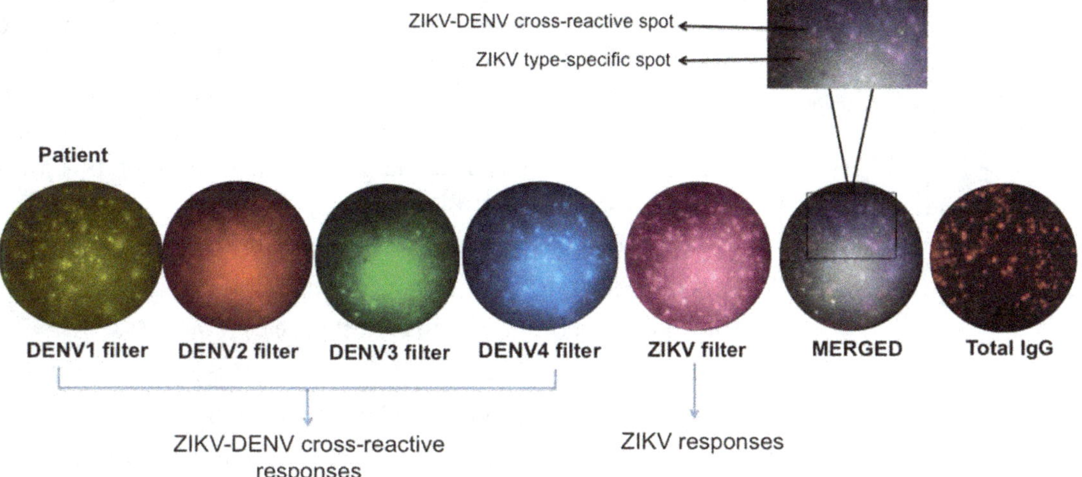

Fig. 2 MCF of an early convalescent PBMC sample (~14 days post-infection) from a Zika patient previously exposed to DENV. The figure shows the results of a single well analyzed with the CTL Analyzer. Each image shows a different filter that captures the emission spectrum from the Qdots conjugated to mAbs against each DENV serotype and ZIKV, labeled according to the antigen specificity. The merged image shows the overlay of the different filters and visualizes type-specific and cross-reactive MBC responses in the same well. The total IgG image shows the total number of activated MBCs in a different dilution of cells; however, this sample was analyzed in a different well, as it requires a different procedure. ZIKV type-specific and ZIKV-DENV cross-reactive spots are indicated in the insert

in serial infections. In our hands, it is being applied to analyze a unique set of longitudinal samples from Zika patients in a cohort study in an area endemic for dengue, where cross-reactive responses could pose a risk for severity in 2° infections, or conversely, could confer protection. Specifically, we are analyzing the MBC response over time in Nicaraguan individuals in our long-term pediatric cohort study with confirmed ZIKV infections, who have experienced either one or more documented DENV infections or are documented to be DENV-naïve. The data generated through the MCF are crucial for understanding the nature of MBC/antibody responses and their role in pathogenesis and/or protection in 2° infections and could have important implications for dengue and Zika vaccine development.

2 Materials

2.1 Virus Growth and Purification

1. *Aedes albopictus* C6/36 cells.

2. Isolated DENV1, DENV2, DENV3, DENV4, and ZIKV.

3. Culture medium: DMEM (Life Technologies) supplemented with 1% GlutaMAX™ Supplement (Life Technologies), 1% Hepes (Life Technologies), 1% Penicillin/Streptomycin (Sciencell).

4. Infection Medium I: RPMI 1640 complete culture medium (Gibco) supplemented with 4% heat-inactivated fetal bovine serum (FBS) (Corning, Fisher), 1% GlutaMAX™ Supplement (Life Technologies), 1% Hepes (Life Technologies), 1% Penicillin/Streptomycin (Sciencell).

5. Infection Medium II has the same components of Infection Medium I but lacking the FBS.

6. 150 cm^2 vented tissue culture flasks (Fisher).

7. CO_2 cell incubator.

8. 100-kDa Amicon filter units (Millipore).

9. OptiPrep (Sigma-Aldrich).

10. Centrifuge for spinning 50-ml tubes at 3740 × *g*.

11. Ultracentrifuge for spinning 12-ml tubes at 120,565 × *g* and 4 °C.

2.2 Conjugation of mAbs to Fluorophores

1. Purified mAbs: E95 (anti-DENV1); E96 (anti-DENV2); 5J7 (anti-DENV3); E88 (anti-DENV4); ZKA64 (anti-ZIKV). DENV mAbs E95, E96, and E88 were kindly donated by M. Diamond (Washington University in St. Louis); DENV mAb 5J7—by J. Crowe (Vanderbilt University); ZIKV mAb ZKA64—by D. Corti (Humabs Biomed, subsidiary of Vir Biotechnology, Inc., Bellinzona).

2. SiteClick™ Qdot® Antibody Labeling Kits (Life Technologies).

3. Qdot® Streptavidin Conjugates (Life Technologies).

4. EZ-Link sulfo NHS LC Biotinylation kit (ThermoFisher Scientific).

2.3 Isolation of Human PBMCs

1. EDTA tubes.

2. Leucosep tubes.

3. Ficoll Histopaque.

4. Centrifuge for 20-ml tubes.

5. PBS supplemented with 2% FBS and 1% Penicillin/Streptomycin.

6. Freezing medium: 90% FBS and 10% dimethyl sulfoxide.

7. Cryovials (2 ml).

8. Mr. Frosty freezing container (Nalgene).

2.4 Activation of MBCs

1. RPMI Activation Medium: RPMI 1640 complete culture medium supplemented with 10% heat-inactivated FBS, 1% GlutaMAX™ Supplement (Life Technologies), 1% Hepes, 1% Penicillin/Streptomycin.

2. DNaseI at 10 U/µl.

3. 24-well, standard tissue culture flat-bottom plates; Growth area 2 cm², well volume 3.5 ml.

4. Human recombinant IL-2 at 1000 U/µl (NIH AIDS Reagent Program).

5. 1 mg/ml of R848 (Life Technologies).

6. Hemocytometer to count lymphocytes under the microscope.

7. Trypan Blue Dye.

8. Cell incubator at 37°C, 5% CO_2.

2.5 Multi-Color FluoroSpot Assay

1. 96-well FluoroSpot plate (Mscrn HTS IP-FL 0.45UM CLEAR, Millipore).

2. 70% ethanol (EtOH).

3. Sterile Dulbecco's Phosphate-buffered saline (DPBS) 1×, no calcium, no magnesium.

4. Phosphate-buffered saline (PBS) plus 1×-Tween 0.05% (PBS-T).

5. OptiPrep®-purified DENV serotypes.

6. Anti-human IgG capture antibody (Fc-specific) (Jackson Immunology).

7. Human serum immunoglobulin (Jackson Immunology).

8. Qdot-conjugated detection mAbs.

9. S6 Universal-V Analyzer, ImmunoSpot Software, CTL Analyzers, LLC.

---

3 Methods

3.1 Virus Growth and Purification

1. Grow C6/36 cells to 80% confluence in a T-150 flask in culture medium.

2. Wash the 80% confluent flask two times with 10 ml of Infection Medium II.

3. Add to the flask 10 ml of Infection Medium II containing the virus at a multiplicity of infection (MOI) of 0.02 and leave it on a rocking platform for 2 h (*see* **Note 1**).

4. After the 2-h infection, add 10 ml of Infection Medium I with a final concentration of 2% FBS in 20 ml.

5. Harvest the 20 ml of medium containing virus on days 5–6 after infection and transfer into a 50-ml conical tube. Centrifuge at 3740 × g at 4°C for 10 min to separate cells from the infectious supernatant.

6. Add the supernatant to 100-kDa Amicon filters and centrifuge at 3740 × g for 30 min or until the final volume is ~250 μl.

7. Collect the concentrated virus in a 1.5-ml Eppendorf tube. Store the concentrated virus at −80°C until purification or purify immediately.

8. To purify the virus, use a discontinuous OptiPrep® 20/55% density gradient and carefully pipette the 250 μl of concentrated virus on top of the 20% gradient. Ultracentrifuge at 120,565 × g for 2 h at 4°C.

9. Collect the virus layer in the interphase between the 20% and 55% densities and make 50–100 μl aliquots. Measure the protein concentration after purification. Keep at −80°C.

10. After harvesting the virus from C6/36 cells, perform quality control on the purity of the virus by extracting RNA from the infectious supernatant and performing RT-PCR for DENV and ZIKV. Purified virus can also be analyzed by SDS-PAGE to discard the possibility of having acquired protein contaminants during the purification process (*see* **Notes 2** and **3**).

3.2 Conjugation of mAbs to Fluorophores

1. SiteClick technology can be used to conjugate Qdots directly to the Fc region of purified mAbs. This technology involves the use of a galactosidase that cleaves the galactose residue on the glycosylation chain, leaving an N-acetylglucosamine group used in the next step by a β-1,4-galactosyltransferase to attach an azide group. Finally the azide group is able to bind to a dibenzocyclooctynol-modified Qdot. According to the manufacturer's instructions, it is possible to conjugate 100–125 μg of the purified mAb. The different Qdots used for this protocol are Qdot®525, Qdot®625, Qdot®700, and Qdot®800, which we use to conjugate four of the different MCF mAbs (*see* **Note 4**).

2. Another way to label the mAbs with Qdots is via Biotin-Streptavidin conjugation. We use the EZ-Link sulfo NHS LC Biotinylation kit that leverages the capacity of NHS esters to react with primary amino groups (−NH2) and form stable amide bonds, leaving several biotin molecules conjugated to the different amino groups of the mAbs. Later, the biotinylated mAbs are bound to Qdots with a Qdot® Streptavidin Conjugate. We label the fifth MCF mAb with Qdot®565 using this protocol.

3. Quality control performed as follows. Before conjugation, it is crucial to assess the serotype specificity of the different mAbs by performing an indirect ELISA using the OptiPrep®-purified viruses (*see* **Notes 4** and **5**). Briefly, plates are coated with a dilution of the OptiPrep-purified DENV and ZIKV (10 μg/ml) in coating buffer at 37°C for 2 h. After three washes with PBS 0.05% Tween (PBS-T), plates are blocked with blocking buffer (5% milk in PBS-T) for 2 h at 37°C. Detection mAbs are incubated with the primary antibody at a 1:100 dilution in blocking buffer at 37°C for 2 h. After three washes with PBS-T, the plates are incubated with either anti-human-HRP or anti-mouse-HRP secondary antibody, depending on the origin of the primary antibody, at 37°C for 2 h. Plates are then washed three times with PBS-T and developed with 3,39,5,59-tetramethylbenzidine. The type specificity of the mAb should be confirmed by testing it against all the different viruses (*see* **Notes 5–7**).

3.3 Isolation of Human PBMCs

1. Collect 5 ml of blood samples in EDTA tubes.

2. Transfer the collected blood into a Leucosep tube containing 3 ml of Ficoll Histopaque and centrifuge at $500 \times g$ for 20 min at room temperature.

3. Collect the PBMC fraction and wash three times in PBS containing 2% FBS and 1% Penicillin/Streptomycin.

4. To freeze an average of 3×10^6 cells per aliquot in freezing medium, place in cryovial tubes in a Mr. Frosty container at −80°C overnight, and transfer to liquid nitrogen for long-term storage.

3.4 Activation of MBCs

1. Use 30 ml of RPMI complete medium previously warmed to 37°C and add 30 μl DNaseI. DNaseI prevents the DNA released from lysed cells from binding to healthy cells, as this can trigger cell death.

2. Thaw the PBMC sample in a water bath for 2–3 min at 37°C and transfer the sample to a 50-ml conical tube. Tilt the conical tube to about 45° and slowly add the RPMI Activation Medium while maintaining a constant and slow rotation of the tube. This prevents an abrupt osmotic change and consequent cell lysis.

3. Centrifuge the PBMCs for 5 min at $1000 \times g$ and resuspend the cells in fresh RPMI Activation Medium.

4. Take 10 μl of the cells and determine the cell concentration and viability using Trypan blue and a hemocytometer.

5. Plate 1×10^6–2×10^6 cells/ml in 1 ml of medium in one well of a 24-well plate (*see* **Note 8**).

6. For activation of MBCs, add 1000 U/ml of IL-2 and 2.5 μg/ml of R848, a TLR7/8 antagonist, to 10 μl of RPMI complete medium and add this cocktail to the cells (*see* **Note 9**).

7. Incubate the plate at 37 °C for 5 days.

3.5 Multi-Color FluoroSpot Assay

1. Activate a 96-well FluoroSpot plate by adding 50 µl/well of 70% EtOH for 2 min.

2. Discard the EtOH and wash three times with sterile 1 × DPBS.

3. Coat the plate with 2 µg/well of the capture anti-human IgG in a 50 µl final volume/well and incubate at 4°C overnight or at 37°C for 2 h.

4. Discard the coating antibody and repeat the washes as in **step 2**.

5. Block the plate with 200 µl/well of RPMI complete culture medium and incubate at 4°C overnight or at 37°C for 2 h.

6. Collect the activated PBMCs and centrifuge at $1000 \times g$ for 5 min.

7. Resuspend the cell pellet in 1 ml of RPMI complete culture medium and take 10 µl of the cells to determine the cell concentration and viability with trypan blue and a hemocytometer.

8. Centrifuge the cells at $1000 \times g$ for 5 min and resuspend the cell pellet in 1 ml of fresh RPMI complete medium and repeat the step one more time.

9. To seed the cells, perform a total of eight 2-fold serial dilutions starting with $5 \times 10^5 – 1 \times 10^6$ cells in the first tube (*see* **Note 10**). Use RPMI complete culture medium and make the dilutions in a final volume of 200 µl.

10. Incubate the plate at 37°C, 5% CO_2 for 48 h.

11. To develop the plate, remove the seeded PBMC cells by washing the plate three times with 200 µl of PBS-T. At the second wash, leave the PBS-T for 5–10 min.

12. Dilute each Optiprep®-purified antigen in 1 × DPBS to 20 µg/ml in a final volume of 50 µl/well and incubate the plate for 1 h at 37°C.

13. Wash 3× with 200 µl/well of PBS-T.

14. Perform an extra blocking step using human gamma globulin diluted 1:500 in PBS and incubate 50 µl/well for 1 h at 37°C. This step blocks the capture antibodies that have not bound to an MBC-secreted antibody and prevents the human mAb 5J7 from being captured. Wash 3× with 200 µl/well of PBS-T.

15. Qdots can aggregate, producing high background in the assay. In order to remove the aggregates, dilute the Qdot-labeled mAb 1:1000 in DPBS. Perform two centrifugations at $18,000 \times g$ for 5 min, transferring the supernatant to a new tube after each centrifugation and pipetting from the surface without disrupting the pellet at the bottom of the tube. Leave the last 30–50 µl and the pellet in the tube and discard, as it

will contain the aggregates. Add 50 μl/well of the final supernatant containing the Qdot-conjugated mAbs and incubate for 1 h at 37 °C.

16. Wash 3× with 200 μl/well of PBS-T.

17. Add 200 μl/well of ddH$_2$O and use the vacuum manifold. This will decrease any possible background and will increase the accuracy of the reading.

18. Use a FluoroSpot reader with the necessary laser and filters that will allow capture of the Qdots' signals most efficiently. In Table 1, we describe the characteristics of our CTL Analyzer.

3.6 Analysis of Results Using the CTL Analyzer

1. Scan the plate using the CTL Analyzer with the filters that correspond to each Qdot-conjugated mAb (Table 1).

2. The MBCs that reacted with the antigen(s) are visualized as spots representing single cells. The different DENV serotype- and ZIKV-specific spots are identified according to the specific mAb Qdot-conjugated emission spectra. Count the spots from each filter using the ImmunoSpot software.

3. Manually review the spots counted on each of the filters, as the software is not completely accurate and it is necessary to check manually well by well to ensure accurate spot counts.

4. Five different images from each of the corresponding filters will be generated by the CTL Analyzer per well, which will allow the software to count the cross-reactivity among the spots visualized by all the filters. When merging the images from an analyzed sample, the ImmunoSpot software is able to distinguish type-specific responses versus cross-reactive responses and can identify the cross-reactivity present among the different filters (e.g., DENV1-DENV2 cross-reactivity, DENV2-DENV3-DENV4 cross-reactivity; cross-reactivity among all four DENV serotypes; DENV1-ZIKV cross-reactivity). This information will be stored in an Excel document that can subsequently be used for analysis.

5. The ImmunoSpot Analyzer has a function for quality control that allows re-counting of the images taken from each filter for each well. Within this function, there is the possibility to fine-tune the machine to count the spots more accurately, and it is also possible to adjust the cross-reactivity analysis.

---

4 Notes

1. It is important to grow a large amount of virus, so that when the virus is concentrated, the final volume is at least 9 ml of concentrated virus. This will enable obtention of ~2–4 ml of purified virus. Ideally, the final concentration should be at least

0.5 mg/ml for the antigen to work properly. The viral prep has to be as pure as possible, as the total protein concentration will include potential contaminants.

2. After virus purification, the quality control procedures include: measuring the protein concentration by BCA assay, performing SDS-PAGE for verification of size and integrity, and conducting ELISAs to confirm antigen specificity. Ideally, an OD of 2–3 should be obtained for each viral antigen with its corresponding mAb to ensure that the viral antigen works when performing the MCF.

3. Make sure to make a large stock of virus that passes the QC tests and that works in the MCF; then, run a set of your samples. Note that every batch of antigen can behave slightly differently.

4. mAbs have to be grown and purified to a final concentration of at least 1 mg/ml, and they have to be of high quality. Perform QC by SDS-PAGE and native PAGE to make sure the mAbs are pure and not degraded.

5. After purifying the mAbs, ensure that in a direct ELISA, the binding of the mAb to its specific antigen will result in an OD of 2–3 to ensure they will work well in the MCF.

6. The site-click conjugation kit can result in unstable conjugations. The percentage of conjugated mAb can vary from assay to assay, and sometimes the mAb has a very low signal and can not be used in the MCF. To improve the conjugation efficiency, make sure to get rid of the unconjugated antibody by performing the last washing step as indicated in the protocol.

7. Be sure to have all the Qdot-conjugated mAbs working well before analyzing samples, as Qdots can spontaneously lose their brightness.

8. Make sure to always use the same medium to culture and to activate the PBMCs. Changing the medium can alter the PBMC growth and will affect the results.

9. Always use the same reagents to activate the MBCs. The cocktail of IL-2 and R848 has been widely studied and optimized for this assay as the best activation cocktail for MBCs and not naïve B cells [12].

10. When working with non-human primate (NHP) or human samples, start the twofold dilutions with at least 1×10^6 cells and prepare at least eight dilutions. This gives a window to capture the best dilutions to most accurately count spots and to analyze results.

Acknowledgements

We thank members of the study team based at the Centro de Salud Sócrates Flores Vivas, the Hospital Infantil Manuel de Jesús Rivera, the National Virology Laboratory in the Centro Nacional de Diagnóstico y Referencia, and the Sustainable Sciences Institute in Nicaragua for their dedication and high-quality work, as well as the children who participated in the studies and their families. We thank Daniela Michlmayr for her contribution to the biotinylation of mAbs and for her support during the quality control process of the conjugated mAbs. Finally we thank Richard Caspell from CTL for his unconditional support with technical matters required to adjust the CTL analyzer, the ImmunoSpot Analyzer and analysis of the data. This work was supported by the following grants from the National Institutes of Health: P01 AI106695, R01 AI099631, and U19 AI118610.

References

1. Bhatt S, Gething PW, Brady OJ et al (2013) The global distribution and burden of dengue. Nature 496(7446):504

2. Faria NR, da Silva Azevedo RDS, Kraemer MU et al (2016) Zika virus in the Americas: early epidemiological and genetic findings. Science 352(6283):345–349

3. Oehler E, Watrin L, Larre P et al (2014) Zika virus infection complicated by Guillain-Barre syndrome—case report, French Polynesia, December 2013. Euro Surveill:19(9)

4. PAHO, Regional Zika Epidemiological Update (Americas), 25 May 2017. Available at http://www.paho.org/hq/index.php?option=com_content&id=11599&Itemid=41691

5. Ahmed R, Gray D (1996) Immunological memory and protective immunity: understanding their relation. Science 272(5258):54–59

6. Radbruch A, Muehlinghaus G, Luger EO et al (2006) Competence and competition: the challenge of becoming a long-lived plasma cell. Nat Rev Immunol 6(10):741–750

7. Guzman MG, Alvarez M, Rodriguez-Roche R et al (2007) Neutralizing antibodies after infection with dengue 1 virus. Emerg Infect Dis 13(2):282

8. Halstead SB (1990) Dengue and dengue hemorrhagic fever. Curr Opin Infect Dis 3(3):434–438

9. Sangkawibha N, Rojanasuphot S, Ahandrik S et al (1984) Risk factors in dengue shock syndrome: a prospective epidemiologic study in Rayong, Thailand: I. The 1980 outbreak. Am J Epidemiol 120(5):653–669

10. Dejnirattisai W, Supasa P, Wongwiwat W et al (2016) Dengue virus sero-cross-reactivity drives antibody-dependent enhancement of infection with Zika virus. Nat Immunol 17(9):1102–1108

11. Hadjilaou A, Green AM, Coloma J, Harris E (2015) Single-cell analysis of B cell/antibody cross-reactivity using a novel multicolor FluoroSpot assay. J Immunol 195(7):3490–3496

12. Pinna D, Corti D, Jarrossay D et al (2009) Clonal dissection of the human memory B-cell repertoire following infection and vaccination. Eur J Immunol 39(5):1260–1270

Chapter 14

Cultured ELISpot Assay to Investigate Dengue Virus Specific T-Cell Responses

Chandima Jeewandara, Graham S. Ogg, and Gathsaurie Neelika Malavige

Abstract

The cultured Enzyme-Linked ImmunoSpot (ELISpot) assay is a functional T cell assay, which is commonly used to assess virus-specific T cell responses. The use of an in vitro expansion step before the ELISpot distinguishes such "cultured" ELISpots from "ex vivo" ELISpots. Cultured ELISpots have the advantage that lower frequency responses can be analyzed compared to ex vivo ELISpots, but do carry the associated potential distortions of the expansion phase. Cultured ELISpot assays are of value to determine silent and symptomatic transmission of the Dengue virus (DENV) in the community and to identify the correlates of a DENV-specific protective immune response. We have evaluated T cell responses to the DENV using cultured ELISpot assays with serotype-specific T cell epitopes to determine past infecting dengue virus (DENV) serotypes. The peptides used in this assay do not cross react with the Japanese encephalitis virus nor other flaviviruses. Therefore, this assay is likely to be useful in determining the past infecting DENV serotype in immune-epidemiological studies and in dengue vaccine trials.

Key words Cultured ELISpot assay, Dengue virus, Serotype-specific T cell responses, Short-term T cell cultures

1 Introduction

ELISpot assays are amongst the most widely used functional T cell assays, which are employed to enumerate T cell responses and define functional capacity. Virus-specific T cells secrete IFN-γ and many other cytokines upon antigen stimulation and can be detected by single-color or multi-color ex vivo ELISpots assays. However ex vivo ELISpot assays may not pickup low frequency responses which might require an in vitro "cultured" expansion step before the ELISpot assay. Therefore, cultured ELISpot assays are an ideal tool to quantify virus-specific T cells, particularly when low frequency responses are to be analyzed [1–3].

Cultured ELISpots assays have been used to identify T cell responses to various DENV proteins [4–7]. Although secondary den-

Alexander E. Kalyuzhny (ed.), *Handbook of ELISPOT: Methods and Protocols*, Methods in Molecular Biology, vol. 1808, https://doi.org/10.1007/978-1-4939-8567-8_14, © Springer Science+Business Media, LLC, part of Springer Nature 2018

gue infections are known to associate with more severe disease, the majority of both primary and secondary dengue infections lead to asymptomatic disease [8, 9]. Therefore, in order to understand how previous dengue infections contribute to clinical disease severity, it would be crucial to determine memory T cell responses to the past infecting serotype and also subsequent DENV-specific T cell responses in naturally infected individuals who develop symptomatic and asymptomatic infection. Although the current most widely used method to determine past infecting serotype in DENV-seropositive individuals is the plaque reduction neutralization assay (PRNT) [10, 11], there have been many concerns regarding the reliability of the PRNT, especially in those who had been infected with multiple DENV serotypes. We have developed a cultured ELISpot assay to determine the past infecting DENV serotype by using a panel of serotype-specific peptides, from highly conserved regions of the DENV, which did not share any homology with other flaviviruses [6]. We found that 93.4% DENV seropositive individuals respond to at least one of these peptides, whereas none of the DENV seronegative individuals or those who received the Japanese Encephalitis vaccine responded. Therefore, this is a useful tool in determining the past infecting DENV serotype in immune-epidemiological studies and in dengue vaccine trials. The materials and methods presented herein use sourced reagents that we have found to work well, but there are many other suppliers and in most cases we have not done direct comparisons.

2   Materials

2.1 Separation of Human Peripheral Blood Mononuclear Cells (PBMCs)

1. Lymphoprep (Axis Shield, Oslo, Norway).
2. 50 mM Phosphate-buffered saline (PBS), pH 7.2.
3. RPMI 1640: supplemented with 2 mM L-glutamine, 100 IU/ml penicillin (R0).
4. Centrifuge allowing spinning of 50 ml culture tubes at $500 \times g$.
5. Trypan blue.
6. Counting slides.
7. Fetal bovine serum: Heat inactivated. 50 ml of heat inactivated and filtered FBS is used to prepare RPMI (R0) supplemented with 10% FBS (R10).

2.2 Preparation of Dengue Peptides

1. Dengue virus peptides consisting of 14 to 17mer peptides.
2. DMSO: Sterile, filtered, endotoxin tested and suitable for cell culture.
3. RPMI: supplemented with 2 mM L-glutamine, 100 IU/ml penicillin.
4. 0.2 μm sterile filters.

<table>
<tr><td valign="top">

2.3 Generation of Short-Term T Cell Cultures

</td><td valign="top">

1. 24 well tissue culture plates.

2. Male AB blood group negative human serum. Heat inactivated. 50 ml of heat inactivated and filtered human serum is used to prepare RPMI (R0) supplemented with 10% human serum (hR10).

3. Recombinant human IL-2.

</td></tr>
<tr><td valign="top">

2.4 Cultured ELISpot Assays

</td><td valign="top">

1. ELISpot plates: Millipore Corp., Bedford, MA, USA.

2. 0.3% alcohol.

3. Distilled water.

4. Multichannel pipette.

5. Commercially ready to use human IFNγ ELISpot kits (Mabtech, Sweden).

6. Fetal Bovine Serum: Heat inactivated.

7. Paraffin film: DuraSeal laboratory stretch film.

8. Upright microscope equipped with bright-field illumination and phase contrast condenser.

9. PHA (Lectin from *Phaseolus vulgaris*): lyophilized powder, BioReagent, suitable for cell culture.

10. CO_2 incubator set at 37 °C with 5% CO_2.

11. ELISpot development substrate: BCIP NBT substrate (Mabtech, Sweden).

</td></tr>
</table>

---

3   Methods

<table>
<tr><td valign="top">

3.1 Separation of PBMCs

</td><td valign="top">

1. Collect blood into heparinized or EDTA tubes.

2. Dilute the fresh heparinized blood 1:1 with RPMI 1640 supplemented with 2 mM L-glutamine, 100 IU/ml penicillin (R0).

3. Layer 15–25 ml diluted blood on top of 14–15 ml of lymphoprep and centrifuge at $500 \times g$ for 20 min without brake. The PBMC layer is seen between the lymphoprep and the plasma layer.

4. Pipette out the PBMC layer and wash the cells in an equal volume of R0 at $300 \times g$ for 10 min and resuspend the cell pellet in RPMI 1640 supplemented with 2 mM L-glutamine, 100 IU/ml penicillin and 100 μg/ml plus 10% fetal calf serum (R10) or human serum (hR10).

5. Resuspend cells in R10 for use in ex vivo ELISpot assays and in hR10 for short-term T cell cultures.

</td></tr>
</table>

3.2 Peptides

1. Use a panel of serotype-specific peptides synthesized in-house in an automated synthesizer using F-MOC chemistry, or purchased.

2. The purity of the peptides should be greater than 90% by high-pressure liquid chromatography analysis and mass spectrometry. These peptides have been previously described [6] and were found to be serotype specific (SS) originating from highly conserved regions of the four DENVs.

3. Use the FEC control peptides which contain a panel of 23, 8–11 amino acid CD8+ T cell epitopes of Epstein Barr virus (EBV), Flu and CMV viruses which have been used as quality control in ELISpot assays [12].

3.3 Dilution of Peptides

1. To dissolve approximately 1 mg of peptide initially dilute with 75–100 μl of DMSO.

2. Once the peptide is fully dissolved, then further dilute it with R0 to make a 1 mM concentration stock solution, which should be stored at −20 °C until further use.

3. The peptides should be diluted to a final concentration of 10 μM for use in ELISpots and short-term T cell cultures after filtered to ensure sterility.

4. If peptides will be tested in peptide pools, the peptides should be pooled in 1 mM concentrations and should be further diluted and filtered to a 10 μM concentration.

3.4 Counting of Cells

1. Use a plastic calibrated counting chamber for counting cells.

2. Dilute 10 μl of the cell suspension with an equal volume of trypan blue and 10 μl of this can be taken for counting.

3. Cells that are alive will be seen as bright while dead cells will be visualized as black spots.

4. Count 16 small squares and then the concentration (counts/ml) is given by:

Counts/ml = total counts in a 4×4 grid $\times\ 10^4 \times$ sample dilution factor.

3.5 Generation and Maintenance of Cell Cultures

1. Four to five million PBMCs of each donor are incubated in a 24 well plate with 200 μl of 40 μM pooled DENV serotype specific peptides for 10 days.

2. Add IL-2 on day 3 and 7 at a concentration of 100 IU/ml (1 ml of media is taken off and 1 ml of hR10 with IL-2 was added).

3. Maintain all cell lines in RPMI 1640 supplemented with 2 mM L-glutamine, 100 IU/ml penicillin and 100 μg/ml plus 10% human serum (hR10) at 37 °C, in 5% CO_2 (*see* **Note 1**).

4. Wash the cells with RPMI and resuspended in hR 10 and rest for 1–2 days before testing. Individual peptide responses for T cell lines can be identified using the panel of peptides after 10 days culture in a 96 well plate (Fig. 1).

5. The cultured ELISpot method is similar to that of ex vivo ELISpot assay, except that instead of 100,000 PBMCs, 40,000 T cells are used in each well (*see* **Note 2**).

6. Consider all peptides that induced an IFN-γ response of more than mean + 2 standard deviations of the negative control as a detectable response.

3.6 Cultured ELISpot Assays

1. Coating of the ELISpot plate can be done on the lab bench at room temperature.

2. Before the ELISpot plates (Millipore Corp., Bedford, MA, USA) are coated with the antibody, the membrane should be activated by adding 100 μl of 35% ethanol into each well for 1–2 min.

3. Wash the wells with distilled water six times using a multichannel pipette.

4. Dilute the primary anti-IFNγ antibody at 15 μl per 1 ml of PBS of sterile PBS and add 50 μl of this to each ELISpot well. In the case of using another cytokine, that particular antibody should be diluted at a concentration specified by the manufacturer. In order to make sure that the antibody is evenly spread over the membrane, gently tap the plate on either side.

5. Wrap the plate in paraffin film to prevent evaporation of antibody solution.

6. The following day, wash the plate six times with R0 and incubate for 1 h with R10 at 37 °C to block the plate.

7. After the incubation, gently tap the solution out of the wells.

8. Prepare the cultured T cells in either R10 or hR10, so that 0.04×10^6 PBMCs are in 150 μl of media. Add the cultured T cells gently into each well, to encourage an even spread of cells.

9. Add 50 μl of 40 μM peptide to each well, so that the peptide concentration of each well is at a final concentration of 10 μM. It is best that responses to each peptide/peptide pool are done in duplicates or in triplicates.

10. As a positive control add 20 μl of PHA at concentration of 40 μg/L, so that the final concentration of PHA is 10 μg/ml and add media alone as a negative control.

A

D1 1	D1 1	D1 11	D1 11	D1 16	D1 16	D1 20	D1 20	D2 1	D2 1	D2 11	D2 11
D2 17	D2 17	D2 18	D2 18	D2 33	D2 33	D3 3	D3 3	D3 11	D3 11	D321	D321
D3 28	D3 28	D4 5	D4 5	D4 10	D4 10	D4 12	D4 12	D4 19	D4 19	Nil	Nil
JEL	JEL	NS3	NS3	FEC	FEC	PHA	PHA	NIL	NIL	Blank	Blank

B

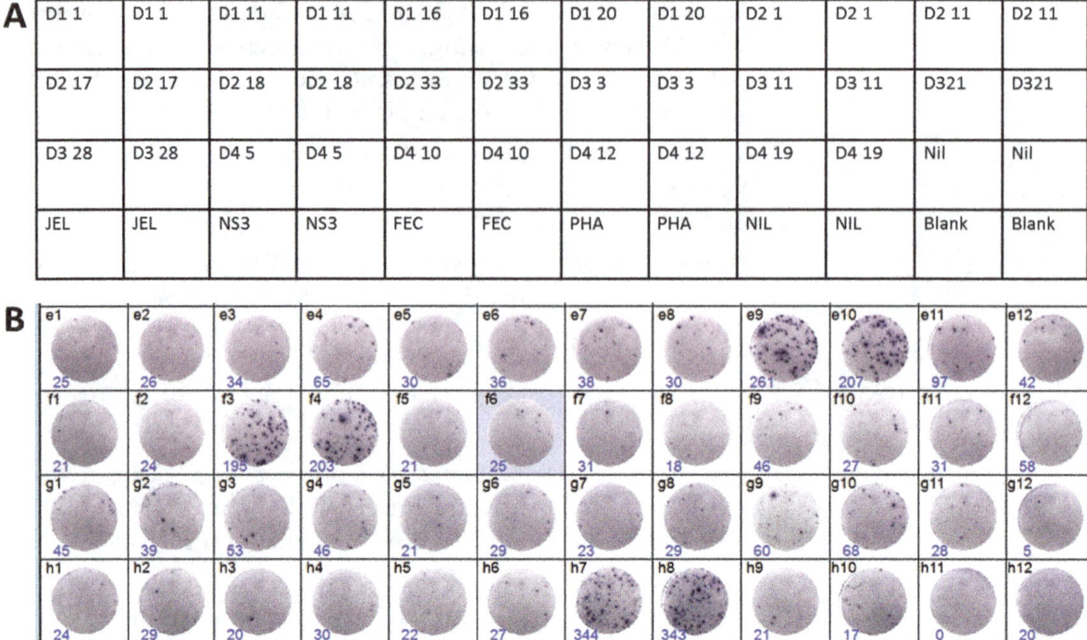

Fig. 1 A typical cultured ELISpot response to the panel of DENV serotype specific peptides. (**a**) The layout of the ELISpot for the 17 DENV serotype specific peptides is shown, with each peptide response done in duplicate. (**b**) A response to these peptides from one dengue seropositive donor is shown with responses to DENV2 peptide 11 and 18, DENV4 peptide 5 and 19 and PHA. Therefore, as this individual responds to SS peptides of DENV2 and DENV4, it is likely that he/she has been infected with these two DENV serotypes in the past

11. Incubate the ELISpot plates overnight at 37 °C in 5% CO_2. The following day the cells are removed by tipping the plate and washing six times with 0.05% PBS tween (500 μl of Tween in 1 L of PBS). Then add the detection antibody (7-B6-1-biotin) at 1 μg/ml in sterile PBS and add 100 μl to each well and incubate at room temperature for 2–4 h.

12. Wash the plates again six times with 0.05% PBS tween. Then add Streptavidin ALP 100 μl diluted at 1:1000 to each well and incubate for a further 1–2 h at room temperature.

13. Then wash the plates again six times with 0.05% PBS tween and develop the plates by adding 100 μl of the substrate solution (BCIP/NBT) to each well. Keep observing the plates for development of spots (5–15 min) and when spots are seen, tip the development solution and wash the plates with normal water under a running tap. Then air dry the plates and then read the plates using an automated ELISpot reader (AID, Germany).

14. The number of spots for each peptide is calculated by counting the number of spots in each well and subtracting the background (cells with media or irrelevant peptide).

4   Notes

1. If the wells turn deep yellow or the cells appear too crowded, the cells need to be split. Basically in such instances, the well is mixed well and half of the contents of the well (1 ml) is transferred to another well and diluted with media.

2. Since T cells cultured for a specific peptide are used in cultured T cell ELISpot assays, there may be a high frequency of peptide-specific T cells. As a result, the whole well might turn black, or one may observe too many spots that cannot be counted. In such instances, lesser number of cells can be used per well.

References

1. Todryk SM, Pathan AA, Keating S, Porter DW et al (2009) The relationship between human effector and memory T cells measured by ex vivo and cultured ELISPOT following recent and distal priming. Immunology 128(1):83–91

2. Keating SM, Bejon P, Berthoud T et al (2005) Durable human memory T cells quantifiable by cultured protection against malaria 1. J Immunol 175:5675–5680

3. Calarota SA, Baldanti F (2013) Enumeration and characterization of human memory t cells by enzyme-linked immunospot assays. Clin Dev Immunol 2013:637649

4. Jeewandara C, Adikari TN, Gomes L et al (2015) Functionality of dengue virus specific memory T cell responses in individuals who were hospitalized or who had mild or subclinical dengue infection. PLoS Negl Trop Dis 9(4):1–17

5. Kurane I, Innis BL, Nisalak et al (1989) Human T cell responses to dengue virus antigens. Proliferative responses and interferon gamma production. J Clin Invest 83(2):506–513

6. Malavige GN, McGowan S, Atukorale V et al (2012) Identification of serotype-specific T cell responses to highly conserved regions of the dengue viruses. Clin Exp Immunol 168:215–223

7. Mangada MM, Endy TP, Nisalak A et al (2002) Dengue-specific T cell responses in peripheral blood mononuclear cells obtained prior to secondary dengue virus infections in Thai schoolchildren. J Infect Dis 185(12):1697–1703

8. Mongkolsapaya J, Dejnirattisai W, Xu X et al (2003) Original antigenic sin and apoptosis in the pathogenesis of dengue hemorrhagic fever. Nat Med 9(7):921–927

9. Guzmán MG, Kourí G, Valdés L et al (2002) Enhanced severity of secondary dengue-2 infections: death rates in 1981 and 1997 Cuban outbreaks. Rev Panam Salud Publica 11(4): 223–227

10. van Panhuis WG, Gibbons RV, Endy TP et al (2010) Inferring the serotype associated with dengue virus infections on the basis of pre- and postinfection neutralizing antibody titers. J Infect Dis 202(7):1002–1010

11. Thomas SJ, Nisalak A, Anderson KB et al (2009) Dengue plaque reduction neutralization test (PRNT) in primary and secondary dengue virus infections: how alterations in assay conditions impact performance. Am J Trop Med Hyg 81(5):825–833

12. Currier JR, Kuta EG, Turk E et al (2002) A panel of MHC class I restricted viral peptides for use as a quality control for vaccine trial ELISPOT assays. J Immunol Methods 260(1–2):157–172

Chapter 15

Ex Vivo ELISpot Assay to Investigate Dengue Virus Specific T-Cell Responses

Gathsaurie Neelika Malavige

Abstract

Enzyme-Linked ImmunoSpot (ELISpot) assay is a functional T cell assay which is commonly used to assess virus-specific T cell responses. We have used ex vivo ELISpot responses to investigate the role of dengue virus (DENV) specific T cells in acute dengue infection, to evaluate their role in possible disease pathogenesis and protection. We have also used ex vivo IFNγ ELISpot assays to determine the functionality of T cell responses in those who were previously naturally infected with dengue and we have determined the frequency of DENV-specific memory T cells responses in relation to past clinical disease severity. We have also evaluated ELISpot supernatants to study multiple cytokines produced by DENV-specific T cells, in instances where there are fewer numbers of cells available for multiple assays. ELISpot assays are likely to be helpful in large-scale dengue vaccine trials to assess the immunogenicity of the vaccines.

Key words Ex vivo ELISpot assays, Dengue virus, NS3, Interferon gamma, Cytokines, ELISpot supernatant

1 Introduction

ELISpots are one of the widely used techniques used functional T cell assays which are used to enumerate antigen-specific T cells. It has many advantages over many other techniques of investigating antigen-specific T cells as it uses fewer number of cells, needs relatively less sophisticated equipment, and can be used to screen many antigens in a single sample or screen many samples at a time [1]. Ex vivo ELISpot assays have been used to identify T cell responses to various dengue viral (DENV) proteins [2] and it has also been used to evaluate T cell responses to the DENV to understand the association of DENV-specific T cells in relation to clinical disease severity [3–5].

The majority of studies have used ex vivo IFNγ ELISpots in order to study T cell responses to DENV proteins [2] and also to understand the role of DENV T cells in acute disease [3, 4] and in naturally infected individuals [5]. However, ex vivo ELISpot assays

Alexander E. Kalyuzhny (ed.), *Handbook of ELISPOT: Methods and Protocols*, Methods in Molecular Biology, vol. 1808,
https://doi.org/10.1007/978-1-4939-8567-8_15, © Springer Science+Business Media, LLC, part of Springer Nature 2018

can also be used to study virus-specific T cell responses to other cytokines such as granzyme B, perforin, and TNFα. Although ex vivo ELISpot assays have not been used to study other cytokine specific DENV-specific T cell responses, they have been used successfully in studying such T cell responses in other viral infections such as in HIV, cytomegalovirus, and influenza [6, 7]. Instead of using many plates for different types of ex vivo ELISpot cytokine assays, especially when the number of cells is limited, antigen-specific cytokine responses can also be assessed in ELISpot supernatants [5, 8]. We have evaluated DENV antigen specific granzyme B and TNFα responses both healthy individuals [5] and TNFα, IL-10, IL-4, IL-13, and IL-17 in DENV NS3 specific T cells in patients with acute infection, in ELISpot culture supernatants [3].

Ex vivo ELISpot assays have been widely used to assess the efficacy of many vaccines such as influenza and have also been proposed to be used in vaccine trials to evaluate immunogenicity of hepatitis C and HIV vaccines [9–11]. There are several dengue vaccines currently undergoing clinical trials and one vaccine which has been licenced [12]. Since the immunogenicity of a vaccine also depends on inducing robust T cell responses to the vaccine, assessment of DENV-specific T cell responses by ex vivo IFNγ ELISpot assays would be helpful tool in these clinical trials to assess functional T cell responses to the DENV following vaccination.

2 Materials

2.1 Separation of Human PBMCs

1. Lymphoprep (Axis Shield, Oslo, Norway).
2. 50 mM Phosphate-buffered saline (PBS), pH 7.2.
3. RPMI 1640: supplemented with 2 mM L-glutamine, 100 IU/ml penicillin.
4. Centrifuge allowing spinning 50 ml culture tubes at $500 \times g$.
5. Trypan blue dye.
6. Counting slides.
7. Heat inactivated Fetal Bovine Serum (FBS).

2.2 Preparation of Dengue Peptides

1. Dengue virus peptides consisting of 14 to 17mer peptides.
2. DMSO: Sterile, filtered, endotoxin tested and suitable for cell culture.
3. RPMI: supplemented with 2 mM L-glutamine, 100 IU/ml penicillin.
4. 0.2 μm sterile filters.

2.3 Ex Vivo ELISpot Assays

1. ELISpot plates (Millipore Corp., Bedford, Massachusetts, USA).

2. 0.3% alcohol.

3. Distilled water.

4. Multichannel pipette.

5. Commercially ready to use human IFNγ ELISpot kit (Mabtech AB, Sweden).

6. Heat inactivated Fetal Bovine Serum (FBS).

7. DuraSeal laboratory sealing film.

8. Upright microscope equipped with bright-field illumination and phase contrast condenser.

9. PHA (Lectin from *Phaseolus vulgaris*): lyophilized powder suitable for cell culture.

10. CO_2 incubator set at 37 °C with 5% CO_2.

11. Streptavidin conjugated to Alkaline Phosphatase (ALP).

12. ELISpot development substrate: BCIP NBT substrate (Mabtech, Sweden).

3   Methods

3.1   Separation of PBMCs

1. Collect blood into heparinized or EDTA tubes.

2. Dilute the fresh heparinized blood 1:1 with RPMI 1640 supplemented with 2 mM L-glutamine, 100 IU/ml penicillin (R0).

3. Layer 15–25 ml diluted blood on top of 14–15 ml of lymphoprep and centrifuge at $500 \times g$ for 20 min without breaks. The PBMC layer is seen between the lymphoprep and the plasma layer.

4. Pipette out the PBMC layer and wash the cells in an equal volume of R0 at $300 \times g$ for 10 min and resuspend the cell pellet in RPMI 1640 supplemented with 2 mM L-glutamine, 100 IU/ml penicillin and 100 µg/ml plus 10% fetal bovine serum (R10) or human serum (hR10).

5. Resuspend cells in R10 for use in ex vivo ELISpot assays and in hR10 for short-term T cell cultures.

3.2   Dilution of Peptides

1. To dissolve the peptide, initially dilute with 75–100 µl of DMSO.

2. Once the peptide is fully dissolved, then further dilute it with R0 to make a 1 mM concentration stock solution, which should be stored at −20 °C until further use.

3. The peptides should be diluted to a final concentration of 10 µM for use in ELISpots and short-term T cell cultures after filtering to ensure sterility.

4. If peptides will be tested in peptide pools, the peptides should be pooled in 1 mM concentrations and this 1 mM of peptides should be further diluted and filtered to a 10 µM concentration.

5. The working concentration can be stored for approximately 1 month at 4 °C and it should be discarded if the solution is cloudy or if the indicator is turning orange or yellow.

3.3 Ex Vivo ELISpot Assays

1. Coating of the ELISpot plate can be done on the lab bench at room temperature.

2. Before ELISpot plates are coated with the antibody, the membrane should be activated by adding 100 µl of 35% ethanol into each well for 1–2 min.

3. Wash the wells with distilled water six times using a multichannel pipette.

4. Dilute anti-IFNγ antibody at 15 µl per 1 ml of PBS of sterile PBS and add 50 µl of this to each ELISpot well. In order to make sure that the antibody is evenly spread over the membrane, gently tap the plate on either side.

5. Wrap the plate in DuraSeal film to prevent evaporation of antibody solution.

6. The following day, wash the plate six times with R0 inside a class II safety cabinet and incubated for 1 h with R10 at 37 °C to block the plate.

7. After the incubation, tap the solution out of the wells.

8. Prepare the PBMCs in either R10 or hR10 so that 0.1×10^6 PBMCs are in 150 µl of media. Add the PBMCs into each well, while being careful not to spurt the solution so that cells are gathered in one side of the well (*see* **Note 1**).

9. Add 50 µl of 40 µM peptide to each well so that the peptide concentration in each well is at a final concentration of 10 µM. It is best that responses to each peptide/peptide pool are done in duplicates or in triplicates.

10. As a positive control add 20 µl of PHA at 40 µg/ml so that the final concentration of PHA is 10µg/ml and add media alone as a negative control.

11. Incubate ELISpot plates overnight at 37 °C in 5% CO_2. The following day the cells are removed by tipping the plate and washed six times with 0.05% PBS tween. Then add the detection antibody (7-B6-1-biotin) at 1 µg/ml in sterile PBS and add 100 µl to each well and incubate at room temperature for 2–4 h.

12. Wash the plates again six times with 0.05% PBS tween. Then add 100 µl of Streptavidin ALP diluted at 1:1000 to each well and incubate for 1–2 h at room temperature.

13. Wash the plates again six times with 0.05% PBS tween and develop the plates by adding 100 µl of the substrate solution (BCIP/NBT) to each well. Keep observing the plates for development of spots (5–15 min) and when spots are seen tip the development solution and wash the plates with normal water under a running tap. Then air dry the plates until the membranes have dried up and then read the plates using an automated ELISpot reader.

14. The number of spots for each peptide is calculated by counting the number of spots in each well and subtracting the background (cells with media) (Fig. 1) (*see* **Notes 2–4**).

4   Notes

1. If the PBMCs have been kept in the incubator for a long time, make sure that they have been mixed properly so that each well will have equal number of PBMCs.

2. The same protocol described above can be used for detection of perforin (Mabtech, Sweden), granzyme B (Mabtech, Sweden) and TNFα (Mabtech, Sweden) producing dengue virus specific T cells. However, with TNFα ELISpots, high background is seen in most instances.

3. The ELISpot culture supernatant can also be used to determine the presence of other cytokines and chemokines either by quantitative ELISAs or by analysis of cytokine multi-bead arrays. If such analysis is planned, instead of discarding the PBMCs after overnight incubation, centrifuge the ELISpot plates and collect the ELISpot culture supernatants into 2 ml tubes or into cryovials and store at −80 °C for further analysis of cytokines.

4. ELISpot assays can also be used to determine the effect of certain cytokines on antiviral responses. For instance, IL-10 has been shown to be high in patients with severe dengue and we have found that serum IL-10 levels inversely correlated with DENV-NS3 specific IFNγ ELISpot responses. We then used IL-10 and IL-10 receptor blocking antibodies in our experiments before adding DENV peptides and found that IL-10 blockade significantly improved DENV-specific T cell responses [4].

5. If ELISpot plate is not coated properly, then the antibody will only be on one side and half-moon shaped stained wells will be seen (Fig. 2a).

6. Once the PBMCs are added to the wells, the plates should not be shaken, or the cells will be rolled to the edges and you will see the spots on the peripheries with the middle of the well clear (Fig. 2b).

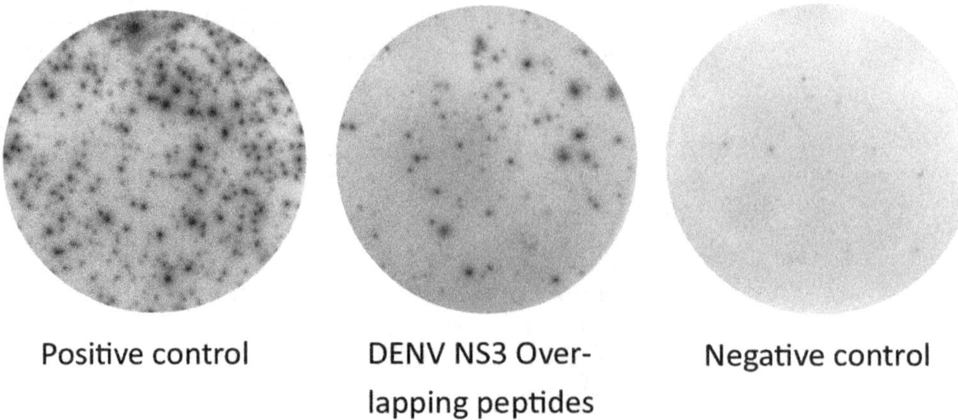

Fig. 1 A typical ex vivo ELISpot assay with PHA as the positive control, DENV NS3 overlapping peptides and media as the negative control

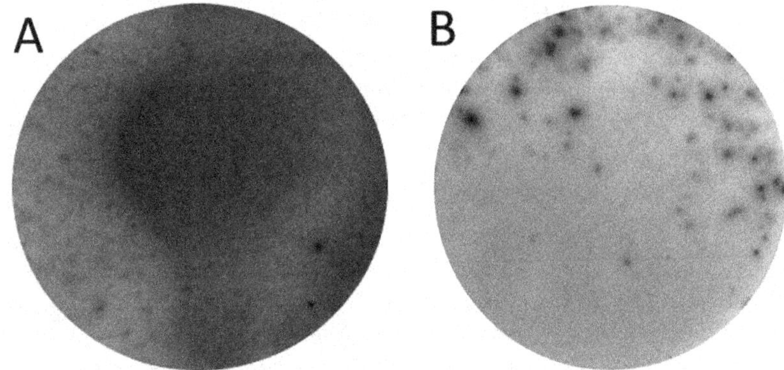

Fig. 2 The spots will not appear uniform if the wells are not coated properly (**a**), or if the cells roll to a side after adding the cells to the well (**b**) (*see* **Notes 5** and **6**)

References

1. Letsch A, Scheibenbogen C (2003) Quantification and characterization of specific T-cells by antigen-specific cytokine production using ELISPOT assay or intracellular cytokine staining. Methods 31(2):143–149

2. Simmons CP, Dong T, Chau NV et al (2005) Early T-cell responses to dengue virus epitopes in Vietnamese adults with secondary dengue virus infections. J Virol 79(9):5665–5675

3. Malavige GN, Huang LC, Salimi M et al (2012) Cellular and cytokine correlates of severe dengue infection. PLoS One 7(11):e50387

4. Malavige GN, Jeewandara C, Alles KM et al (2013) Suppression of virus specific immune responses by IL-10 in acute dengue infection. PLoS Negl Trop Dis 7(9):e2409

5. Jeewandara C, Adikari TN, Gomes L et al (2105) Functionality of dengue virus specific memory T cell responses in individuals who were hospitalized or who had mild or subclinical dengue infection. PLoS Negl Trop Dis 9(4):e0003673

6. Yue FY, Cohen JC, Ho M et al (2017) HIV-specific granzyme B-secreting but not gamma interferon-secreting T cells are associated with reduced viral reservoirs in early HIV infection. J Virol 91(8). https://doi.org/10.1128/JVI.02233-16

7. Theeten H, Mathei C, Peeters K (2016) Cellular interferon gamma and granzyme B responses to cytomegalovirus-pp65 and influenza N1 are positively associated in elderly. Viral Immunol 29(3):169–175

8. Goovaerts O, Jennes W, Massinga-Loembe M et al (2014) Antigen-specific interferon-gamma responses and innate cytokine balance in TB-IRIS. PLoS One 9(11):e113101

9. van Doorn E, Pleguezuelos O, Liu H et al (2017) Evaluation of the immunogenicity and safety of different doses and formulations of a broad spectrum influenza vaccine (FLU-v) developed by SEEK: study protocol for a single-center, randomized, double-blind and placebo-controlled clinical phase IIb trial. BMC Infect Dis 17(1):241

10. Ahlen G, Frelin L (2016) Methods to evaluate novel hepatitis C virus vaccines. Methods Mol Biol 1403:221–244

11. Fiore-Gartland A, Manso BA, Friedrich DP et al (2016) Pooled-peptide epitope mapping strategies are efficient and highly sensitive: an evaluation of methods for identifying human T cell epitope specificities in large-scale HIV vaccine efficacy trials. PLoS One 11(2):e0147812

12. Pang T, Mak TK, Gubler DJ (2017) Prevention and control of dengue-the light at the end of the tunnel. Lancet Infect Dis 17(3):e79–e87

Ex Vivo ELISpot Assay to Investigate iNKT Cell Responses in Acute Dengue Infection

Achala Indika Kamaladasa and Gathsaurie Neelika Malavige

Abstract

T cell receptors of the invariant Natural Killer T (iNKT) cells are downregulated with antigen stimulation. Therefore, identification of this cell population with flow cytometry in functionality studies is challenging. iNKT cells are known to produce both Th1 and Th2 cytokines immediately upon antigen stimulation. Therefore, we have used an ELISpot assay to determine the production of IFN-γ and IL-4 after stimulation with KRN7000, which has shown to bind to CD1d molecules and activate iNKTs in a similar fashion as α-GalCer. In this study, we observed that peripheral iNKT cells in patients with acute dengue show distinct production of IFN-γ, but not IL-4 with KRN7000 stimulation.

Key words iNKT cells, α-Galactosylceramide, IFN-γ ELISpot, IL-4 ELISpot

1 Introduction

Invariant Natural Killer T (iNKT) cells are a specialized T cell subset that gets activated by lipid antigens presented by CD1d molecules [1].

There are several self and foreign lipid antigens identified in the recent past that can activate iNKT cells. However, α-Galactosylceramide (α-GalCer) which was identified from a marine sponge extract is the prototypical iNKT cell agonist that can activate these cells to react immediately [2, 3]. Studies have shown that of the cells in the peripheral blood mononuclear (PBMC) fraction only the iNKT cells respond to α-GalCer in humans [4, 5]. Enumerating cytokine producing iNKT cells with flow cytometry could be challenging as the Vα24Jα18 T cell receptor, which is used to identify iNKTs, is significantly downregulated upon stimulation with α-GalCer and to lesser extent with IL-12 and PMA/Ionomycin [5, 6]. Therefore determining iNKT cells functionality with an ex vivo ELISpot assay would be a more suitable.

Alexander E. Kalyuzhny (ed.), *Handbook of ELISPOT: Methods and Protocols*, Methods in Molecular Biology, vol. 1808, https://doi.org/10.1007/978-1-4939-8567-8_16, © Springer Science+Business Media, LLC, part of Springer Nature 2018

Table 1
Secretion of IFN-γ and IL-4 from peripheral iNKT cells in dengue patients and healthy individuals

	Dengue patients Mean Median Interquartile range	Controls Mean Median Interquartile range
IFN-γ response (spot forming units/10⁶ PBMC)	78.4 40 2.25–93	107.6 40.5 8.5–131
IL-4 response (spot forming units/10⁶ PBMC)	5.4 2.5 0–10.75	4.7 3.0 0.25–9.5

A synthetic analogue for α-GalCer known as KRN7000 has been developed for use in research and clinical trials, which has shown to bind to the CD1d molecule and activate iNKT cells in a similar fashion as α-GalCer [7]. In this ELISpot protocol we have used KRN7000 to stimulate peripheral iNKT cells from patients with acute dengue infection, and PBMCs of healthy individuals were used as controls. We observed that when PBMCs of both patients and healthy individuals were stimulated with α-GalCer (KRN7000), although IFN-γ by iNKT cells were clearly observed, the IL-4 production was extremely low (Table 1).

2 Materials

2.1 Separation of Human PBMCs

1. Lymphoprep (Axis Shield, Oslo, Norway).

2. RPMI 1640: supplemented with 2 mM L-glutamine, 100 IU/ml penicillin (R0).

3. 50 ml centrifuge tubes.

4. Centrifuge allowing spinning 50 ml centrifuge tubes at $500 \times g$.

5. Trypan blue.

6. Counting slides.

7. Fetal bovine serum: Heat inactivated. 50 ml of heat inactivated and filtered FBS is used to prepare RPMI (R0) supplemented with 10% FBS (R10).

8. Upright microscope equipped with bright-field illumination and phase contrast condenser.

2.2 Preparation ***of KRN7000***	1. KRN7000 (Cayman Chemicals, USA). 2. 100% dimethyl Sulfoxide (DMSO). 3. 2. 50 mM Phosphate-buffered saline (PBS).

2.3 Ex Vivo ELISpot Assays

1. ELISpot plates (Millipore Corp., Bedford, MA, USA).
2. Absolute Ethanol.
3. Distilled water.
4. Commercially ready to use human IFNγ ELISpot kit (Mabtech, Sweden).
5. Commercially ready to use human IL-4 ELISpot kit (Mabtech, Sweden).
6. Fetal Bovine Serum heat inactivated.
7. Parafilm.
8. PHA (Lectin from Phaseolus vulgaris): lyophilized powder suitable for cell culture.
9. Tween 20.
10. ELISpot development substrate: BCIP NBT substrate.
11. CO_2 incubator set at 37 °C with 5% CO_2.
12. Multichannel pipette.
13. ELISpot reader (AID, Germany).

---

3   Methods

3.1 Separation of PBMCs

1. Collect blood into heparinized or EDTA tubes.
2. Dilute the fresh heparinized blood 1:1 with RPMI 1640 supplemented with 2 mM L-glutamine, 100 IU/ml penicillin (R0).
3. Add 15 ml of lymphoprep in 15 ml of centrifuge tubes and very slowly layer 15–25 ml of diluted blood over the lymphoprep layer (*see* **Note 1**).
4. Centrifuge the tubes at $500 \times g$ for 20 min without breaks. The PBMC layer is seen between the lymphoprep and the plasma layer.
5. Pipette out the PBMC layer and wash the cells in an equal volume of R0 at 250 rpm for 10 min with high breaks.
6. Resuspend the cell pellet in RPMI 1640 supplemented with 2 mM L-glutamine, 100 IU/ml penicillin and 100 μg/ml plus 10% Fetal Bovine serum (R10) (*see* **Note 2**).
7. Mix an aliquot of the cells 1:1 with Trypan Blue dye and pipette 10 ml of that mixture into a counting slide. Count cells under the microscope using 20× lens and phase contrast condenser. Express the living cell count as number of cells per ml.

3.2 Preparation of KRN7000

1. Dissolve KRN7000 in 100% DMSO and store the stock solution at −20 °C (*see* **Note 3**).

2. Dilute the KRN7000 to achieve the stimulating concentration (100 ng/ml) using PBS immediately before the stimulation (*see* **Note 4**).

3.3 Ex Vivo ELISpot Assays

3.3.1 Coating of Plate (Sterile Condition)

1. Before adding the coating antibody, pre-wet the ELISpot plates by adding 100 µl of 30% ethanol (*see* **Note 5**) in to each well for 1 min.

2. Then wash the plate six times with sterile water (200 µl/well) using a multichannel pipette.

3. Dilute the coating antibody (IL4-I for IL-4 and 1D1-K for IFN-γ) with sterile PBS to 15 µl/ml and add 50 µl per well. In order to make sure that the antibody is evenly spread over the membrane, gently tap the plate on either side.

4. Cover the plate with a parafilm to prevent evaporation of antibody solution and store at 4 °C until the plate is used. This plate can be kept at 4 °C for maximum of 1 month.

3.3.2 Incubation of Cells in the Plate (Sterile Condition)

1. Before plating the cells, remove the excess coating antibody and wash the plate six times with sterile PBS (200 µl/well).

2. Then add 200 µl/well of R10 and incubate for at least 30 min at 37 °C.

3. Discard the R10.

4. Add the PBMCs at 5×10^5/well and adjust the total volume of the cell suspension to 200 µl/well with R10 (*see* **Note 6**).

5. Add 2 µl of KRN7000 to each well to achieve a concentration of 100 ng/ml to stimulate iNKT cells. As a positive control add 20 µl of PHA at 40 µg/l so that the final concentration of PHA is 10 µg/ml and media alone as the negative control. Carry out all stimulations in duplicate or triplicate wells.

6. Incubate the IFN-γ plate for overnight and IL-4 plate for 48 h at 37 °C incubator supplemented with 5% CO_2.

3.3.3 Detection of Spots

1. At the end of the incubation period, discard the cells and wash the plate six times with 0.05% PBS-Tween (200 µl/well).

2. Dilute the detection antibody (IL4-II-biotin for IL-4 and 7-B6-I-biotin for IFN-γ) to 1 µg/ml in PBS and add 100 µl/well and incubate for 2 h at room temperature.

3. Discard the antibody solution and wash the plate six times with PBS-Tween, 200 µl/well.

4. Dilute the Streptavidin-APL at 1:1000 with PBS and add 100 µl/well and incubate for 1 h at room temperature.

5. Discard the Streptavidin-APL solution and wash the plate six times with PBS-Tween, 200 µl/well.

6. Add the substrate solution BCIP/NBT as 100 µl/well and observe the plate for spot development.

7. Once spots start to develop, wash the plate extensively with tap water and allow to air dry.

8. Reading and analyze the plate in an ELISpot reader (AID, Germany).

3.3.4 Calculation of Spot Forming Units

The frequency of IFN-γ and IL-4 producing iNKT cells can be determined according to the following calculation as Spot Forming Units/10^6 PMBC for each sample.

$$\text{Spot Forming Units} / 10^6 = \frac{\text{Average spots in } \alpha\text{-GalCer stimulated wells} - \text{Average spots in negative control wells}}{\text{Number of PMBC added to a well}} \times 10^6$$

Spots in the positive control wells are indicating that the ELISpot assay carried out have worked. When PBMCs of both patients and controls (healthy individuals) were stimulated with α-GalCer, IFN-γ responses were clearly observed but the IL-4 responses were extremely low (Fig. 1).

4   Notes

1. When layering blood onto lymphoprep, make sure that the blood does not mix with the lymphoprep to gain the best separation and the highest yield of PBMCs.

2. Before using fetal calf serum, it is important to heat inactivate the serum at 56 °C for 30 min.

3. KRN7000 is shipped in an amber glass vial. It is better to dissolve this in the same glass vial and keep the stock solution in it. Because organic solvents can solubilize some plastics.

4. Do the serial dilution of KRN7000 stock solution with PBS in an approach to minimize the amount of DMSO (from the stock KRN7000) added to the PBMCs.

5. Dilute the absolute ethanol with distilled water to make 30% ethanol. This can be made in large quantity and stored for a maximum of 1 month. If the spots don't appear nicely make a fresh batch of 30% ethanol because most probably this could be due to ethanol being degraded.

6. Mix the PBMCs well before adding the cells in each to ensure equal number of cells added to each well.

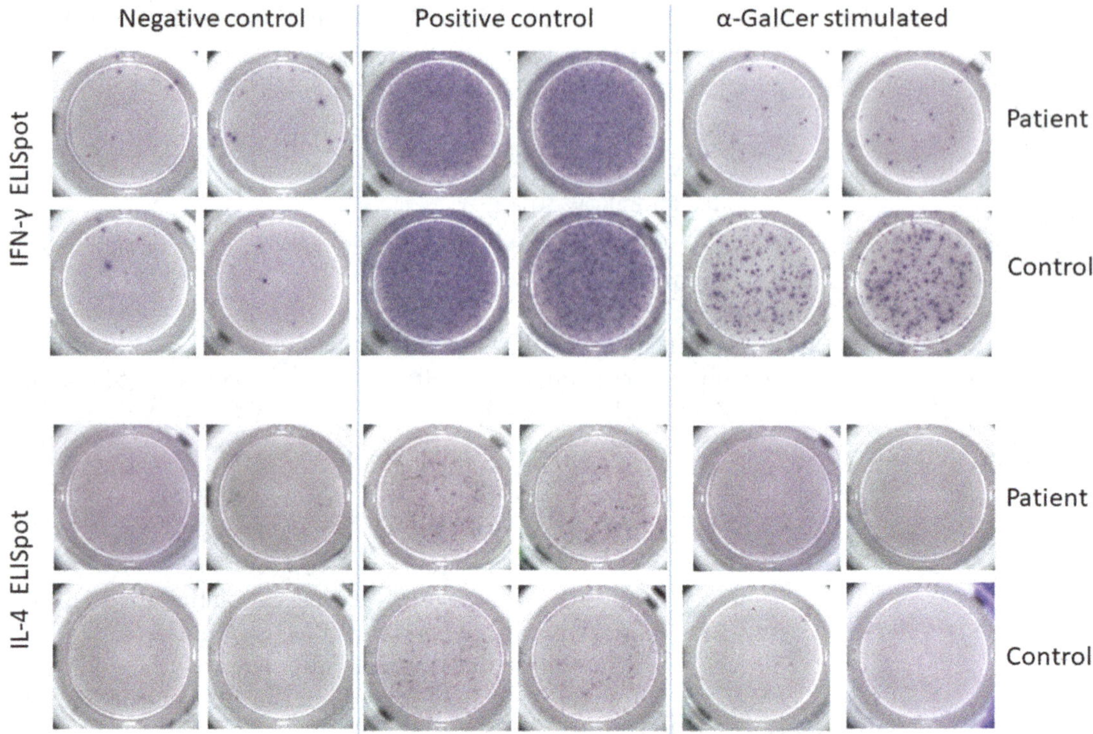

Fig. 1 Representative wells for IFN-γ and IL-4 ELISpots carried out for dengue patients and controls. When PBMCs of both patients and controls (healthy individuals) were stimulated with α-GalCer, IFN-γ responses were clearly observed but the IL-4 responses were extremely low

References

1. Brennan PJ, Brigl M, Brenner MB (2013) Invariant natural killer T cells: an innate activation scheme linked to diverse effector functions. Nat Rev Immunol 13(1):101–117

2. Kawano T, Cui J, Koezuka Y et al (1997) CD1d-restricted and TCR-mediated activation of valpha14 NKT cells by glycosylceramides. Science 278(5343):1626–1629

3. Tessmer MS, Fatima A, Paget C et al (2009) NKT cell immune responses to viral infection. Expert Opin Ther Targets 3(2):153–162

4. Dhodapkar MV, Geller MD, Chang DH et al (2003) A reversible defect in natural killer T cell function characterizes the progression of pre-malignant to malignant multiple myeloma. J Exp Med 197(12):1667–1676

5. Gumperz JE, Miyake S, Yamamura T et al (2002) Functionally distinct subsets of CD1d-restricted natural killer T cells revealed by CD1d tetramer staining. J Exp Med 195(5):625–636

6. Wilson MT, Johansson C, Olivares-Villagómez D et al (2003) The response of natural killer T cells to glycolipid antigens is characterized by surface receptor down-modulation and expansion. Proc Natl Acad Sci U S A 100(19):10913–10918

7. Van Der Vliet HJ, Nishi N, Koezuka Y et al (1999) Effects of alpha-galactosylceramide (KRN7000), interleukin-12 and interleukin-7 on phenotype and cytokine profile of human Valpha24+ Vbeta11+ T cells. Immunology 98:557–563

Dendritic Cell-Based ELISpot Assay for Assessing T-Cell IFN-γ Responses in Human Peripheral Blood Mononuclear Cells to Dengue Envelope Proteins

Peifang Sun and Monika Simmons

Abstract

Dengue envelope (E) protein is a dominant antigen for vaccine development and E-based vaccines have shown partial or full protection against live-virus challenge in non-human primates. Generally, T cell responses can be investigated with peptides. However, hundreds of over-lapping peptides need to be synthesized to cover the whole sequence of a protein, which brings the cost up to a much higher level than purchasing a protein. We have developed an enzyme-linked immunospot (ELISpot) assay that uses intact E proteins instead of peptides for assessing IFN-gamma (IFN-γ) responses. The assay relies on professional antigen presenting cells, dendritic cells, to process and present the E proteins to stimulate T cells.

Peripheral blood mononuclear cells (PBMCs) from dengue-exposed and naïve subjects were selected for the assay development. IFN-γ production ranged from 53 to 513 spot forming units (SFUs) and 0–45 SFUs per million PBMCs in dengue-exposed and naive subject groups, respectively. The assay allowed quantification of E-specific IFN-γ secreting memory T cells in subjects 9 years after exposure to a live-attenuated virus vaccine and live-virus challenge. Our results suggest that the dendritic cell-based IFN-γ assay is a useful tool for assessing immunological memory for clinical research.

Key words ELISpot, Dengue virus envelope protein, IFN-γ, Peripheral blood, Mononuclear cells, PBMCs, Dendritic cells

1 Introduction

The dengue viruses (DENVs) consist of four antigenically distinct but related serotypes, DENV 1, 2, 3, and 4, and belong to the family *Flaviviridae*, genus *Flavivirus* and species *Dengue virus*. Each serotype can cause febrile disease with symptom severity ranging from mild dengue fever to severe dengue hemorrhagic fever (DHF) and dengue shock syndrome (DSS). DENV is endemic in more than 100 countries in tropical and sub-tropical regions of the world; about 2.5 billion people or 40% of the world's population live in risk areas of dengue exposure, and 50–100 million people are infected yearly, including 500,000 DHF cases and 22,000

Alexander E. Kalyuzhny (ed.), *Handbook of ELISPOT: Methods and Protocols*, Methods in Molecular Biology, vol. 1808, https://doi.org/10.1007/978-1-4939-8567-8_17, © Springer Science+Business Media, LLC, part of Springer Nature 2018

deaths, mostly among children [1–3]. The recently licensed dengue vaccine on the market, Dengvaxia, developed by Sanofi Pasteur, does provide equal protection to all for serotypes. The vaccine efficacy is modest and varies widely between age groups. The pooled vaccine efficacy against PCR confirmed symptomatic dengue infection of any serotype in the year starting 1 month after the third dose is around 60% [4–6]. At least six additional dengue candidates are in clinical development including live-attenuated vaccines, purified inactivated vaccines, and an E protein subunit vaccine [7]. The E glycoprotein is the major virion surface antigen (494–501 amino acids) and is responsible for virus attachment to target cells, such as human dendritic cells and macrophages, and virus fusion [8, 9]. It is also a strong immunogen capable of eliciting long-lasting neutralizing antibodies (Abs) and cell-mediated immunity (CMI) [10]. The FDA-accepted primary endpoint of vaccine immunogenicity for DENV vaccines is neutralizing Ab titer. However, human and non-human primate vaccine trials, including clinical trials for the vaccine Dengvaxia, suggest that neutralizing Ab only mildly correlates with protection, raising concerns that it may not be a perfect predictive marker for immune protection [7, 11]. Therefore other possible mechanisms including CMI may play a protective role in the absence of neutralizing Ab.

Dengue-specific CMI is characteristically a long-term immune response found in endemic individuals with confirmed dengue infection. T cell responses can be detected 20 years after only one DENV exposure [12, 13]. Dengue-specific cytotoxic T cells (CTLs) are found in endemic donors during or after the convalescent period as well as in dengue vaccinated donors [1, 14]. This chapter describes an ELISPOT assay that uses human dendritic cells as antigen presenting cells and E proteins as antigens to stimulate memory CD4 and CD8 T cells for IFN-γ production.

The assay is primarily designed for clinical vaccine immunogenicity evaluation, but can also be used for basic clinical research. Using this assay, IFN-γ responses were detected in subjects 9 years after exposure to dengue viruses or vaccines (Fig. 3).

2   Materials

2.1 Supplies and Equipment

1. Phosphate buffered saline (pH 7.4 with 9.0 g/L NaCl. Without Ca^{2+} and Mg^{2+}).

2. Fetal Bovine Serum (FBS), tissue culture grade, sterile filtered, heat-inactivated 56 °C for 30 min.

3. RPMI 1640.

4. Tween-20.

5. 50 and 15 mL conical tubes.

6. Multichannel pipette (1–50 and 10–300 μL).

7. Disposable 1, 5, and 10 mL pipettes and tips sized from 1 μL to 1 mL.

8. 96-well round bottom tissue culture plates.

9. Centrifuge with adapters for test tubes and tissue culture plates.

10. Water bath 37 °C.

11. 37 °C humidified 5% CO_2 water jacket incubator.

12. Cellometer Auto 2000 Fluorescent Viability Counter for Primary Cells (Nexcelom, or equivalent). The cell counter should be able to count nucleated cells, live and dead cells and give viability. Record total cell number, viable cell number, and percent viability.

13. Cellometer AO/PI (acridine orange/propidium iodide) staining solution (Nexcelom, Cat.CS1-0106-5 mL, or equivalent).

14. Cellometer Disposable Counting Chamber PD300 (Nexcelom, Cat.CHT4-PD300-002, or equivalent).

2.2 Isolation and Freezing Human PBMCs

1. Heparinized blood specimens in blood collection tubes or unit packs.

2. Ficoll-Paque™ or an equivalent product.

3. Freezing medium: FBS with 10% Dimethyl Sulfoxide (DMSO), prepared freshly before cell freezing.

4. CryoTubes™ or an equivalent cryovial.

5. Mr. Frosty cell freezing units prepared according to the manufacturer's instructions, stored at room temperature.

2.3 Preparation of Dendritic Cells

1. Complete medium (CM): RPMI 1640 1× Modified with L-Glutamine containing 10% Fetal Bovine Serum (Heat inactivated at 56 °C for 30 min), 1% Penicillin-Streptomycin, and 1% Non-essential Amino Acid.

2. Recombinant human IL-4(rhIL4) and GM-CSF (rhGM-CSF), (R&D Systems, Cat. 204-IL-050 and 215-GM-050, respectively). Reconstitute with PBS (1% BSA) to 10 μg/mL. Aliquot the stock solution and store aliquots in −80 °C and thaw before use. Keep the thawed aliquot in 4 °C for <15 days.

3. Corning™ Primaria™ Tissue Culture Dish, 100 × 20 mm.

4. Corning™ Primaria 6-well plates.

2.4 Stimulation of PBMCs and ELISpot Plate Setup

1. RPMI 1640 Complete Medium (see above).

2. ELISpot plate: Millipore Plate (Millipore, Cat. MAIPSWU10).

3. Human IFN-γ ELISpot Kit, Cat. 3420-2H (Mabtec Lab).

4. DENV E protein of all four dengue serotypes (special order from Hawaii Biotech), stock 1 mg/mL in PBS, pH 7.4, aliquots in −80 °C, thaw before use.

5. Killed *Staphylococcus aureus* Cowan strain I (SAC), (Sigma Aldrich, Cat. 507861).

2.5 Develop the ELISpot Plate

1. IFN-γ ELISPOT Kit, Cat. 3420-2H, Mabtec Lab.
2. AEC substrate, Vector Laboratories, Cat. SK-4200.
3. ELISPOT Reader, Autoimmun Diagnostika GmbH (AID), or equivalent.

3   Methods

3.1 Isolation and Freezing Human PBMCs

1. Obtain fresh heparinized blood. Invert tubes to mix immediately after blood draw.
2. Place the blood into a 50-mL tube and centrifuge 10 min at $400 \times g$. Separate plasma from cells using a Pasteur pipette. Dilute cells in PBS at a ratio of 1.5:1 (PBS:blood).
3. Aliquot Ficoll-Paque into 50-mL centrifuge tubes at 20 mL per tube.
4. Carefully and slowly overlay 22.5 mL diluted blood sample on top of the 20-mL Ficoll-Paque. Centrifuge the blood tubes at $400 \times g$ at room temperature for 30 min (turn the centrifuge brake off).
5. Carefully pipet off a large portion of the top (buffer) layer. Do not disturb the interface.
6. Carefully collect PBMCs banded at the interface between the top layer and Ficoll-Paque into a 50-mL tube (pool 2 interfaces per tube).
7. Adjust the PBMC volume to 50 mL with PBS. Centrifuge the PBMCs at $400 \times g$ for 10 min at room temperature.
8. Decant or aspirate supernatant from the PBMC tube. Flick cell pellet to resuspend. Adjust the tube volume to 50 mL with PBS. Centrifuge the tube at $300 \times g$ for 10 min at room temperature. Repeat this step two more times.
9. After last wash, remove supernatant from the tube. Loosen cell pellet by tapping the side of tube.
10. Resuspend cell pellet in PBS, in 1/10 volume of whole blood collected. Count cells using the Cellometer Auto 2000.
11. Prepare freezing medium and filter-sterilize through a 0.22 μm filter. Keep the freezing medium cold on ice until ready to use.
12. Immediately before freezing, centrifuge cell solution at $300 \times g$ for 10 min to pellet the cells. Flick cell pellet to resuspend.
13. On ice, add ice-cold freezing medium slowly and resuspend cell pellet to a final concentration of 10×10^6 cells/

mL. Carefully aliquot the cell suspension into cryovials at 1 mL/vial.

14. Place cryovials in commercially available Mr. Freezy® container for at least 2 h, but no longer than 24 h at −80 °C freezer before transfer to liquid nitrogen.

3.2 Preparation of Dendritic Cells

1. Thaw a PBMC sample in a 37 °C water bath until just thawed, then gently and slowly transfer the content into 10 mL cold RPMI in 50-mL conical tubes, gently shake the tube to mix the cells while transferring.

2. Spin the cells at $300 \times g$ for 10 min at room temperature.

3. Discard supernatant and wash with cold RPMI.

4. Resuspend cells in 10 mL of CM and count the cells using the Cellometer Auto 2000. Record total cell number, viable cell number and viability.

5. Adjust cells to 5×10^6 cells/mL and add 10 mL of cells to a Primaria tissue culture dish or to wells of a Primaria 6-well plate at $5–10 \times 10^6$ cells/well.

6. Gently swirl the dish or the plate to even the distribution of the cell suspension and incubate the plate at 37 °C, 5% CO_2 for 2 h.

7. Examine cell adherence under an inverted microscope.

8. Gently pipet the culture medium to loosen the non-adherent cells. Aspirate all the culture medium to remove non-adherent cells. Gently add 10 mL of RPMI 1640 along the edge of the plate or the well. Pipet the medium gently and remove the medium. Repeat this step several times until a few floating cells can be spotted under the microscope.

9. Add 10 mL of fresh CM into the plates. Add 10 µL rhIL-4 (stock 10 µg/mL) and 10 µL GM-CSF (stock 10 µg/mL).

10. Incubate the plate at 37 °C, 5% CO_2 incubator for 3 days.

11. Remove 1/3 of the medium and add the same volume of fresh medium containing rhGM-CSF and rhIL-4 and keep the culture for 3 more days.

12. During the 6 days of culturing, monocytes undergo a transformation into dendritic cells (*see* **Note 1**) and detach from the plastic plates. At day 6, dendritic cells are ready to use (*see* **Note 2**).

3.3 Stimulation of PBMCs and ELISpot Plate Setup

1. The day before harvesting the dendritic cells, coat a Millipore ELISpot plate with coating antibody from the Mabtech IFN-γ ELISpot kit at 10 µg/mL and 100 µL/well. Place the plate overnight at 4 °C. The plate should be pre-wet with 30 µL/ well 35% ethanol for <1 min and washed three times with PBS before antibody coating.

2. In the hood, wash the plate five times with PBS and block the plate with CM for at least 1 h at 37 °C.

3. Decant the blocking medium.

4. Harvest dendritic cells from the Primaria dish or plate. Spin the dendritic cells at $300 \times g$ for 5 min to remove the culture medium and wash the cells with complete medium once.

5. Resuspend the dendritic cells in CM and check cell viability and count. Adjust cells to 1×10^6/mL in CM.

6. Take the amount of dendritic cells required and add them into six 15-mL conical tubes. Pulse dendritic cell with E protein by adding the E protein one serotype per tube (stock 1 mg/mL) to dendritic cells at a concentration of 20 µg/mL. Add the same amount of CM to one tube of cells as the negative control and 1 µg/mL SAC as the positive control.

7. Place dendritic cells in the 37 °C incubator and allow 4–6 h of antigen internalization and processing. During this time, perform **step 10**.

8. Adjust the dendritic cells to 2.0×10^5/mL after antigen pulsing.

9. Add 100 µL of dendritic cells to the ELISpot plate. Make at least triplicates for each condition.

10. Thaw vials of frozen PBMCs (*see* Subheading 3.1, **steps 1–4**) (*see* **Note 3**). Count the cells and resuspend cells to 2×10^6/mL.

11. Add 100 µL of PBMC cell suspension to the ELISpot plate pre-seeded with antigen-pulsed dendritic cells (*see* **Note 4**).

12. Place both plates in 5% CO_2 incubator for 20–24 h.

13. Following incubation, remove cells from the ELISpot plate by washing the plate six times with PBS-T (Tween-20, 0.05%).

14. Decant the plate right before adding the secondary antibody from the Mabtech kit. Don't let the plate dry. Add 100 µL/well of biotinylated anti-IFN-γ antibody at a 1:1000 dilution.

15. Incubate the secondary Ab for 2 h at room temperature.

16. Wash the plate six times with PBS-T and add peroxidase-conjugated streptavidin (KPL) at a 1:500 dilution in PBS.

17. Incubate the plate 1.5 h at room temperature.

18. Wash the plate six times with PBS-T.

19. Prepare AEC substrate according to the manufacturer's instructions right before use. Add AEC substrate to the plate.

20. Develop plates in the dark for 15–30 min, wash thoroughly with H_2O to stop the reaction and wait for the plate to dry.

21. Count the plate on the AID ELISpot counter. Examine the spots and record the number. Figure 1 shows typical ELISpot images.

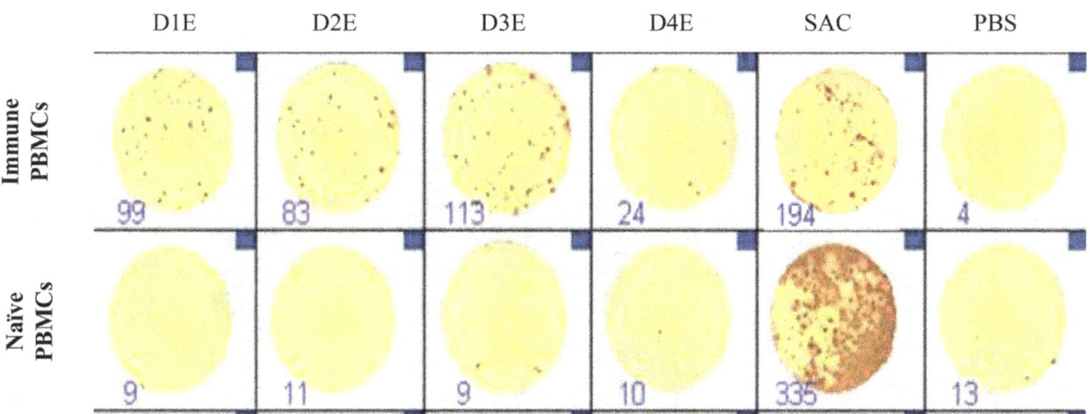

Fig. 1 Typical IFN-γ ELISpot images showing antigen-specific responses to serotypes of DENV E protein from a representative DENV-immune and a DENV-naïve subject

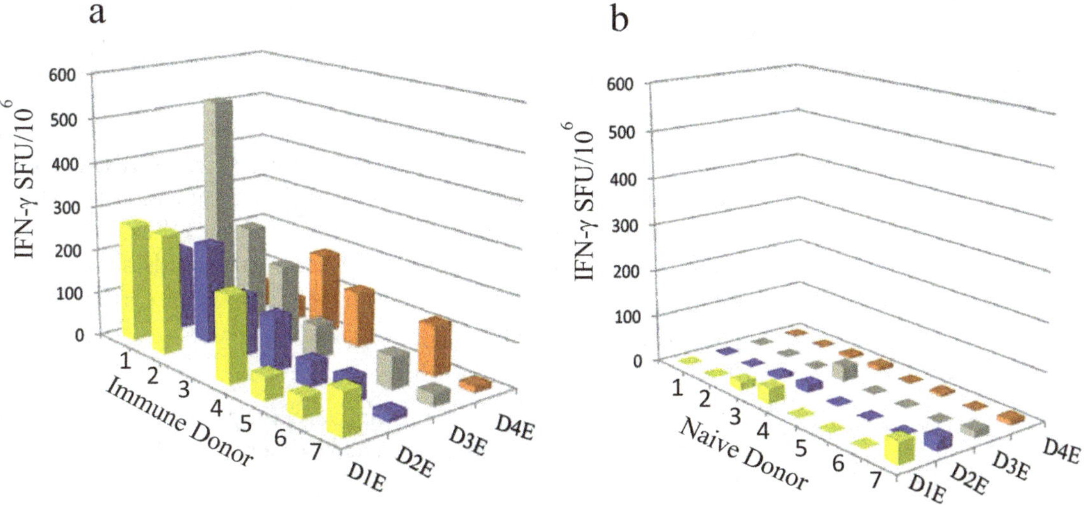

Fig. 2 IFN-γ responses measured by the dendritic cell-based ELISpot correlated with the immune status of the subjects suggesting the assay is antigen specific. SPUs to dengue serotype-specific E proteins in seven immune subjects (**a**) and seven naïve subjects (**b**)

3.4 Data Analysis

1. ELISpot data is presented as spot forming units (SFU) per million PBMCs. The SFU from triplicate wells are averaged. The SFU from negative control (PBS control) is considered as background response and is subtracted from that of E protein-stimulated cultures. The background-subtracted values are considered as E protein-specific SFU.

2. The E protein-specific SFU/well is further multiplied based on the input cells/well to yield a standardized value: $SFU/10^6$ PBMCs. Figure 2 shows the IFN-γ ELISpot results from seven dengue-immune and seven dengue-naive subjects (10).

3. This assay was used to detect IFN-γ responses (Fig. 3) in subjects 9 years after exposure to dengue viruses or vaccines (10).

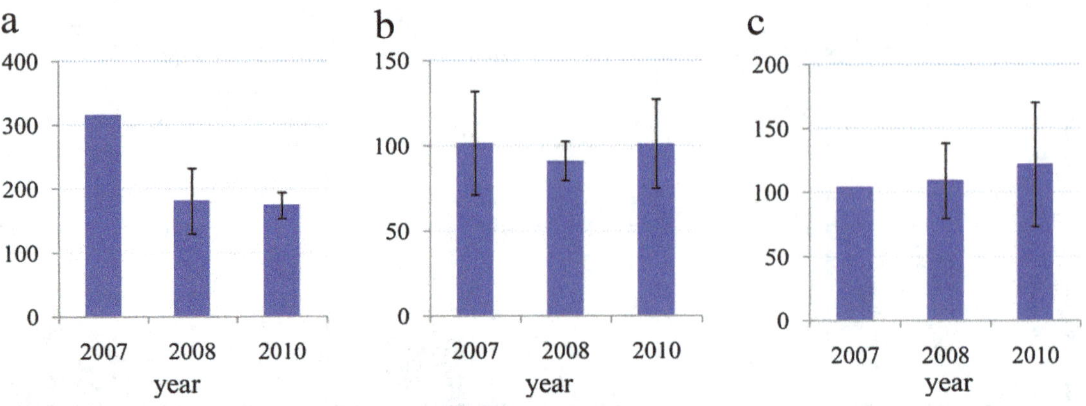

Fig. 3 IFN-γ memory response was detected 9 years after the exposure to dengue infection. Three dengue-immune subjects (**a**, **b**, and **c**) received live-attenuated dengue vaccine in year 2001 and IFN-γ response was measured in samples obtained in 2007, 2008, and 2010

4   Notes

1. The yield of dendritic cells is critical for the assay. It is recommended to use non-relevant cells to practice CD14-cell isolation and dendritic cell cultivation. At the end of the cultivation, phenotype the dendritic cells. The dendritic cells should not have CD14 expression, and should have CD1a expression.

2. Dendritic cells can be ready either on day 5 or day 6. Choose the best day and keep it consistent for your own study.

3. Some individuals can have fewer percentages of monocytes to begin with. Always make sure there are enough PBMCs to use for the assay.

4. For T cell stimulation, the ratio of dendritic cells to PBMCs in this assay is 1:10. It is recommended to practice with your own antigens to find the best ratio.

Disclaimer

The views expressed in this chapter are those of the authors and do not necessarily reflect the official policy or position of the Department of the Navy, Department of Defense, the U.S. Government or the Henry Jackson Foundation (HJF). MS is an employee of the U.S. Government and PS is a HJF government contract employee. Title 17 U.S.C. article 105 provides that "Copyright protection under this title is not available for any work of the United States Government." Title 17 U. S.C. article 101 defines a U.S. Government work as a work prepared by a military service member or employee of the U.S. Government as part of that person's official duties. The study protocol was approved by the Naval Medical Research Center Institutional Review Board in compliance with all applicable federal regulations governing the protection of human subjects.

Financial Support

This work was funded by a grant from the Military Infectious Disease Research Program (MIDRP), U.S. Army Medical Research and Materiel Command, Fort Detrick, MD, work unit number A0311.

References

1. Mukhopadhyay S, Kuhn RJ, Rossmann MG (2005) A structural perspective of the flavivirus life cycle. Nat Rev Microbiol 3(1):13–22. https://doi.org/10.1038/nrmicro1067

2. Guzman MG, Harris E (2015) Dengue. Lancet 385(9966):453–465. https://doi.org/10.1016/S0140-6736(14)60572-9

3. Bhatt S, Gething PW, Brady OJ, Messina JP, Farlow AW, Moyes CL, Drake JM, Brownstein JS, Hoen AG, Sankoh O, Myers MF, George DB, Jaenisch T, Wint GR, Simmons CP, Scott TW, Farrar JJ, Hay SI (2013) The global distribution and burden of dengue. Nature 496(7446):504–507. https://doi.org/10.1038/nature12060

4. Simmons CP (2015) A candidate dengue vaccine walks a tightrope. N Engl J Med 373(13):1263–1264. https://doi.org/10.1056/NEJMe1509442

5. Capeding MR, Tran NH, Hadinegoro SR, Ismail HI, Chotpitayasunondh T, Chua MN, Luong CQ, Rusmil K, Wirawan DN, Nallusamy R, Pitisuttithum P, Thisyakorn U, Yoon IK, van der Vliet D, Langevin E, Laot T, Hutagalung Y, Frago C, Boaz M, Wartel TA, Tornieporth NG, Saville M, Bouckenooghe A, Group CYDS (2014) Clinical efficacy and safety of a novel tetravalent dengue vaccine in healthy children in Asia: a phase 3, randomised, observer-masked, placebo-controlled trial. Lancet 384(9951):1358–1365. https://doi.org/10.1016/S0140-6736(14)61060-6

6. Villar L, Dayan GH, Arredondo-Garcia JL, Rivera DM, Cunha R, Deseda C, Reynales H, Costa MS, Morales-Ramirez JO, Carrasquilla G, Rey LC, Dietze R, Luz K, Rivas E, Miranda Montoya MC, Cortes Supelano M, Zambrano B, Langevin E, Boaz M, Tornieporth N, Saville M, Noriega F, Group CYDS (2015) Efficacy of a tetravalent dengue vaccine in children in Latin America. N Engl J Med 372(2):113–123. https://doi.org/10.1056/NEJMoa1411037

7. Nedjadi T, El-Kafrawy S, Sohrab SS, Despres P, Damanhouri G, Azhar E (2015) Tackling dengue fever: Current status and challenges. Virol J 12:212. https://doi.org/10.1186/s12985-015-0444-8

8. Chen Y, Maguire T, Hileman RE, Fromm JR, Esko JD, Linhardt RJ, Marks RM (1997) Dengue virus infectivity depends on envelope protein binding to target cell heparan sulfate. Nat Med 3(8):866–871

9. Wahala WM, Silva AM (2011) The human antibody response to dengue virus infection. Virus 3(12):2374–2395. https://doi.org/10.3390/v3122374

10. Sun P, Beckett C, Danko J, Burgess T, Liang Z, Kochel T, Porter K (2011) A dendritic cell-based assay for measuring memory T cells specific to dengue envelope proteins in human peripheral blood. J Virol Methods 173(2):175–181. https://doi.org/10.1016/j.jviromet.2011.01.023

11. Sabchareon A, Wallace D, Sirivichayakul C, Limkittikul K, Chanthavanich P, Suvannadabba S, Jiwariyavej V, Dulyachai W, Pengsaa K, Wartel TA, Moureau A, Saville M, Bouckenooghe A, Viviani S, Tornieporth NG, Lang J (2012) Protective efficacy of the recombinant, live-attenuated, CYD tetravalent dengue vaccine in Thai schoolchildren: a randomised, controlled phase 2b trial. Lancet 380(9853):1559–1567. https://doi.org/10.1016/S0140-6736(12)61428-7

12. Sierra B, Garcia G, Perez AB, Morier L, Rodriguez R, Alvarez M, Guzman MG (2002)

Long-term memory cellular immune response to dengue virus after a natural primary infection. Int J Infect Dis 6(2):125–128

13. Mongkolsapaya J, Dejnirattisai W, Xu XN, Vasanawathana S, Tangthawornchaikul N, Chairunsri A, Sawasdivorn S, Duangchinda T, Dong T, Rowland-Jones S, Yenchitsomanus PT, McMichael A, Malasit P, Screaton G (2003) Original antigenic sin and apoptosis in the pathogenesis of dengue hemorrhagic fever. Nat Med 9(7):921–927. https://doi.org/10.1038/nm887

14. Kurane I, Meager A, Ennis FA (1989) Dengue virus-specific human T cell clones. Serotype crossreactive proliferation, interferon gamma production, and cytotoxic activity. J Exp Med 170(3):763–775

Utilization of Feline ELISpot to Evaluate the Immunogenicity of a T Cell-Based FIV MAP Vaccine

Bikash Sahay, Alek M. Aranyos, Andrew McAvoy, and Janet K. Yamamoto

Abstract

The prototype and the commercial dual-subtype feline immunodeficiency virus (FIV) vaccines conferred protection against homologous FIV strains as well as heterologous FIV strains from the vaccine subtypes with closely related envelope (Env) sequences. Such protection was mediated by the FIV neutralizing antibodies (NAbs) induced by the vaccines. Remarkably, both prototype and commercial FIV vaccines also conferred protection against heterologous FIV subtypes with highly divergent Env sequences from the vaccine strains. Such protection was not mediated by the vaccine-induced NAbs but was mediated by a potent FIV-specific T-cell immunity generated by the vaccines (Aranyos et al., Vaccine 34: 1480–1488, 2016). The protective epitopes on the FIV vaccine antigen were identified using feline interleukin-2 (IL-2) and interferon-γ (IFNγ) ELISpot assays with overlapping FIV peptide stimulation of the peripheral blood mononuclear cells (PBMC) from cats immunized with prototype FIV vaccine. Two of the protective FIV peptide epitopes were identified on FIV p24 protein and another two protective peptide epitopes were found on FIV reverse transcriptase. In the current study, the multiple antigenic peptides (MAPs) of the four protective FIV peptides were combined with an adjuvant as the FIV MAP vaccine. The laboratory cats were immunized with the MAP vaccine to evaluate whether significant levels of vaccine-specific cytokine responses can be generated to the FIV MAPs and their peptides at post-second and post-third vaccinations. The PBMC from vaccinated cats and non-vaccinated control cats were tested for IL-2, IFNγ, and IL-10 ELISpot responses to the FIV MAPs and peptides. These results were compared to the results from CD4$^+$ and CD8$^+$ T-cell proliferation to the FIV MAPs and peptides. Current study demonstrates that IL-2 and IFNγ ELISpot responses can be used to detect memory responses of the T cells from vaccinated cats after the second and third vaccinations.

Key words Feline immunodeficiency virus, MAP, Vaccine peptides, T-cell peptides

1 Introduction

The antigen-specific cytokine production by the re-stimulated peripheral blood mononuclear cells (PBMC) has been used for rapid screening of the mounted immunity in a vaccinated human or animal population [1–4]. The immune cells responsible for the cytokine production can be determined by the nature of cytokines produced post vaccination. Interferon-γ (IFNγ) is mainly produced

Alexander E. Kalyuzhny (ed.), *Handbook of ELISPOT: Methods and Protocols*, Methods in Molecular Biology, vol. 1808, https://doi.org/10.1007/978-1-4939-8567-8_18, © Springer Science+Business Media, LLC, part of Springer Nature 2018

by CD4$^+$ T cells, CD8$^+$ T cells, and NK cells [5, 6], while the release of interleukin-2 (IL-2) is mostly limited to T cells (both CD4$^+$ T cells and CD8$^+$ T cells) [7, 8]. In contrast, cytokines such as IL-6 and IL-10 are constitutively produced by cells of myeloid origin (macrophages, monocytes, and dendritic cells (DC)); however, stimulation induces the release of cytokines mentioned earlier by T and B cells along with the myeloid cells in the PBMC [5, 9–12]. Although macrophages/monocytes and NK cells respond to the immunogenic antigens but lack immunological memory (amnestic) to the vaccinated peptides or antigens, cytokines produced may play a role in the T-cell responses in the adjuvant-based vaccination [5, 13, 14]. T cells, but not NK cells and macrophages/monocytes, recognize the peptides from the previous vaccinations and respond to the peptides with equivalent or enhanced magnitude upon subsequent recognition, demonstrating memory responses to these peptides [5, 6]. Thus, IFNγ and/or IL-2 responses from T cells of the vaccinated host are used as the benchmark of acquired immunity post restimulation. Such understanding about the specific cell source(s) of the individual cytokine expressed by the PBMC provides additional value to the cytokine ELISpot results. Furthermore, after determining the source of the cytokine using purified cells from PBMC, total PBMC could be used to determine the amplitude of the response in the subsequent PBMC-based ELISpot analysis. This is particularly important when performing feline cytokine studies where feline-specific reagents (e.g., lack of commercial antibodies to feline macrophage, monocyte, DC, NK cell, CD107a, perforin, and granzymes, and commercial feline immune assay kits) are limited compared to those for humans. In addition, the total amount of blood that can be safely collected from domestic cats is far less than the amount that can be safely collected from humans.

IFNγ ELISpot assay was one of the first cytokine ELISpot commercially available and was extensively used to evaluate antigen-specific immunity developed in humans/felines vaccinated against or infected with HIV or FIV [1, 4, 15–18]. In the initial HIV-1 and FIV vaccine studies, expression of IFNγ in the antigen-specific CD8$^+$ T cells was considered as the marker for the cytotoxic T lymphocytes (CTLs) activity, which are the key cells that kill or lyse the HIV/FIV infected cells in their respective hosts [19, 20]. This view was later rejected by (1) the dissociated CTL activity found in certain studies [21] and (2) the availability of reagents more relevant to the biological CTL activity against HIV-infected cells, such as perforin, granzymes, and/or CD107a [21–23]. Nevertheless, the viral antigen-specific production of cytokines such as IFNγ and IL-2 by the CD8$^+$ and CD4$^+$ T cells is considered an important feature of polyfunctional CD8$^+$ and CD4$^+$ T cells which are equally important against HIV and FIV infections [23–25]. HIV-specific polyfunctional T cells are associated with the control of HIV infection in the long-term nonprogressors and the elite controllers [26, 27]. Furthermore, in recent HIV and SIV vaccine studies, polyfunctional T-cell activities induced in response to vaccination correlated with protection against HIV and SIV [23, 28].

In the current study, the feline IFNγ, IL-2, and IL-10 ELISpot results were compared to the CD4[+] and CD8[+] T-cell proliferation data in the restimulated PBMC obtained from the FIV-vaccinated and non-vaccinated control cats. In the previous studies using prototype FIV vaccine (the prototype to the commercial Fel-O-Vax® FIV vaccine [29]), the FIV vaccine antigen-specific IFNγ and IL-2 (both at transcript and protein levels) in the PBMC from vaccinated cats demonstrated the existence of strong memory responses to FIV antigen by the T cells upon each subsequent FIV vaccination [30]. Although all in vitro stimulant groups (media control, FIV antigen, T-cell mitogen) had substantial levels of TNFα and IL-6, no vaccination or memory responses to FIV antigen were detected by monitoring the TNFα and IL-6 levels. However, FIV antigen-specific IFNγ and IL-2 responses were detected in those animals receiving annual boosts even at second and fourth year of vaccination [25].

Additionally, the FIV vaccine used in the current study contains a novel mix of T cell-based antigens consisting of four multiple antigenic peptides (MAPs) derived from FIV p24 or reverse transcriptase (RT). These FIV peptides have been reported to be recognized by the PBMC and T cells from prototype FIV-vaccinated cats and HIV[+] human subjects [2, 3, 25]. MAP system was used most frequently as an immunogen to stimulate antibody production in the mice or rabbits to the peptide(s) present in the MAP [31–35]. The current study is the first demonstration of strong T-cell responses measured as T-cell proliferation and cytokine release generated in domestic laboratory cats against uniquely constructed four MAPs, serving as the vaccine immunogen.

2 Materials

2.1 Animal Subjects

1. Specific pathogen free (SPF) cats were purchased from Liberty Research, Inc. (Waverly, NY) or were bred in the Laboratory of Comparative Retrovirology and Immunology at the University of Florida. Beginning at 12–13 weeks of age, these cats were vaccinated 3× with FIV MAP vaccine at intervals of 6 weeks. Blood samples were collected in heparin coated tubes on 6 weeks post-second vaccination (i.e., third vaccination immediately before the vaccination) and 6 weeks post-third vaccination.

2. All cats were maintained and utilized according to the policies and protocols approved by Institutional Animal Care and Use Committee (IACUC) of University of Florida (UF).

2.2 FIV MAP Vaccine

1. Vaccine immunogen consisted of four MAPs each containing a single FIV p24 or RT peptide (Fig. 1). Each MAP contained four identical peptides on the amino-end of the lysine backbone and a palmitic acid (Pam) on the carboxyl-end of the lysine chain (Fig. 1). Equal amounts (100 μg each/dose; 400 μg combined total in 1 mL PBS) of Pam-MAPs synthesized by LifeTein LLC (South Plainfield, NJ) were mixed with FD-1 adjuvant supplemented with feline IL-12 [25]. The four Pam-MAPs (hereon called MAPs) consisted of FIV p24 peptides (Fp9-3 and Fp14-3/4) and FIV RT peptides (FRT3-3/4 and FRT7-1/2). Fp14-3/4 was an overlapping peptide of Fp14-3 and Fp14-4 peptides. Similarly, FRT3-3/4 was an overlapping peptide of FRT3-3 and FRT3-4, while FRT7-1/2 was an overlapping peptide of FRT7-1 and FRT7-2. Initial studies determined that these p24 and RT peptides (Fp9, Fp14-3, Fp14-4, FRT3-3, FRT3-4, FRT7-1, FRT7-2) induced immune responses in the PBMC from cats that received the prototype FIV vaccine [25].

2. Vaccine adjuvant consisted of 1 mL of FD-1 adjuvant (Fort Dodge Animal Health, Fort Dodge, IA) which was supplemented with feline IL-12 (R&D Systems, Inc.) at 5 μg per dose [25] (*see* **Note 1**).

2.3 Peripheral Blood Mononuclear Cell Preparation

1. Lymphocyte Separation Medium (LSM or ficoll-hypaque) (Corning/Mediatech, Inc., Manassas, VA).

2. Hanks' Balanced Salt Solution without sodium bicarbonate, calcium, and magnesium.

2.4 IFNγ, IL-2, and IL-10 ELISpot for Cats

1. 96-well polyvinylidene fluoride (PVDF)-membrane white plates (Millipore MultiScreen plates, Merck Millipore, Cork, Ireland).

2. PBMC medium for ELISpot: AIM-V® medium (GIBCO, Grand Island, NY) supplemented with gentamicin (25 μg/mL) and with 5% heat (56 °C, 30 min)-inactivated fetal bovine serum (FBS) (*see* **Note 2**).

3. Phosphate-Buffered Saline (PBS): 11.9 mM phosphate, 137 mM sodium chloride, 2.7 mM potassium chloride, pH 7.4. Endotoxin-low, DNase-free, RNase-free, and protease-free, and sterile filtered (0.2 μm) PBS (Janssen Pharmaceuticalaan 3a, Fair Lawn, NJ) to decrease background.

4. Reagent diluent: PBS supplemented with 1% (w/v) fraction V bovine serum albumin (BSA) for use in reconstituting lyophilized antibodies (*see* **Note 2**).

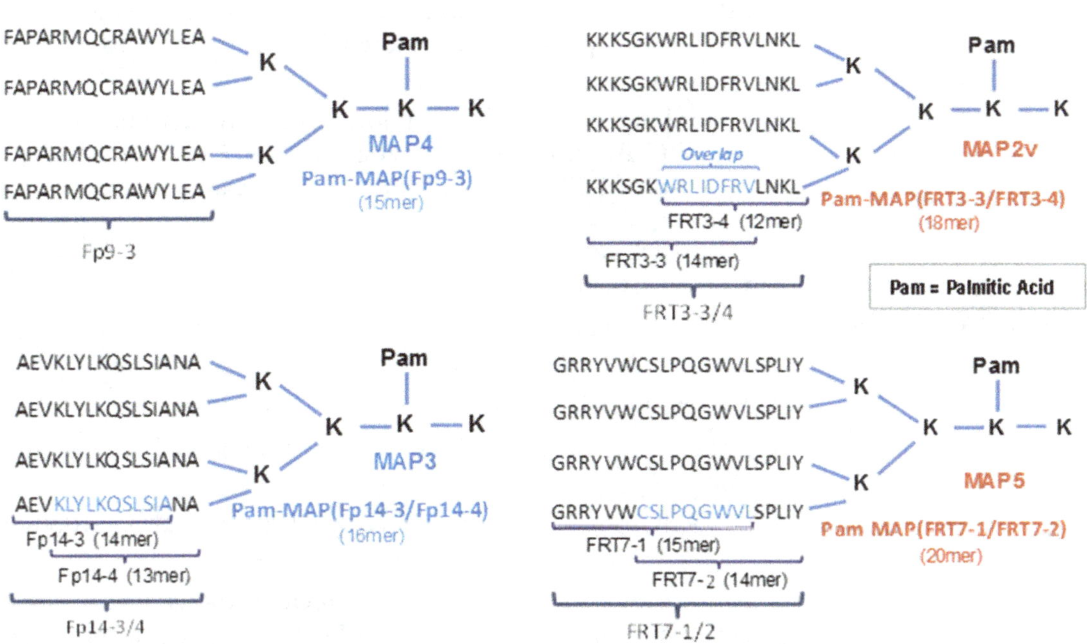

Fig. 1 Structure and sequences of the four multiple antigenic peptides (MAPs). The two MAPs on the left (top and bottom) consist of FIV p24 peptides (Fp9-3 and Fp14-3/4), and those on the right consist of FIV reverse transcriptase (RT) peptides (FRT3-3/4 and FRT7-1/2). The sequences of the long peptide and its smaller overlapping peptides are shown for Fp14-3/4 (Fp14-3, Fp14-4), FRT3-3/4 (FRT3-3, FRT3-4), and FRT7-1/2 (FRT7-1, FRT7-2). Four identical FIV peptides are on the amino-end of the MAP attached to a branched lysine backbone with palmitic acid (Pam) on the carboxyl-end. The final MAP vaccine consisted of all four MAPs at equal amounts (100 μg/dose each; total 400 μg/dose). Each MAP and its long and short peptides were used as FIV peptide stimulants in the IL2, IFNγ, and IL10 ELISpot assays and the RT T-cell proliferation analysis

5. Blocking buffer: 1% BSA, 5% (w/v) sucrose in PBS (*see* **Notes 2** and **3**).

6. AIM-V diluent: AIM-V® medium supplemented with gentamicin (25 μg/mL).

7. Feline (Fe) IFNγ ELISPOT Development Module, FeIL-2 ELISPOT Development Module, and FeIL-10 ELISPOT Development Module (R&D Systems Inc., Minneapolis, MN) included a matching pair of antibodies used for capture and detection of individual feline cytokine and ELISPOT Blue Color Module (R&D Systems Inc.):

   (a) Respective feline cytokine (IFNγ, IL-2, IL-10) Capture Antibody Concentrate reconstituted in 1 mL PBS and diluted 1 in 50 parts PBS.

   (b) Respective feline cytokine (IFNγ, IL-2, IL-10) Detection Antibody Concentrate reconstituted in 1 mL reagent diluent and diluted in 50 parts reagent diluent

8. ELISPOT Blue Color Module (R&D Systems Inc.):

    (a) Streptavidin-AP concentrate (streptavidin conjugated to alkaline phosphatase) diluted 1 in 50 parts with reagent diluent.

    (b) 5-bromo-4-chloro-3′ indolylphosphate *p*-toluidine salt (BCIP)/nitro blue tetrazolium (NBT) chromogen consists of BCIP and NBT chloride in organic solvent.

2.5 CFSE Proliferation of Feline CD4+ and CD8+ T Cells

1. Carboxyfluorescein diacetate succinimidyl ester (CFSE or CFDA) (Invitrogen, Carlsbad, CA).

2. PBMC medium for CFSE assay: AIM-V® medium containing 25 μg/mL gentamicin and 10% heat-inactivated FBS.

3. Dimethyl sulfoxide (DMSO) for diluting CFSE.

4. AIM-V diluent: AIM-V® medium supplemented with gentamicin (25 μg/mL).

5. LIVE/DEAD™ Fixable Yellow Dead Cell Stain kit for 405 nm (LIVE/DEAD reagent) (Invitrogen).

6. Antibodies to feline cell markers include mouse monoclonal antibody (MAb) to feline CD3 (APC labeled) (kindly provided by Dr. Yorihiro Nishimura, The University of Tokyo, Tokyo, Japan), feline CD4 (PE labeled) (SouthernBiotech, Birmingham, AL), and feline CD8 (PE/Cy7 labeled) (kindly provided by Dr. Nazareth Gengozian, University of Tennessee) (*see* **Note 4**).

7. Fluorescence activated cell sorting buffer (FACS buffer) consists of 0.5% BSA and 0.1% sodium azide in PBS.

8. BD LSR II flow cytometer with FACSDiva software.

2.6 FIV Peptides, FIV Antigen, and Mitogens

1. FIV peptides (Fp9-3, Fp14-3, Fp14-4, FRT3-3, FRT3-4, FRT7-1, FRT7-2) for ELISpot and CFSE-proliferation assays were synthesized by RS Synthesis (Louisville, KY), and their sequences shown in Fig. 1. All peptides were amidated on the carboxyl-end.

2. Partially purified and concentrated whole FIV virus (IWV) preparation was inactivated by UV irradiation (15 min) and then by heat inactivation at 56 °C (30 min). Above inactivated FIV IWV preparation was negative for infectious virus when cultured in feline PBMC and monitored every 3 days for at least 2 weeks by RT assay.

3. AIM-V diluent: AIM-V® medium with gentamicin (25 μg/mL).

4. T-cell mitogens: Concanavalin A (ConA) and phytohemagglutinin-M (PHA) diluted in AIM-V diluent for use as a positive control (*see* **Note 5**).

5. Macrophage/monocyte mitogen: Phorbol 12-myristate 13-acetate (PMA) in combination with PHA.

3   Methods

Two approaches have been undertaken to compare the results from feline IFNγ and IL-2 ELISpot assays to those from feline IL-10 ELISpot assay using PBMC from MAP-vaccinated cats and non-vaccinated cats. Both IL-2 and IFNγ are produced predominantly by T cells in response to peptide stimulation [5, 7, 36]. Moreover, T cells in the PBMC of vaccinated cats possess memory responses to vaccine antigens [5, 6]. In contrast, macrophages/monocytes can respond to peptides, but they do not possess memory responses [5, 37–39]. Since IL-10 expression of human PBMC has been reported to possess high spontaneous or constitutive release (i.e., media control) [9, 10], the first approach is to evaluate if the spontaneous release of IL-10 by feline PBMC is much higher than those of IL-2 and IFNγ. If this is the case, the PBMC from the vaccinated cats after the second and the third vaccinations will express IL-10 at similar levels as those expressed by the PBMC from the control cats. The second approach is to evaluate whether FIV peptide-specific memory responses induced by feline T cells are also induced by feline macrophages/monocytes by comparing the results from the second vaccination to those from the third vaccination.

3.1 *Post-Second Vaccination*

1. **Figure 2a, b**: Both IL-2 and IFNγ responses to FIV peptides and MAPs were observed at 6 weeks post-second vaccination (Fig. 2a, b), and these were higher than the low responses at 6 weeks post-first vaccination (data not shown). In Fig. 2, all results shown are after the subtraction of the average responses to each stimulant of the control cat group, with a single exception of the mitogens. The mitogens (ConA, PMA/PHA) were without any subtraction since similar level of responses was expected from the control group based on our previous experience. When compared to the responses of the control cat group, the vaccinated cats displayed significantly elevated IL-2 and IFNγ responses to peptides FRT3-3/4, FRT3-3, Fp14-4, and FRT7-2 (Fig. 2a, b). In addition, IL-2 responses to Fp14-3/4 and Fp9-3 were also significantly elevated in the vaccinated cats, whereas IFNγ responses to MAP2v, MAP3, and FRT7-1 were also significantly elevated.

2. **Figure 2c**: In contrast, IL-10 responses to FIV peptides and MAPs (Fig. 2c) were not significantly elevated when compared to those of the control cat group.

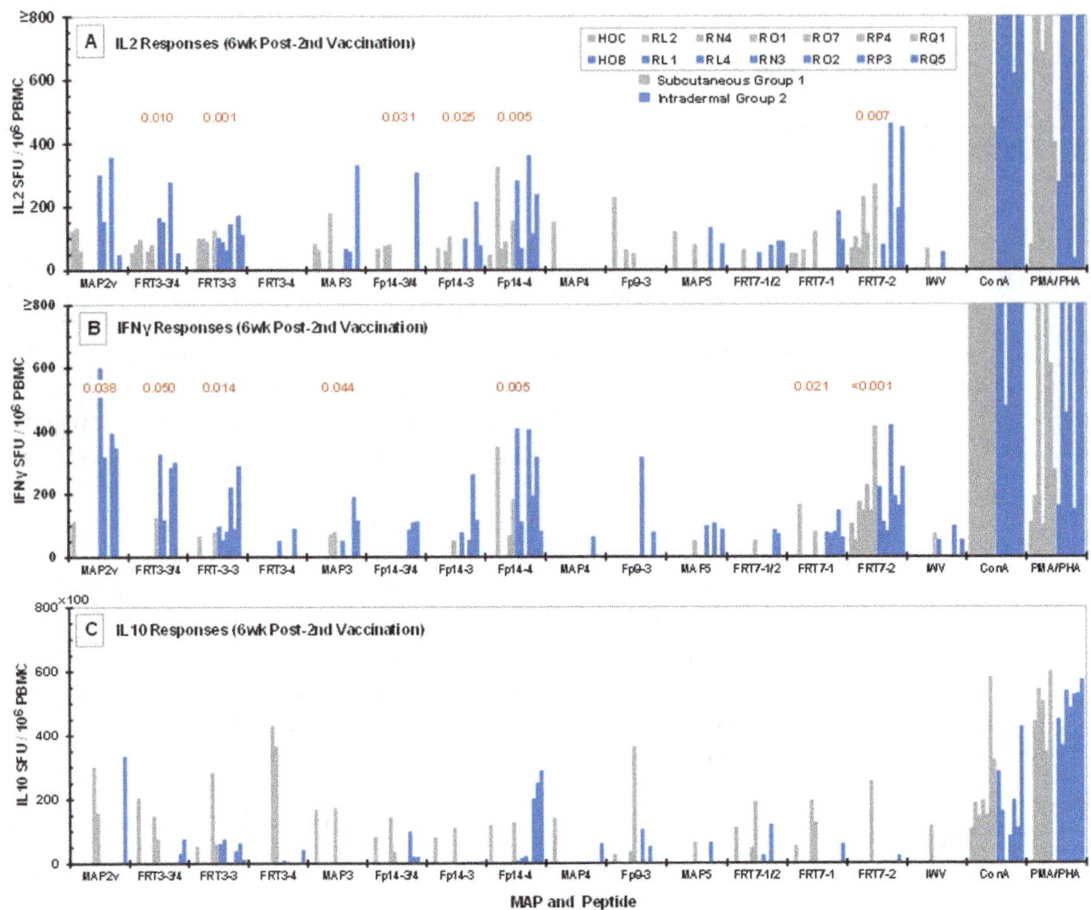

Fig. 2 IL2, IFNγ, and IL10 responses of MAP-vaccinated cats at 6 weeks post-second vaccination. The IL2 (**a**), IFNγ (**b**), and IL10 (**c**) responses were after the in vitro stimulation of the PBMC from the vaccinated cats with FIV MAPs and peptides. One set of seven cats was subcutaneously vaccinated with the MAP vaccine (grey bars), and another set of seven was intradermally vaccinated with MAP vaccine (blue bar). Each bar represents the value after subtraction of the average value of the results from the nine control cats, with the exception of the mitogens (ConA and PMA/PHA). The results for the mitogens (**a–c**) are without any subtraction. The p-value (t-test) in red above the bars of each FIV stimulant indicates that the results from the combined vaccine group are significantly elevated in response to the corresponding FIV stimulant when compared to the results from the control cat group. Note that FIV stimulant IWV, which is inactivated whole viruses, do not stimulate any cytokine responses since no cats were immunized in this study with IWV. Furthermore, T cells from MAP-vaccinated cats can recognize the FIV MAPs and/or the FIV peptides present in the vaccine

3. **Figure 3a–c**: In reanalyzing the IL-10 data, the IL-10 media control or spontaneous release of each cat (Fig. 3c) was extremely high when compared to those of IL-2 and IFNγ (Fig. 3a, b). Hence, a simple subtraction of the average response to each stimulant by the control cat group would result in a misinterpretation of the data due to the high spontaneous release of IL-10.

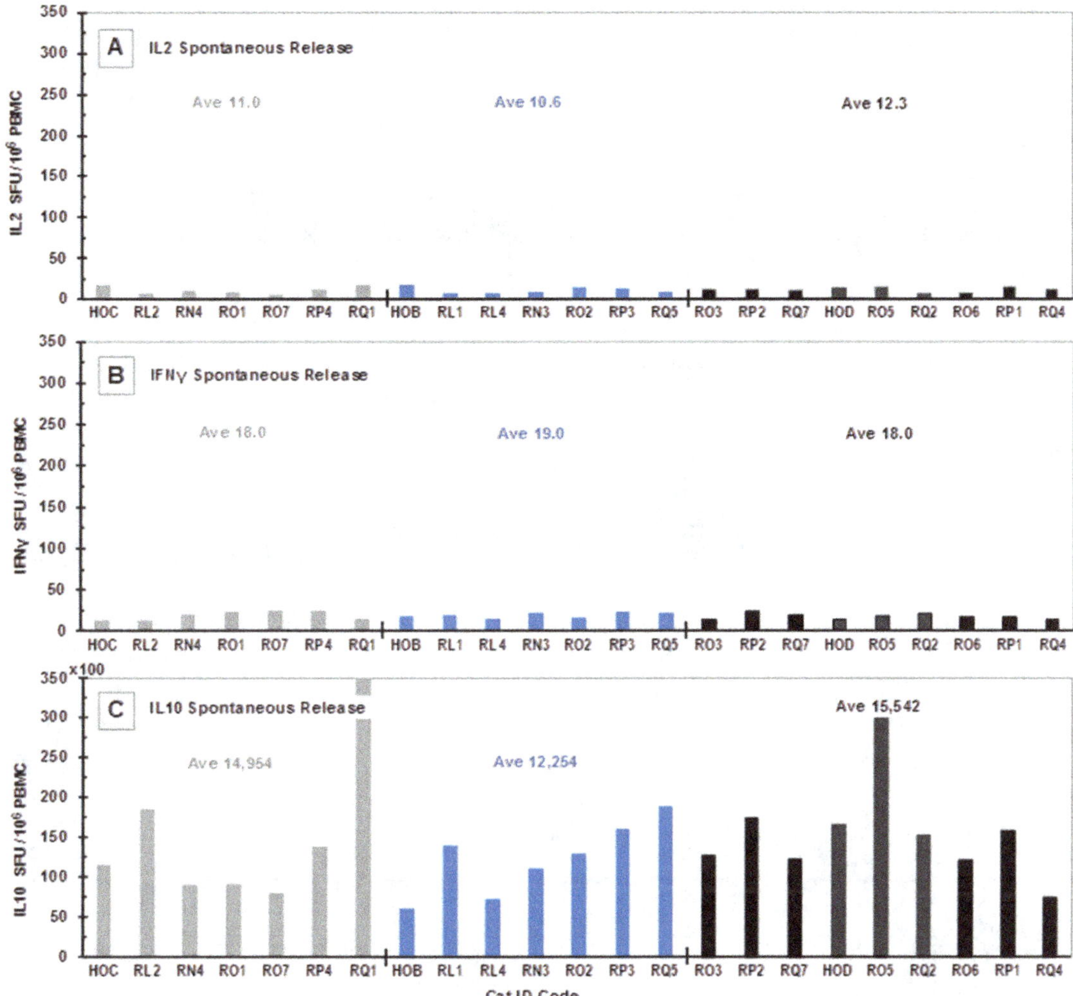

Fig. 3 Constitutive IL2, IFNγ, and IL10 production of the PBMC of vaccinated and non-vaccinated cats. The constitutive production or the spontaneous release of IL2 (**a**), IFNγ (**b**), and IL10 (**c**) are shown for the PBMC of the seven subcutaneous vaccinated cats (Vaccine Group 1, grey bars), seven intradermally vaccinated cats (Vaccine Group 2, blue bars), and nine non-vaccinated control cats (Control Group, black bars) at 6 weeks post-second vaccination. The average (ave) value of each group is shown above the bars of each group. Note that the magnitude of the IL10 spontaneous release is about 1000-fold higher (see *y*-axis) than those of IL2 and IFNγ

4. **Figure 4a, b**: Since MAPs and peptides could suppress IL-10 responses, the IL-10 data were analyzed by subtracting the media control of individual cat (Fig. 4a) and another set without any subtraction (Fig. 4b). These results were compared to the responses from the control cats. The results from the comparison made between combined vaccine group and control group are shown above the bars. Such comparison demonstrated significant IL-10 suppression to MAP5 (Fig. 4a, b) and FIV antigen (IWV) (Fig. 4b) in the vaccinated cats, whereas the

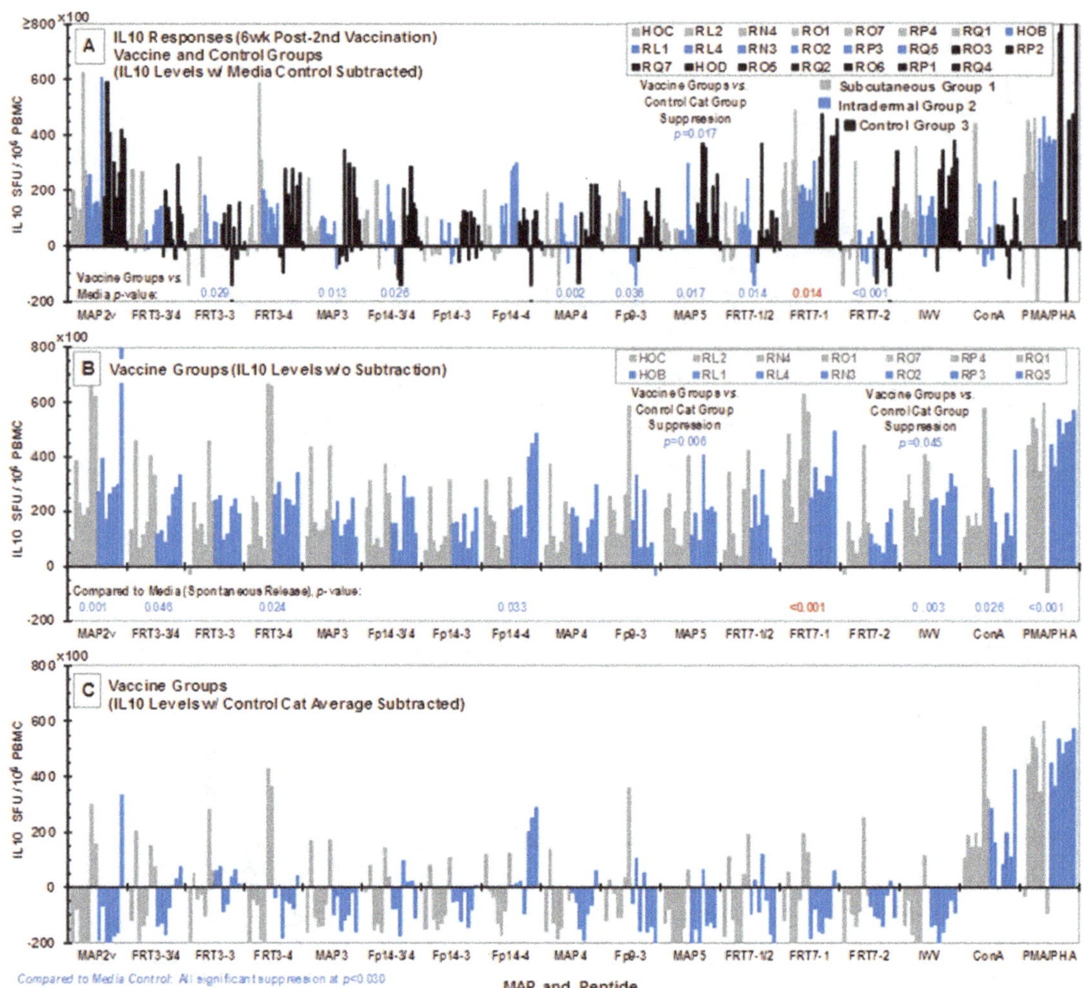

Fig. 4 Analyses of IL10 responses of the PBMC from vaccinated and non-vaccinated cats. The analyses of the IL10 responses of the PBMC from vaccinated and non-vaccinated cats at 6 weeks post-second vaccination are shown in three different formats (**a–c**). The bar results of the two vaccine groups and one control group (**a**) are shown after the subtraction of the media control of each cat. The grey bars represent results from the subcutaneous vaccine group 1; the blue bars represent results from intradermal vaccine group 2; and the black bars represent results from non-vaccinated control group 3. The bar results of the two vaccine groups (**b**) are without any subtraction and are shown without control group. The bar results of the two vaccine groups (**c**) are after the subtraction of the average value of the IL10 responses of the control group and as a result cannot be statistically compared to the control group. The p-values (t-test) on the top of the bars represent statistical comparison made between the combined vaccine group and the control group, and the p-values on the bottom of the bars are based on the statistical comparison between the combined vaccine group and their media controls. The p-values in red represent significant increase or elevation, whereas those in blue represent significant decrease or suppression. The results of the combined vaccine group in panel (**c**) are significantly decreased when compared to their spontaneous release (i.e., media control)

others had no significant suppression or enhancement of IL-10. However, when the responses by the combined vaccine group were compared to their media control, the responses to FRT7-1 (Fig. 4a, b, red p-value below the bars) were significantly higher than the media control. Conversely, a significant suppression was observed to FRT3-3, MAP3, Fp14-3/4, MAP4, Fp9-3, MAP5, FRT7-1/2, and FRT7-2 in Fig. 4a (blue p-values below the bars) and to MAP2v, FRT3-3/4, FRT3-4, Fp14-4, and IWV in Fig. 4b (blue p-values below the bars).

5. **Figure 2c vs. Fig. 4c:** In the previous Fig. 2c, the lower negative bars were not shown to be consistent with the IL-2 and IFNγ results where all were subtracted with the average of the control cats for each stimulant. Figure 4c displays Fig. 2c with the negative values upon subtraction of the average of the control cats for each stimulant. Figure 4c clearly demonstrated that each IL-10 response should not be subtracted with the average value of the control cat group nor with their media control. This conclusion is based on the high spontaneous release in each media control of the vaccinated and the control cats.

6. **Figure 4c:** However, upon subtraction of the average of the IL-10 responses from the control cats (Fig. 4c), all IL-10 responses displayed a significant decrease when compared to the media controls. This observation indicated that the IL-10 responses of the control cats may be similar to the responses made by the vaccinated cats. Hence, the vaccination did not significantly enhance or suppress the FIV MAP/peptide-specific IL-10 expression of the vaccinated cats.

7. **Figure 5:** Since FIV MAP/peptide-specific IL-2 and IFNγ responses were observed in the ELISpot assays, the next study indirectly determined whether T cells specifically the CD3+CD4+ and the CD3+CD8+ T cells in the CFSE-proliferation assay were responding to the similar FIV stimulants as those from the IL-2 and IFNγ ELISpot assays (Fig. 5). Four FIV stimulants (MAP2v, FRT7-1/2, FRT7-1, FRT7-2) were significantly elevated in CD4+ T-cell proliferation when compared to the control cats (Fig. 5a). However, no significant CD8+ T-cell proliferation was observed to all FIV stimulants except for MAP2v (Fig. 5b). The possibility existed that the T-cell proliferation of CFSE assay may be less sensitive than the ELISpot assay. CFSE proliferation is affected by the affinity of the selected T-cell antibodies as well as by the length of stimulation (3–6 days). The post-third vaccination results of the CFSE proliferation could determine if the T-cell proliferation is somewhat delayed in their responses to FIV stimulants.

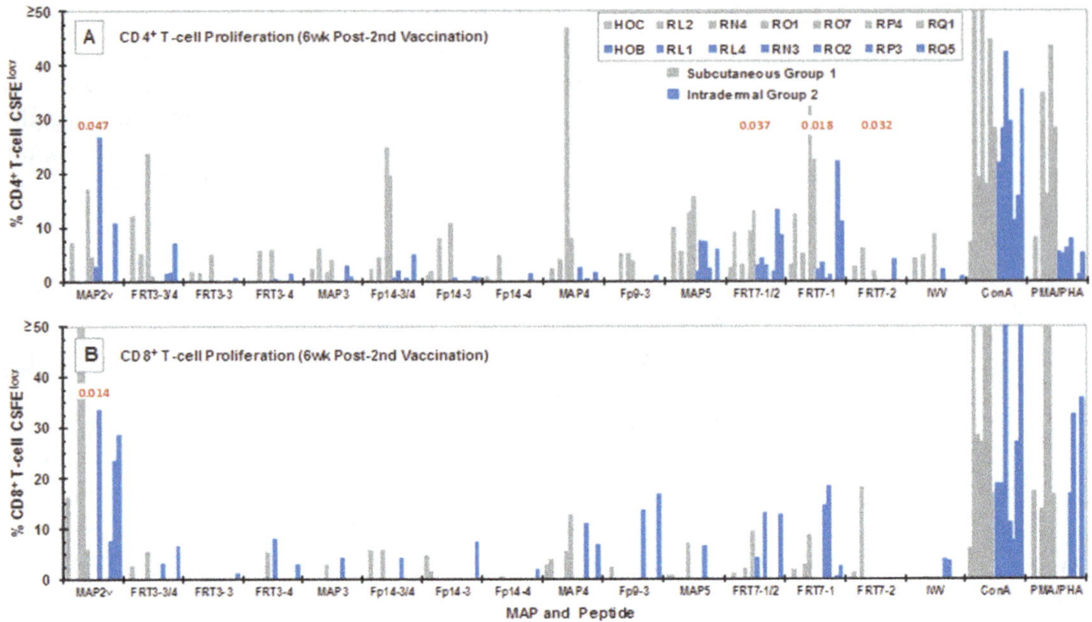

Fig. 5 FIV MAP/peptide-specific T-cell proliferation of the PBMC from vaccinated cats at 6 weeks post-second vaccination. The CD4⁺ (**a**) and the CD8⁺ (**b**) T-cell proliferation of the PBMC from vaccinated cats are shown with the subcutaneous vaccine group 1 in grey bars and with the intradermal vaccine group 2 in blue bars. The *p*-value (*t*-test) on the top of the bars of the vaccine group represents significant increase in proliferation when compared to the non-vaccinated control group. Hence, the CD4⁺ T-cell proliferation to MAP2v, FRT7-1/2, FRT7-1, and FRT7-2 are significantly elevated when compared to those of the control group, whereas the CD8⁺ T-cell proliferation to MAP2v is the only FIV stimulant with significant elevation compared to that of the control group

3.2 Post-Third Vaccination

1. **Figure 2a vs. Fig. 6a:** After the third vaccination, a potential IL-2 memory response of the vaccine groups was observed only to FRT3-4 and a little to MAP3 (Fig. 2a vs. Fig. 6a). Those previously detected IL-2 responses to six peptides (FRT3-3/4, FRT3-3, F14-3/4, FRT7-1/2, FRT7-1, FRT7-2 of Fig. 2) and to MAP2v were minimal to undetectable after the third vaccination (Fig. 2a vs. Fig. 6a). When compared to post-second vaccination, major IFNγ memory responses to FRT3-3/4, FRT3-4, MAP3, Fp14-3/4, and Fp14-3 were observed.

2. **Figure 2b vs. Fig. 6b:** However, IFNγ responses to MAP5, FRT7-1, and FRT7-2 were minimal to undetectable after the third vaccination (Fig. 2b vs. Fig. 6b). Such loss in IL-2 and IFNγ responses was not caused by the loss of MAP/peptide activities.

3. **Figure 7a:** In fact, five of the six FIV stimulants (FRT3-3/4, FRT14-3/4, FRT7-1/2, FRT-7-1, FRT7-2), which gave rise to low or undetectable in IL-2 responses after the third vaccination, stimulated CD4⁺ T-cell proliferation after the third vaccination (Fig. 7a). In addition, the IFNγ responses to

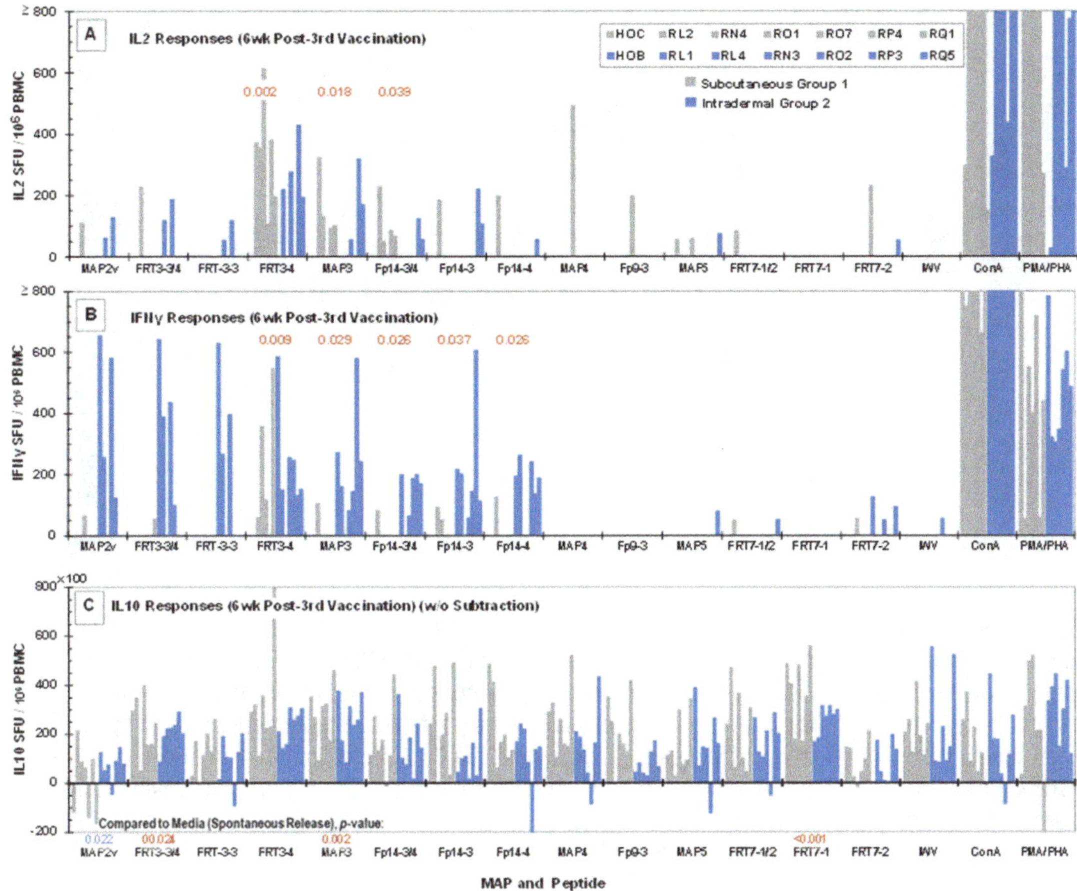

Fig. 6 IL2, IFNγ, and IL10 responses of MAP-vaccinated cats at 6 weeks post-third vaccination. The IL2 (**a**), IFNγ (**b**), and IL10 (**c**) responses were after the in vitro stimulation of the PBMC from vaccinated cats with FIV MAPs and peptides. One set of seven cats was subcutaneously vaccinated with the MAP vaccine (grey bars), and another set of seven was intradermally vaccinated with MAP vaccine (blue bars). Each bar for the IL2 (**a**) and the IFNγ (**b**) responses represents the value after the subtraction of the average value of the results from the nine control cats, with the exception of the mitogens (ConA and PMA/PHA). Each bar for the IL10 responses (**c**) represents the value without any subtractions. The results for the mitogens (**a–c**) are shown without any subtraction. The *p*-value (*t*-test) in red above the bar(s) for the FIV stimulant indicates that the results from the combined vaccine group were significantly elevated in response to the corresponding FIV stimulant when compared to the results from the control cat group. The *p*-values on the bottom of the bars represent the statistical comparison between combined vaccine group and their media controls. The *p*-values in red represent significant increase or elevation, whereas those in blue represent significant decrease or suppression

MAP5, FRT7-1, and FRT7-2 in the vaccinated cats were minimal to undetectable after the third vaccination; however, they stimulated CD4⁺ T-cell proliferation after the third vaccination. Hence, the activity of the FIV stimulants was intact.

4. **Figure 7a vs. b**: More importantly when compared to the control group, significant CD4⁺ T-cell proliferation was observed to nine FIV MAPs/peptides, resulting in additional

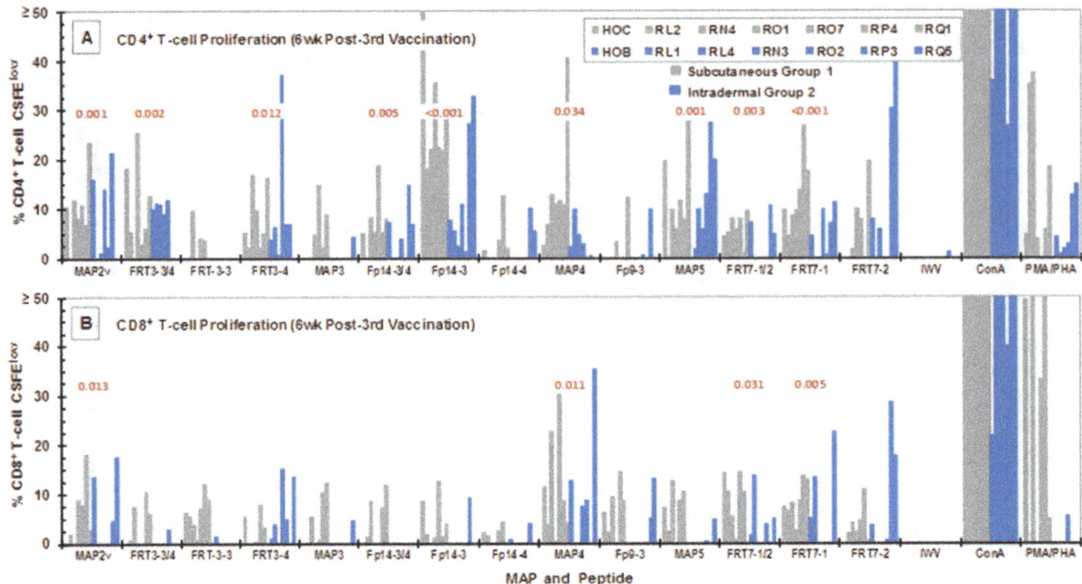

Fig. 7 FIV MAP/peptide-specific T-cell proliferation of the PBMC from vaccinated cats at 6 weeks post-second vaccination. The CD4+ (**a**) and the CD8+ (**b**) T-cell proliferation of the PBMC from vaccinated cats are shown with the subcutaneous vaccine group 1 in grey bars and with the intradermal vaccine group 2 in blue bars. The *p*-value (*t*-test) on the top of the bars of the vaccine group represents a significant increase in proliferation when compared to the non-vaccinated control group. Hence, the CD4+ T-cell proliferation to MAP2v, FRT3-3/4, FRT3-4, Fp14-3/4, Fp14-3, MAP4, MAP5, FRT7-1/2, and FRT7-1 are significantly elevated when compared to those of the control group, whereas the CD8+ T-cell proliferation to MAP2v, MAP4, FRT7-1/2, and FRT7-1 are significantly elevated when compared to those of the control group

five FIV stimulants with significant CD4+ T-cell proliferation after the third vaccination (Fig. 7a). Furthermore, after the third vaccination significantly more CD8+ T-cell proliferation responses were observed to several MAPs and peptides compared to post-second vaccination (Fig. 7b). Overall, the significant increases in T-cell proliferation to nine MAP/peptides for CD4+ T cells and four MAPs/peptides for CD8+ T cells suggest memory responses to the T-cell proliferation augmented with additional vaccination.

5. **Figure 6c:** Remarkably, the IL-10 responses after the third vaccination were similar to the levels of control cats for each FIV stimulant (e.g., no statistical difference between vaccine group and control group) (Fig. 6c). Based on the IL-10 results from post-second vaccination, the IL-10 responses in the post-third vaccination are shown without any subtraction (Fig. 6c).

6. **Figure 8:** The spontaneous release of IL-10 was high (Fig. 8) in the control cats, and the release did not elevate post vaccination (Fig. 6c, no significant comparison to the control group).

7. **Summary on IL-10 (Figs. 4b and 6c):** The latter observation indicated lack of IL-10 memory responses to FIV MAPs/

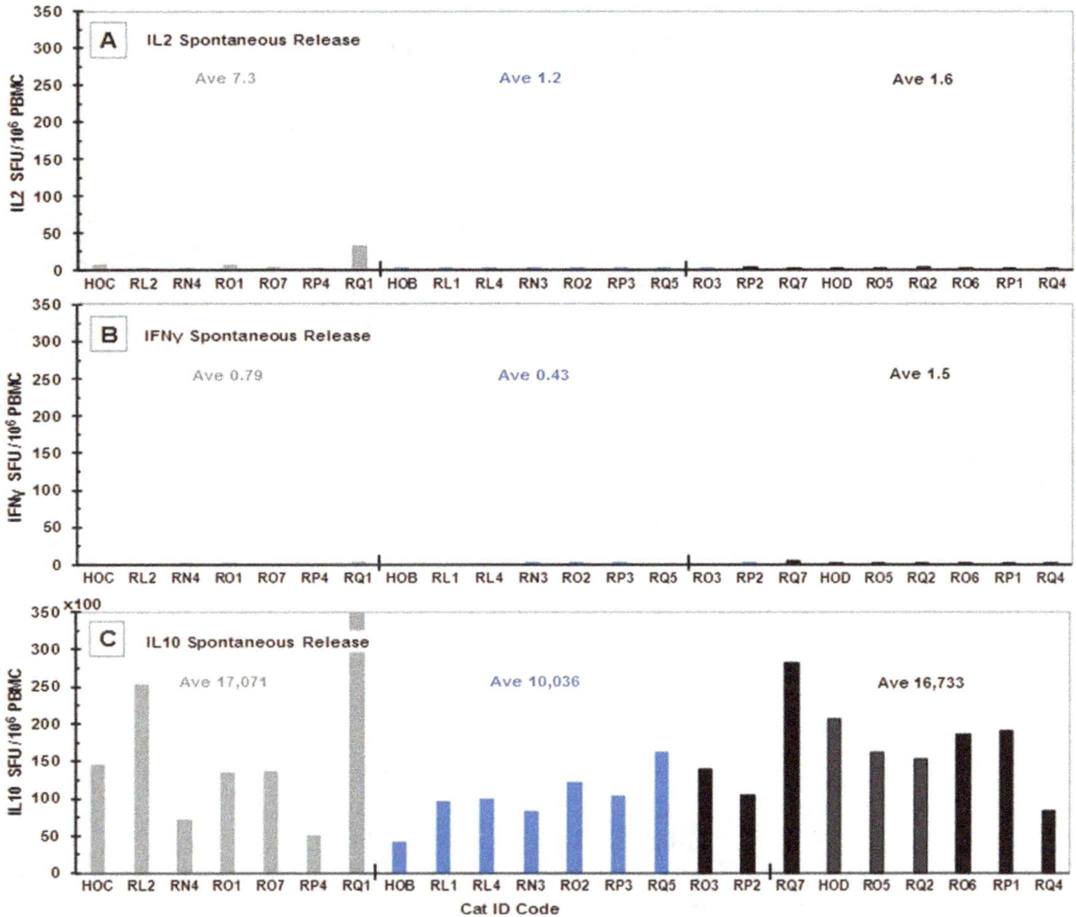

Fig. 8 Constitutive IL2, IFNγ, and IL10 production of the PBMC of vaccinated and non-vaccinated cats at post-third vaccination. The constitutive production or the spontaneous release of IL2 (**a**), IFNγ (**b**), and IL10 (**c**) are shown for the PBMC of the seven subcutaneous vaccinated cats (Vaccine Group 1, grey bars), seven intradermally vaccinated cats (Vaccine Group 2, blue bars), and nine non-vaccinated control cats (Control Group, black bars) at 6 weeks post-third vaccination. The average (ave) value of each group is shown above the bars of each group. Note that the magnitude of the IL10 spontaneous release is 2000-fold to 20,000-fold higher (see *y*-axis) than those of IL2 and IFNγ, respectively

peptides in the combined vaccine group. Instead, the vaccinated cats (Figs. 4b and 6c) were responding to the direct stimulation to those MAPs and peptides in a similar level as the control cats (data not shown for control cats). One FIV peptide of interest is the Fp7-1 that stimulates significant IL-10 production compared to the individual media control in the combined vaccine group (Figs. 4b and 6c) and the control group (data not shown for the control group) from both post-second and -third vaccinations. Conversely, MAP2v induced significant suppression of IL-10 production in the combined vaccine group of both post-second and -third vaccinations

(Figs. 4b and 6c) and control group from post-third vaccination (data not shown for control group).

8. **Conclusion**: Current results demonstrate that FIV MAP vaccine induces substantial IL-2 and IFNγ memory responses to the MAPs and peptides most likely by the T cells in the vaccinated cats. Both CD4+ and CD8+ T cells displayed potent memory proliferation responses to multiple MAPs and peptides after the third vaccination. Overall, current study demonstrates the valuable use of cytokine ELISpot assays to evaluate the specificity and the magnitude of cytokine production elicited by the vaccine MAPs and their peptides.

3.3 Isolation of Feline PBMC

1. A slight modification of manufacturer's protocol was used to isolate PBMC with lymphocyte separation medium (LSM). The commercial LSM is produced for human cell use and not optimized for feline cell use (*see* **Note 6**).

2. Briefly, the whole blood is diluted with an equal volume of HBSS, and 10–11 mL of diluted blood is layered on 3 mL of LSM in a sterile 15-mL conical culture tube. The tubes containing blood layered LSM are centrifuged at 500 × g for 20 min.

3. Only the PBMC band on the LSM layer is gently pipetted with minimal contamination of the liquid above the band and the LSM below. The collected PBMC preparation is diluted with an equal volume of HBSS and centrifuged at 450 × g for 10 min.

4. The fluid is discarded and the PBMC pellet is resuspended into 10 mL of HBSS, and centrifuged at 400 × g for 5 min. Repeat the final wash step at least 1× or 2× to remove platelet contamination before cell counting.

5. Once the number of cells needed for ELISpot and CFSE assays is determined based on the cell count, place appropriate numbers of PBMC into PBS (15-mL sterile conical tube) for CFSE assay (*see* below Subheading 3.5, **steps 2** and **3**) and resuspend the remaining PBMC into PBMC medium for ELISpot (*see* below Subheading 3.4, **step 5**).

3.4 Feline Cytokine ELISpot Analyses

1. 96-well PVDF membrane plates are primed by adding 30 μL of 35% ethanol in each well and incubating at room temperature for 60 s.

2. The wells are washed 3× with PBS (250 μL per well) using a multichannel pipette or plate washer if available (*see* **Note 7**). Remove any remaining PBS by inverting the plate and blotting it against a clean paper towel (*see* **Note 8**).

3. Once the plates are primed, immediately (*see* **Note 8**) add 100 μL of Capture Antibody Solution at 1:50 dilution to each well, cover, and incubate for at least 10 h at 2–8 °C.

4. Remove the Capture Antibody Solution from each well by aspirating or by inverting the plate and blotting it against a clean paper towel, and then wash 3× with PBS (250 μL per well).

5. Block the membranes by adding 250 μL of blocking buffer to each well, and incubate the plates for 2 h at 37 °C.

6. The blocking buffer is removed by aspiration or by inverting the plates. Subsequently, the wells are washed 1× with AIM-V diluent.

7. AIM-V diluent (50 μL) is added to each well and kept at room temperature until addition of antigen (i.e., stimulant) and PBMC.

8. Each antigen or stimulant (peptide, MAP, inactivated IWV, mitogen) is diluted with AIM-V diluent, and the negative control consisting of diluent alone (without any stimulant) serves as a control for spontaneous release of the cytokine by PBMC (*see* **Note 9**).

9. A total volume of 50 μL per well of each FIV peptide or MAP at 40 μg/mL, IWV at 80 μg/mL, PHA at 20 μg/mL, ConA at 16 μg/mL, PMA at 1 μg/mL, PMA/PHA combination at 0.2 μg PMA plus 4.0 μg PHA per mL, and diluent (AIM-V® medium with gentamicin) was added to 50 μL of AIM-V diluent previously added to the wells to prevent drying (*see* **Note 10**). Each antigen/stimulant or diluent control should have at least duplicate wells. Thus, the final volume per well at this point will be 100 μL.

10. PBMC (100 μL) is added at a concentration of 2.5×10^6 PBMC per mL in PBMC medium for IL-2 and IFNγ ELISpot, and 1×10^5 PBMC per mL for IL-10 ELISpot (*see* **Note 11**). The final volume per well with PBMC/stimulant is 200 μL.

11. Incubate the covered plates for 14–24 h at 37 °C in 5% CO_2 (*see* **Note 12**).

12. The wells are washed 5× with PBS (250 μL per well). After the final wash, remove any remaining liquid by inverting the plate and blotting it against a clean paper towel.

13. Detection Antibody Solution (100 μL) is added at 1:50 dilution to each well and incubated for 12 h or overnight at 2–8 °C.

14. Remove the Detection Antibody Solution by inverting the plates. The wells are washed 5× with PBS (250 μL per well). After the final wash, remove any remaining liquid by inverting the plate and blotting it against a clean paper towel.

15. Streptavidin-AP solution (100 µL) is added to each well and incubated for 2 h at room temperature.

16. Wash the wells 5× with PBS (250 µL per well). After the final wash, remove any remaining liquid by inverting the plate and blotting it against a clean paper towel.

17. BCIP/NBT chromogen solution (100 µL) is added to each well, covered, and incubated for 30–45 min at room temperature in the dark by wrapping the plates in foil.

18. Rinse with deionized water. Invert plate and tap to remove excess water. Allow the plates to dry at room temperature or at 37 °C (~2 h).

19. Once the plates are fully developed and dried, the spots are quantitated by automatic ELISpot reader and photographs taken by the reader (*see* **Note 13**).

20. Following quantification, the average number of spots in the negative diluent controls is subtracted from all sample wells to determine the spot-forming units (SFU) (*see* **Note 14**) and typically reported as SFU per 10^6 PBMC. The average SFU per 10^6 PBMC of the duplicate wells that are >50 SFU per 10^6 PBMC is considered significant for IFNγ and IL-2 ELISpot. However, the data analysis of IL-10 is more difficult to interpret due to the high spontaneous release from feline PBMC as discussed in Subheading 3.1 before the detailed methods of the assays (Fig. 4).

3.5 Feline CFSE-Proliferation Analysis

1. Reconstitute carboxyfluorescein diacetate succinimidyl ester (CFSE) in 90 mL of DMSO and then dilute in sterile PBS at 2 µL CFSE to 50 mL PBS. Warm the CFSE solution at 37 °C immediately before the addition of PBMC.

2. Calculate the number of cells needed per assay as follows: 2.5×10^5 to 5.0×10^5 PBMC per well multiplied by the number of wells per assay. Then, centrifuge ($500 \times g$ for 5 min) to remove PBS from the calculated number of PBMC.

3. Resuspend the PBMC pellet with warm CFSE solution at 1×10^6 PBMC per mL (15-mL sterile conical tube).

4. Incubate CFSE solution with PBMC for 15 min at 37 °C.

5. Centrifuge the CFSE-labeled PBMC for 5 min at $500 \times g$, decant the supernatant, and add an equal volume of warm (37 °C) AIM-V diluent to the CFSE-labeled PBMC pellet.

6. Incubate for 30 min at 37 °C to allow CFSE to leach from the PBMC.

7. Centrifuge the CFSE-labeled PBMC for 5 min at $500 \times g$ to remove free CFSE.

8. Decant and resuspend the CFSE-labeled PBMC with 10 mL of warm (37 °C) PBS.

9. Centrifuge the CFSE-labeled PBMC for 5 min at $500 \times g$ and decant the PBS and resuspend the PBMC at 1.67×10^6 PBMC per mL in PBMC medium for CFSE assay.

10. Plate 300 μL of stimulant in AIM-V diluent in 96-well plate. This procedure should be performed for each stimulant: 300 μL of stimulant at concentrations of FIV peptide or MAP at 40 μg/mL, IWV at 40 μg/mL, PHA at 20 μg/mL, ConA at 4 μg/mL, PMA/PHA combination at 0.1 μg PMA/2 μg PHA per mL, and AIM-V diluent as a negative control (*see* **Note 15**).

11. Add 300 μL of PBMC to each well and incubate the plate in 5% CO_2-incubator for 5 days at 37 °C.

12. Collect the CFSE-labeled PBMC from each well into a 1-mL microfuge tube and centrifuge for 5 min at $500 \times g$.

13. Decant the fluid and resuspend the PBMC in 250 μL PBS and centrifuge for 5 min at $500 \times g$.

14. Meanwhile reconstitute the Live/Dead reagent in 50 μL DMSO, calculate the volume of this reagent needed (250 μL per tube), and dilute 1 μL per mL of Live/Dead reagent in PBS.

15. Resuspend each stimulant and CFSE-labeled PBMC with 250 μL of Live/Dead reagent solution in the microfuge tube and incubate for 30 min at room temperature.

16. Decant the fluid and wash twice with 250 μL PBS.

17. Decant and add 50 μL of FACS buffer containing MAbs to CD3-APC, CD4-PE, and CD8-PE/Cy7 (concentration, *see* **Note 16**).

18. Incubate 30 min at room temperature and wash the PBMC once with 250 μL PBS.

19. Resuspend the PBMC pellet in 50 μL of FACS buffer and perform FACS analysis within 18 h.

---

4   Notes

1. Montanide® ISA 720 VG adjuvant (SEPPIC Inc., Fairfield, NJ) and Ribi adjuvant (Corixa Corporation, Hamilton, MT) can be used safely in cats in place of FD-1 adjuvant, but vaccines formulated with these adjuvants may not induce T-cell responses to FIV antigen in cat to the level detected when vaccine is formulated with FD-1 adjuvant.

2. These reagents should be filter sterilized with a 0.2-μm filter before use.

3. These reagents should be stored at 2–8 °C with caution not to freeze.

4. Both labeled and unlabeled MAb to feline CD8 can be purchased (SouthernBiotech) and rabbit polyclonal antibodies cross-reactive with feline CD3epsilon for FACS usage can be purchased (Novus Biologicals LLC, Littleton CO).

5. PHA is a strong T-cell mitogen for human T cells but not for feline T cells.

6. Feline PBMC prepared by commercial LSM has more neutrophil contamination than similarly prepared human PBMC.

7. Be careful not to damage the membranes during washing.

8. Do not dry the plates before the Capture Antibody Solution is ready.

9. High levels of IL-10 are spontaneously released by PBMC even without stimulant.

10. The concentration of the working solutions for each stimulant is fourfold higher than the final concentration in the well and thus the final concentrations are FIV peptide (10 μg/mL), MAP (10 μg/mL), IWV (20 μg/mL), PHA (5 μg/mL), ConA (4 μg/mL), PMA (0.25 μg/mL), and PMA/PHA (0.05 μg/1 μg/mL).

11. The final volume after addition of antigen and PBMC is 200 μL per well, and the final cell number per well is 2.5×10^5 PBMC for IFNγ and IL-2 ELISpot, and 1×10^4 PBMC for IL-10 ELISpot.

12. Care should be taken not to move, bump, or expose plates to vibrations that may cause the cells to move, as the assay is dependent on cells remaining in place to create a "spot."

13. Automatic readers are quick and able to read each well with the same thresholds and algorithms enhancing consistency. When using an automatic reader, it is imperative to set the thresholds and check spot numbers for each plate or assay to avoid underestimating or overestimating spots. Automatic readers often have problems with artifacts if threads or dust get in the wells; however, built-in algorithms attempt to detect gradients in the spots to distinguish between artifacts and true "spots" as well as subdividing coalescing spots.

14. Each SFU is considered to represent a single cell secreting the cytokine. The SFUs in the positive controls often coalesce and make enumerating individual spots difficult or impossible.

15. The final concentration of some stimulants for CFSE assay is generally higher than those used for the ELISpot assay in

Note 10. In the CFSE assay, the final concentrations in total volume of 0.6 mL (600 μL) per well are FIV peptide (20 μg/mL), MAP (20 μg/mL), IWV (20 μg/mL), PHA (10 μg/mL), ConA (4 μg/mL), and PMA/PHA (0.1 μg/2 μg/mL).

16. Concentration of each of these MAbs feline markers is dependent on the source and should be pretested by titration with feline PBMC by FACS analysis before use in CFSE assay.

Acknowledgment

This work was supported by JKY Miscellaneous Donors Fund. We thank Dr. Ruiyu Pu for his technical assistance. J.K.Y. is the inventor of record on a patent held by the University of Florida and may be entitled to royalties from companies developing commercial products related to the research described in this chapter.

References

1. Rerks-Ngarm S, Pitisuttithum P, Nitayaphan S, Kaewkungwal J, Chiu J, Paris R et al (2009) Vaccination with ALVAC and AIDSVAX to prevent HIV-1 infection in Thailand. N Engl J Med 361:2209–2220

2. Sanou MP, Roff SR, Mennella A, Sleasman JW, Rathore MH, Yamamoto JK et al (2013) Evolutionarily conserved epitopes on human immunodeficiency virus type 1 (HIV-1) and feline immunodeficiency virus reverse transcriptases detected by HIV-1-infected subjects. J Virol 87:10004–10015

3. Roff SR, Sanou MP, Rathore MH, Levy JA, Yamamoto JK (2015) Conserved epitopes on HIV-1, FIV and SIV p24 proteins are recognized by HIV-1 infected subjects. Hum Vaccin Immunother 11:1540–1556

4. Uhl EW, Martin M, Coleman JK, Yamamoto JK (2008) Advances in FIV vaccine technology. Vet Immunol Immunopathol 123:65–80

5. Abbas AK, Lichtman AH, Pillai S (2015) Cellular and molecular immunology, 8th edn. Elsevier, Philadelphia, PA, pp 51–84. 199–229, 231-238, 493-501.

6. Schoenborn JR, Wilson CB (2007) Regulation of interferon-gamma during innate and adaptive immune responses. Adv Immunol 96:41–101

7. Smith KA (2001) IL-2. In: Oppenheim J, Feldmann M (eds) Cytokine reference, Volume 1: Ligands. Academic Press, San Diego, CA, pp 113–125

8. Taniguchi T, Matsui H, Fujita T, Takaoka C, Kashima N, Yoshimoto R et al (1983) Structure and expression of a cloned cDNA for human interleukin-2. Nature 302:305–310

9. Hagiwara E, Abbasi F, Mor G, Ishigatsubo Y, Klinman DM (1995) Phenotype and frequency of cells secreting IL-2, IL-4, IL-6, IL-10, IFN and TNF-alpha in human peripheral blood. Cytokine 7:815–822

10. Barrett L, Dai C, Gamberg J, Gallant M, Grant M (2007) Circulating CD14⁻CD36⁺ peripheral blood mononuclear cells constitutively produce interleukin-10. J Leukoc Biol 82:52–160. (Note that CD14⁻CD36⁺ PBMC is considered to be macrophages and monocytes [5].).

11. Rutz S, Ouyang W (2016) Regulation of interleukin-10 expression. Adv Exp Med Biol 941:89–116

12. Sabat R, Grütz G, Warszawska K, Kirsch S, Witte E, Wolk K et al (2010) Biology of interleukin-10. Cytokine Growth Factor Rev 21:331–344

13. Hunter RL (2002) Overview of vaccine adjuvants: present and future. Vaccine 20(Suppl. 3):S7–S12

14. Gołoś A, Lutyńska A (2015) Aluminium-adjuvanted vaccines--a review of the current state of knowledge. Przegl Epidemiol 69:731–734. 871-874.

15. Buchbinder SP, Mehrotra DV, Duerr A, Fitzgerald DW, Mogg R, Li D et al (2008) Efficacy assessment of a cell-mediated immunity HIV-1 vaccine (the Step Study): a double-blind, randomised, placebo-controlled, test-of-concept trial. Lancet 372:1881–1893

16. Abbott JR, Pu R, Coleman JK, Yamamoto JK (2012) Utilization of feline ELISPOT for mapping vaccine epitopes. Methods Mol Biol 792:47–63

17. Addo MM, Yu XG, Rathod A, Cohen D, Eldridge RL, Strick D et al (2003) Comprehensive epitope analysis of human immunodeficiency virus type 1 (HIV-1)-specific T-cell responses directed against the entire expressed HIV-1 genome demonstrate broadly directed responses, but no correlation to viral load. J Virol 77:2081–2092

18. Novitsky V, Rybak N, McLane MF, Gilbert P, Chigwedere P, Klein I et al (2001) Identification of human immunodeficiency virus type 1 subtype C Gag-, Tat-, Rev-, and Nef-specific elispot-based cytotoxic T-lymphocyte responses for AIDS vaccine design. J Virol 75:9210–9228

19. Lieberman J (2004) Tracking the killers: how should we measure CD8 T cells in HIV infection? AIDS 18:1489–1493

20. Streeck H, Frahm N, Walker BD (2009) The role of IFN-gamma Elispot assay in HIV vaccine research. Nat Protoc 4:461–469

21. Kuerten S, Nowacki TM, Kleen TO, Asaad RJ, Lehmann PV, Tary-Lehmann M (2008) Dissociated production of perforin, granzyme B, and IFN-gamma by HIV-specific CD8(+) cells in HIV infection. AIDS Res Hum Retroviruses 24:62–71

22. Soghoian DZ, Jessen H, Flanders M, Sierra-Davidson K, Cutler S, Pertel T et al (2012) HIV-specific cytolytic CD4 T cell responses during acute HIV infection predict disease outcome. Sci Transl Med 4:123ra25

23. de Souza MS, Ratto-Kim S, Chuenarom W, Schuetz A, Chantakulkij S, Nuntapinit B et al (2012) The Thai phase III trial (RV144) vaccine regimen induces T cell responses that preferentially target epitopes within the V2 region of HIV-1 envelope. J Immunol 188:5166–5176

24. Makedonas G, Betts MR (2006) Polyfunctional analysis of human t cell responses: importance in vaccine immunogenicity and natural infection. Springer Semin Immunopathol 28:209–219

25. Aranyos AM, Roff SR, Pu R, Owen JL, Coleman JK, Yamamoto JK (2016) An initial examination of the potential role of T-cell immunity in protection against feline immunodeficiency virus (FIV) infection. Vaccine 34:1480–1488

26. O'Connell KA, Bailey JR, Blankson JN (2009) Elucidating the elite: mechanisms of control in HIV-1 infection. Trends Pharmacol Sci 30:631–637

27. Owen RE, Heitman JW, Hirschkorn DF, Lanteri MC, Biswas HH, Martin JN et al (2010) HIV+ elite controllers have low HIV-specific T-cell activation yet maintain strong, polyfunctional T-cell responses. AIDS 24:1095–1105

28. Hansen SG, Sacha JB, Hughes CM, Ford JC, Burwitz BJ, Scholz I et al (2013) Cytomegalovirus vectors violate CD8+ T cell epitope recognition paradigms. Science 340:1237874

29. Uhl EW, Heaton-Jones TG, Pu R, Yamamoto JK (2002) FIV vaccine development and its importance to veterinary and human medicine: a review FIV vaccine 2002 update and review. Vet Immunol Immunopathol 90:113–132

30. Omori M, Pu R, Tanabe T, Hou W, Coleman JK, Arai M et al (2004) Cellular immune responses to feline immunodeficiency virus (FIV) induced by dual-subtype FIV vaccine. Vaccine 23:386–398

31. Zhang J, Yang JM, Wang HJ, Ru GQ, Fan DM (2013) Synthesized multiple antigenic polypeptide vaccine based on B-cell epitopes of human heparanase could elicit a potent anti-metastatic effect on human hepatocellular carcinoma in vivo. PLoS One 8:e52940

32. Zhao G, Sun S, Du L, Xiao W, Ru Z, Kou Z et al (2010) An H5N1 M2e-based multiple antigenic peptide vaccine confers heterosubtypic protection from lethal infection with pandemic 2009 H1N1 virus. Virol J 7:151

33. Amexis G, Young NS (2007) Multiple antigenic peptides as vaccine platform for the induction of humoral responses against dengue-2 virus. Viral Immunol 20:657–663

34. Mägerlein M, Hock D, Adermann K, Neidlein R, Forssmann WG, Strein K (1998) Production of sequence specific polyclonal antibodies to human parathyroid hormone 1-37 by immunization with multiple antigenic peptides. Arzneimittelforschung 48:783–787

35. Cruz LJ, Quintana D, Iglesias E, Garcia Y, Huerta V, Garay HE et al (2000) Immunogenicity comparison of a multiantigenic peptide bearing V3 sequences of the human immunodeficiency virus type 1 with TAB9 protein in mice. J Pept Sci 6:217–224

36. Moldovan I, Targoni O, Zhang W, Sundararaman S, Lehmann PV (2016) How frequently are predicted peptides actually recognized by CD8 cells? Cancer Immunol Immunother 65:847–855

37. Wessely-Szponder J, Szponder T, Bobowiec R (2017) Different activation of monocyte-derived macrophages by antimicrobial peptides at a titanium tibial implantation in rabbits. Res Vet Sci 115:201–210

38. Pantic JM, Mechkarska M, Lukic ML, Conlon JM (2014) Effects of tigerinin peptides on cytokine production by mouse peritoneal macrophages and spleen cells and by human peripheral blood mononuclear cells. Biochimie 101:83–92

39. Bangert M, Wright AK, Rylance J, Kelly MJ, Wright AD, Carlone GM et al (2013) Immunoactivating peptide p4 augments alveolar macrophage phagocytosis in two diverse human populations. Antimicrob Agents Chemother 57:4566–4569

Detection and Quantification of Influenza A/H1N1 Virus-Specific Memory B Cells in Human PBMCs Using ELISpot Assay

Iana H. Haralambieva, Inna G. Ovsyannikova, Richard B. Kennedy, and Gregory A. Poland

Abstract

Immune response following subsequent encounter of viruses (and vaccines) relies largely on the pool and frequencies of antigen-specific memory B cells. In addition to antibody titers, the reliable measurement of these cells in human blood (peripheral blood mononuclear cells/PBMCs or purified B cells) provides valuable information on the preparedness of the adaptive immune system to respond to infection or vaccines, and potentially supports the discovery of new quantitative correlates of protection. The Mayo Clinic Vaccine Research Group has developed and optimized a high-throughput ELISPOT-based assay for the quantification of influenza A/H1N1 virus-specific memory B cells in human PBMCs. Here, we present the materials and detailed methodology for using this assay on cryopreserved cells for the measurement of recall humoral immunity readiness (antigen-specific memory B cell frequencies) after influenza vaccination. This assay could be readily adapted to other influenza virus strains and other respiratory viruses and vaccines for use in systems biology and larger population-based studies.

Key words B cell ELISPOT, Influenza A/H1N1 virus, Influenza vaccine, PBMCs, Humoral immunity

1 Introduction

Seasonal influenza causes significant morbidity and mortality in the United States and worldwide. It is estimated that between 3000 and 49,000 Americans die of influenza annually [1]; many more suffer from influenza-related complications and undergo hospitalization with an annual cost of >$90 billion in the United States alone [2]. Influenza can be prevented through annual seasonal influenza vaccination with antigenically matched strains/antigens. Considering the significant public health impact of the disease, it is essential to monitor influenza vaccine-induced immunity and identify additional correlates of protective immunity. Previous studies in humans have demonstrated the importance of activated influenza

Alexander E. Kalyuzhny (ed.), *Handbook of ELISPOT: Methods and Protocols*, Methods in Molecular Biology, vol. 1808, https://doi.org/10.1007/978-1-4939-8567-8_19, © Springer Science+Business Media, LLC, part of Springer Nature 2018

virus-specific memory B cells—specific for conserved epitopes—as a source of influenza A virus subtype H1N1-specific plasmablasts for production of broadly cross-reactive and protective neutralizing antibodies in the course of infection [3]. Similarly, the humoral immune response to the pandemic influenza A/H1N1 vaccine has been shown to be largely a recall response derived from cross-reactive memory B cells in vaccinated individuals [4]. While the currently accepted correlate of protection from influenza relies on the measurement of hemagglutination-inhibition (HAI) antibody titers [5], it is apparent that reliable methods for quantification of influenza virus-specific memory B cells after infection/vaccination are also needed for in-depth assessment of influenza-specific humoral immunity. The Mayo Clinic Vaccine Research Group has developed and optimized an ELISPOT assay for the measurement of influenza A/H1N1-specific IgG-secreting memory B cells, using cryopreserved PBMCs, which has been used in a relatively large systems biology study to monitor influenza vaccine-induced humoral immunity in a cohort of older individuals [6]. The dynamics of influenza A/H1N1-specific memory B cell frequencies in the course of vaccination (Baseline, Day 3, Day 28, and Day 75) is depicted in Fig. 1 [7, 8].

Several strengths of this ELISPOT assay exist: it offers reliable and sensitive detection and quantification of influenza virus-specific IgG memory-like B cells; the method provides consistent information on a single-cell antigen-specific analyte (IgG) secretion; the method is readily applicable for high-throughput testing and immune monitoring in the course of vaccination and/or infection (and therefore is useful in systems biology and other vaccine studies); the method is economic and sample/cell sparing (uses PBMCs); the method uses cryopreserved cells and is convenient for use in larger studies, where the usage of fresh cells is not feasible; the method provides an additional correlate/surrogate of influenza-specific protective immunity; and the method can be modified for other viruses/vaccines. The main challenges are related to the reliable counting and interpretation of ELISPOT results, particularly when measurements are performed a long time after specific antigenic stimulation (vaccination). This is at least partially overcome by the use and availability of automated ELISPOT readers for scanning and counting, appropriate software, and stringent QA/QC procedures for data quality assessment. Another challenge is the use of cryopreserved cells, which necessitates the use of standardized procedures for sample collection, cell isolation, cryopreservation, and thawing of viable cells to avoid sample handling-related variation and assure consistency of results.

In conclusion, the described influenza virus-specific memory B cell ELISPOT method can be used for comprehensive assessment of humoral immunity in systems biology and other influenza

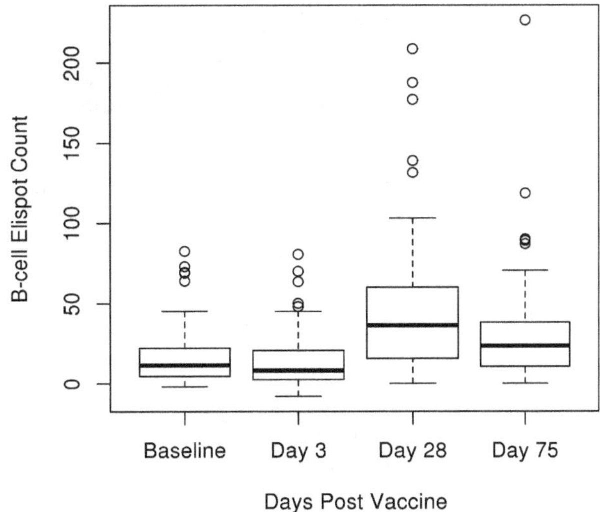

Fig. 1 Influenza A/H1N1-specific memory B cell response pre- and post-influenza vaccination. Figure 1 demonstrates the dynamics of influenza-specific memory B cell ELISPOT response after influenza vaccination (in a cohort of 106 healthy older adults, 50–74 years old) and has been previously published in Viral Immunology [7] and Plos One [8]. The top (bottom) of the box indicates the 75th (25th) percentiles, respectively, while the bold line within the box indicates the median. The "whiskers" extend up to 1.5 times the interquartile range above or below the 75th or 25th percentiles, respectively. Beyond that point, individual points are plotted. B cell ELISPOT counts representing the influenza A/H1N1-specific IgG-producing memory-like B cell response plotted for each timepoint as spot forming units (SFUs) per 2×10^5 PBMCs

vaccine studies to provide better insights into the development and maintenance of protective immunity after vaccination [7, 9–11].

We have previously published some of the materials and methods for this or other ELISPOT procedures [7, 8, 12–14].

2 Materials

2.1 Propagation and Harvesting of Influenza A/H1N1 Virus in Embryonated Eggs

1. 9–11-day-old Specific Pathogen-Free (SPF), fertile hen eggs (Charles River, Flock S23).

2. Penicillin-Streptomycin (10,000 U/mL).

3. Influenza virus stock ~1×10^3 TCID$_{50}$/mL: influenza A/California/7/2009/H1N1-like virus (Centers for Disease Control and Prevention, CDC, Atlanta, GA).

4. 70% ethanol.

5. Glue or melted paraffin.

6. 34–37 °C Egg incubator, 82% humidity.

7. Centrifuge.

8. Candling light.

9. Engraving tool or rotating drill.

10. Syringe with a 23 gauge 1 in. needle.

11. Sterile pointed scissors, forceps, spatula.

12. Lab supplies: 50 mL conical tubes, 1 mL cryovials, Pasteur pipettes or 5 mL pipettes, disinfecting solution.

2.2 Titration of Influenza A/H1N1 Virus

1. 1.6% agarose prepared by autoclaving or microwaving. Aliquots are pre-warmed in 56 °C water bath before use.

2. L15 medium: 100 mL 2× L15, 4 mL 1 M HEPES, 1 mL Penicillin-Streptomycin [×10], 1 mL of 200 mM Glutamine, 100 μL of 50 μg/mL Gentamycin, 2 mL $NaHCO_3$.

3. DMEM.

4. Dilution media: 3% bovine serum albumin (BSA)/DMEM.

5. Madin Darby Canine Kidney Cell line (MDCK) (ATCC #CCL-34; American Type Culture Collection, Manassas, VA, PTA-6500).

6. l-(tosylamido-2-phenyl)ethylchloromethylketone (TPCK)-treated trypsin (Sigma-Aldrich, St. Louis, MO).

2.3 Collection and Isolation of Peripheral Blood Mononuclear Cells (PBMCs)

1. HISTOPAQUE-1077 (Sigma).

2. Accuspin™ tube (Sigma).

3. 1× sterile PBS.

4. ACK lysis buffer (Invitrogen—Life Technologies, Carlsbad, CA).

5. Cell strainers (BD Falcon).

6. Trypan blue.

7. Hemocytometer.

8. RPMI freezing medium (RPMI 1640 with L-glutamine supplemented with 20% FCS and 10% DMSO).

9. 1.8 mL cryogenic freezing tubes.

2.4 Thawing of Cryopreserved PBMCs

1. 15 mL sterile conical centrifuge tubes.

2. RPMI culture medium supplemented with DNAse: RPMI 1640 with L-glutamine supplemented with 10% FCS, 100 U/mL penicillin-100 μg/mL streptomycin, 1 mM sodium pyruvate, 10 μg/mL DNase.

3. RPMI culture medium: RPMI 1640 with L-glutamine supplemented with 5% FCS, 100 U/mL penicillin-100 μg/mL streptomycin, and 1 mM sodium pyruvate.

4. Cell strainers (BD Falcon).

5. 50 mL sterile conical centrifuge tubes.

6. Trypan Blue.

7. 1× sterile PBS.

2.5 Resting PBMCs in the Presence of IL-2 and R848

1. 24-well sterile tissue culture plates.

2. Recombinant human IL-2 (rhIL-2) and R848 are provided as reagents for B cell pre-stimulation in the Mabtech ELIspot^PLUS kit for human IgG (Mebtech Inc., Cincinnati, OH).

3. RPMI culture medium: RPMI 1640 with L-glutamine, supplemented with 5% FCS, 100 U/mL penicillin-100 µg/mL streptomycin and 1 mM sodium pyruvate.

4. Trypan Blue.

5. 1× sterile PBS.

2.6 Coating of ELISPOT Plates

1. Millipore Immobilon-P-Membrane Multiscreen filter plate, cat. No. S2EM004M99.

2. Influenza virus stock (e.g., the influenza A/California/7/2009/H1N1-like strain, obtained from the Centers for Disease Control and Prevention, CDC, Atlanta, GA).

3. Anti-human total IgG capture antibody: mAb MT91/145 provided in the Mabtech ELIspot^PLUS kit for human IgG.

4. PBS, pH 7.4.

2.7 Human B Cell ELISPOT Assay Setup: Plating and Culture

1. Mabtech ELIspot^PLUS kit for human IgG (Mebtech Inc., Cincinnati, OH, product Code: 3850-2H).

2. RPMI culture medium: RPMI 1640 with L-glutamine supplemented with 5% FCS, 100 U/mL penicillin-100 µg/mL streptomycin, and 1 mM sodium pyruvate.

3. 0.25% Trypsin-EDTA.

4. Trypan Blue.

5. 1× sterile PBS.

6. Aluminum foil.

2.8 Assay Development

1. Mabtech ELIspot^PLUS kit for human IgG (Mebtech Inc., Cincinnati, OH, product Code: 3850-2H).

2. Tetramethylbenzidine (TMB) substrate solution.

3. Automated ELISPOT reader or stereomicroscope.

2.9 Determination of Memory B Cell Frequencies (in SFUs per 2 × 10^6 cells)

1. An automated scanning/counting on an ELISPOT reader: ImmunoSpot® S6Macro696 Analyzer (Cellular Technology Ltd., Cleveland, OH, USA) with the ImmunoSpot® version 5.1 software or manually using a stereomicroscope.

3   Methods

The following methods describe the steps required to detect and quantify influenza A/H1N1-specific memory B cells and total IgG-expressing B cells in human PBMCs.

3.1   Propagation and Harvesting of Influenza A/H1N1 Virus in Embryonated Eggs

1. Before receiving eggs, set egg incubator to proper temperature and humidity based on virus strain (for influenza A viruses: −37 °C with 82% humidity).

2. Incubate fertile hen eggs until they reach 9–11 days old; at this point, identify viable and fertile eggs using a candling light. Any unfertilized (or not viable) eggs are discarded.

3. Locate air sacs using the candling light and mark with "x" on the shell opposite the embryo location.

4. Wipe eggs with 70% ethanol.

5. Using an engraving tool (or rotating drill), make a hole in the shell on the "x" mark without going through the egg membranes.

6. Add 50 μL of 10,000 U/10 mg/mL Pen/Strep using a 23 gauge 1 in. needle.

7. Inject each egg with 100 μL of influenza virus into the allantoic sac. Needle should be inserted vertically or at a slight angle to its full length before inoculation.

8. Seal the hole with drop of white glue or melted paraffin.

9. Place eggs in incubator and incubate for desired length of time (e.g., 2 days for influenza A H1/H3 viruses).

10. After incubation, transfer eggs from incubator to 4 °C overnight or −20 °C for 20 min to kill embryos and achieve constriction of blood vessels.

11. Place the eggs in a biosafety hood. All remaining steps should be conducted in the biosafety hood.

12. Wipe eggs with 70% ethanol for the virus harvest.

13. Starting at the puncture hole, remove shell above the air sac with sterile scissors or sterile forceps.

14. Puncture membranes to access the allantoic fluid, using a sterile spatula (or a forceps) to hold down embryo. Remove clear allantoic fluid using a Pasteur pipette and transfer to a sterile 50 mL conical tube.

15. Place the egg contents and shell in a disinfecting solution.

16. After harvest, centrifuge allantoic fluid at $600 \times g$, 4 °C for 10 min.

17. Aliquot allantoic fluid into labeled cryovials and freeze at −80 °C. Thaw a vial and determine the virus titer in plaque forming units (PFU) per mL.

3.2 Titration of Influenza A/H1N1 Virus

All steps should be performed in a biosafety hood.

1. Grow MDCK cells in a 6-well plate (till 95–100% confluency).

2. Aspirate grown medium MDCK cell monolayers.

3. Wash cells twice with DMEM media.

4. Add 200 μL of virus dilutions (10–3 to 10–7 [or 10–2 to 10–6] in 3% BSA-DMEM dilution media). Include at least one well with PBS only as a cell "no virus" control.

5. Allow virus absorption for 1 h at 37 °C; rock/gently rotate the plate every 20 min to prevent cells from drying out.

6. After 1 h, remove the inoculum by aspiration and rinse the cells once with 0.5 mL DMEM.

7. Add 18 μL TPCK-Trypsin to L15/2×MEM medium and mix (for PR).

8. Mix L15/2×MEM/TPCK-Trypsin to pre-warmed 1.6% Agarose.

9. Quickly add 2 mL to each well. Allow agar to solidify in hood.

10. Invert plates and incubate them in 5% CO_2 incubator at 37 °C for 48–72 h.

11. To fix and stain cells, carefully remove agar plug from wells.

12. Add ~2 mL 70% ethanol to fix cells for 5–10 min.

13. Remove ethanol.

14. Add ~2 mL crystal violet solution to cover the bottom of the plate and stain for 30 min.

15. Wash once with water and air dry the plates.

16. The viral titer is a quantitative measurement of the biological activity of the harvested virus and is expressed as plaque forming units (PFU) per mL. To calculate the viral titer, count the number of well-isolated plaques, then use the following formula to determine the titer (PFU/mL) of your viral stock:

$$\frac{\#\,plaques}{d \times V} = PFU\,/\,mL$$

d = dilution factor

V = volume of diluted virus added to the well

3.3 Collection and Isolation of Peripheral Blood Mononuclear Cells (PBMCs)

The protocol is based on the manufacturer's procedure for separating PBMCs using Accuspin™ tubes and has been previously published [12]. Blood is collected in tubes treated with anticoagulant (heparin or EDTA) to prevent coagulation.

1. Warm HISTOPAQUE-1077 to room temperature using a 37 °C water bath. Keep HISTOPAQUE-1077 out of direct light.

2. Pipet 15 mL of HISTOPAQUE-1077 into the upper chamber of each Accuspin™ tube.

3. Centrifuge tubes at 800 × g for 30 s to move HISTOPAQUE-1077 into the lower chamber of the tube.

4. Gently pipette whole blood into the upper chamber of the tube (15–20 mL/tube, *see* **Note 1**).

5. Add sterile 1× PBS into the tube up to 45 mL.

6. Gently mix blood and PBS, being careful not to drive blood below the frit.

7. Centrifuge tubes at 1000 × g for 15 min at 25 °C with the centrifuge brake OFF.

8. After centrifugation, carefully remove approximately half of the plasma layer using a sterile Pasteur pipette. Do not disturb the buffy coat (white layer) of PBMCs located above the frit.

9. Using a sterile Pasteur pipette, carefully remove the layer of PBMCs (white hued layer directly above the frit) and transfer it to a 15 mL sterile conical centrifuge tube.

10. To wash cells, add 1× sterile PBS to PBMCs, bringing the volume of liquid in the 15 mL conical centrifuge tube up to the 10 mL mark.

11. Resuspend PBMCs by inverting the tube several times.

12. Centrifuge at 500 × g for 10 min at 25 °C with brake ON.

13. Remove supernatant without disturbing the cell pellet.

14. Add 5 mL of ACK lysis buffer to the cell pellet. Resuspend cells by pipetting cell suspension up and down.

15. Allow cells to incubate at room temperature for 5 min in the ACK lysis buffer.

16. Add 1× sterile PBS to the cells + ACK lysis buffer, to bring the volume of liquid in the 15 mL conical centrifuge tube up to the 10 mL mark.

17. Centrifuge at 500 × g for 10 min at 25 °C with brake ON.

18. Remove supernatant without disturbing the cell pellet, then resuspend pellet in 5 mL of 1× sterile PBS.

19. Place a cell strainer on top of a 50 mL conical centrifuge tube. Transfer the cell suspension from the 15 mL conical centrifuge tube to the 50 mL conical centrifuge through the cell strainer.

20. To count the number of live and dead cells, place 200 μL of 1× PBS, 37.5 μL of Trypan blue, and 12.5 μL of cell suspension into a 5 mL falcon tube; mix well, then fill a hemocytometer

with 10 μL of sample. Count and record the number of unstained (live) cells in the outer four quadrants of the hemocytometer.

21. Total number of cells = number of live cells/4 × 10,000 × 20 (dilution factor [250/12.5]) × total volume of cells (5 mL or pooled total).

22. Centrifuge cell suspension at 500 × g for 10 min at 25 °C with brake ON.

23. Adjust cell concentration to 1 × 10^7 cells/mL with cold (4 °C) RPMI freezing medium (*see* **Note 2**).

24. Aliquot 1 mL of cell suspension into prelabeled cryogenic freezing tubes.

25. Place cryogenic freezing tubes into a −80 °C freezer in a controlled-rate freezing container overnight.

26. Transfer cells into a liquid nitrogen storage tank for long-term storage (*see* **Note 3**).

3.4 Thawing of Cryopreserved PBMCs [12]

Our protocol for detection of influenza virus-specific IgG memory B Cells by ELISPOT is based on using cryopreserved PBMCs. This method allows testing of previously stored samples in larger batches (i.e., the method is more convenient for larger studies), thus minimizing assay drift/variability and batch effects. Alternatively, freshly isolated PBMCs can be also used in the ELISPOT assay.

1. Warm RPMI culture medium supplemented with DNAse in a 37 °C water bath for a minimum of 15 min.

2. Add 100 μL of RPMI culture medium supplemented with DNAse into a 15 mL conical centrifuge for each sample being thawed.

3. Remove one vial of PBMCs (cell concentration 1 × 10^7) for each sample from liquid nitrogen storage tank.

4. Rapidly thaw PBMCs stored in cryogenic freezing tubes using a 37 °C water bath by swirling the vial in the water bath until a small amount of ice remains.

5. Quickly wipe the vial with 70% ethanol and place in a sterile tissue culture hood.

6. Pipette each sample from the cryogenic freezing tube into a 15 mL conical centrifuge tube containing 100 μL of RPMI culture medium supplemented with DNAse.

7. Mix the cells and medium by gently shaking the 15 mL conical centrifuge tube.

8. Slowly add 500 μL of RPMI culture medium supplemented with DNAse while swirling the tube gently to mix the cells and medium together.

9. In 1 min, add double the amount (1 mL) of RPMI culture medium supplemented with DNAse to the cell suspension in the 15 mL conical centrifuge tube.

10. Continue adding double the amount of RPMI culture medium supplemented with DNAse every minute until the cell suspension reaches a final volume of 10 mL.

11. Cap each conical tube and invert it 5 times to mix the cells; do not vortex cell suspension.

12. Centrifuge at $300 \times g$ for 7 min at 25 °C with brake ON.

13. Remove supernatant, then resuspend cells in 10 mL of RPMI culture medium supplemented with DNAse.

14. Cap each conical tube and invert it five times to mix the cells; do not vortex cell suspension.

15. Incubate cells at 37 °C for 20 min by placing the 15 mL conical centrifuge tubes in a 37 °C water bath. Invert tubes once 10 min into the incubation period.

16. After 20-min incubation, place cells on ice for 7 min.

17. Centrifuge cells at $300 \times g$ for 7 min at 4 °C with brake ON.

18. Carefully remove all supernatant and resuspend cells in 1 mL of RPMI culture medium supplemented with 5% FCS.

19. Place a cell strainer on top of a 50 mL conical centrifuge tube. Transfer the cell suspension from the 15 mL conical centrifuge tube to the 50 mL conical centrifuge through the cell strainer (*see* **Note 4**).

20. To count the number of live and dead cells, place 200 µL of 1× PBS, 37.5 µL of Trypan blue, and 12.5 µL of cell suspension into a falcon tube. Mix well and fill a hemocytometer with 10 µL of sample. Count and record the number of unstained (live) cells in the outer four quadrants of the hemocytometer.

21. Total number of cells = Number of live cells/4 × 10,000 × 20 (dilution factor [250/12.5]) × total volume of cells (1 mL or pooled total).

22. Adjust the cell concentration to 2×10^6 cells/mL by adding RPMI culture medium supplemented with 5% FCS.

3.5 Resting PBMCs in the Presence of IL-2 and R848 (Nonspecific Stimulation of B Cells)

Antigen-specific memory B cells have low frequencies; this is particularly true if quantification is performed years after vaccination/infection. For this reason, protocols for their quantification via ELISPOT assay rely on in vitro nonspecific pre-stimulation of B cells to promote activation of memory B cells, cell proliferation, and to increase cell viability (if cryopreserved cells are used). Multiple stimulants have been commonly used in human vaccine studies, including CpG, pokeweed mitogen (PWM), and *Staphylococcus aureus* Cowan, but one of the most efficient combinations for memory B cell pre-stimulation reported was a combination including the Toll-like receptor (TLR) agonist R848 and recombinant human Interleukin (IL)-2 (rhIL-2) [15]. The use of this combination is also recommended as per the manufacturer's specifications for the Mabtech ELIspot^{PLUS} kit for human IgG. Note that rhIL-2 and R848 are provided as reagents in the above kit.

1. Add 2 mL of PBMC suspension in RPMI with 5% FCS (from a concentration of 2×10^6 cells/mL) into each well of a 24-well sterile tissue culture plate (final 4×10^6 cells/well) (*see* **Note 5**).

2. Add 20 μL of rhIL-2 to each well to obtain 10 ng/mL concentration (*see* **Note 6**).

3. Add R848 at 1 μg/mL (i.e., add 2 μL of R848 to each well of 2 mL).

4. Incubate plate with cells at 37 °C in a 5% CO_2 humidified incubator for 72 h.

3.6 Coating of ELISPOT Plates

The antigen coating of plates should be performed the day before assay setup.

1. Dilute the available influenza virus stock (e.g., influenza A/ H1N1 virus stock with a titer 5×10^6 PFF/mL) at 1/10 (optimal coating is achieved with 50,000 PFUs per well) in phosphate-buffered saline (PBS, pH 7.4).

2. Dilute the anti-human total IgG capture mAb MT91/145 at 15 μg/mL (optimal coating is achieved with 1.5 μg per well; for antibody concentration/dilution, please refer also to the insert of the Mabtech ELIspot^{PLUS} kit for human IgG).

3. Coat the wells of a Millipore Immobilon-P-Membrane multi-screen filter (PVDF) plate with the diluted antigens at 100 μL/ well. Include one control well coated with PBS, pH 7.4 only, to represent a subject-specific background measure (negative control).

4. Seal the plate with appropriate plate sealer and incubate overnight at 4 °C.

3.7 Human B Cell ELISPOT Assay Setup: Plating and Culture

1. After the pre-stimulation step, remove medium from wells and pool all media/cells from one subject into a single 15 mL conical centrifuge tube (or one 50 mL tube if more cells).

2. Add 0.5 mL of pre-warmed (*see* **Note 7**) 0.25% Trypsin-EDTA to each well.

3. Place plate at 37 °C in a 5% CO_2 humidified incubator for ~10 min until cells detach. Confirm detachment using a microscope.

4. Remove cells/trypsin suspension from each well and add to the corresponding 15 mL conical centrifuge tube that contains medium/cells harvested from the same wells.

5. Repeat the procedure. Add another 0.5 mL of pre-warmed 0.25% Trypsin-EDTA to each well, incubate plate for 10 min at 37 °C in a 5% CO_2 humidified incubator, and harvest the cells/trypsin suspension.

6. Add 0.5 mL of RPMI culture medium supplemented with 5% FCS to each well and mix by pipetting up and down. Pool suspension from each well and add to the corresponding 15 mL conical centrifuge tube that contains cells harvested from the same well/wells (subject).

7. Bring the volume of each 15 mL conical centrifuge tube up to 10 mL by adding RPMI culture medium supplemented with 5% FCS.

8. Centrifuge cells at 300 × g for 7 min at 4 °C with the centrifuge brake ON.

9. Remove supernatant without disturbing the cell pellet, then resuspend cell pellet in 0.5 mL of RPMI culture medium supplemented with 5% FCS. Keep cells on ice.

10. Count the number of live and dead cells by placing 200 μL of 1× PBS, 37.5 μL of Trypan blue, and 12.5 μL of cell suspension into a falcon tube. Mix well and fill a hemocytometer with 10 μL of sample. Count and record the number of unstained (live) cells in the outer four quadrants of the hemocytometer.

11. Total number of cells = Number of live cells/4 × 10,000 × 20 (dilution factor [250/12.5]) × total volume of cells (0.5 mL).

12. Adjust the cells to the desired concentration (2 × 10^6 cells/mL) by adding RPMI culture medium supplemented with 5% FCS (*see* **Note 8**).

13. Keep cells on ice until they are ready to be plated (*see* **Note 9**).

14. One hour before plating the cells, remove the **pre-coated** B cell ELISPOT plate from 4 °C (cold room) in order to perform the blocking step.

15. For the blocking step, first discard the coating reagents. Wash 5× with sterile PBS (250 μL/well) to remove excess antibody/coating reagents. Add 200 μL/well blocking solution (RPMI with 10% FCS) and incubate for 1 h at room temperature (in a biosafety hood).

16. Remove the blocking solution and pat the plate dry on paper towels until there is no media remaining in the ELISPOT plate (in a biosafety hood).

17. Add aliquots of cells (200,000 cells/well) from 2 × 10^6 cells/mL cell suspension into influenza virus-coated wells (e.g., four

wells per subject) and into the empty (no antigen) cell control (one well) (*see* **Notes 8** and **10**).

18. Perform 1:10 additional dilution of the cell suspension by adding 900 µL of media to 100 µL of cells. Add 50 µL cells (10,000 cells/well) into the total IgG-coated wells (e.g., three wells per subject). Add 50 µL of media (RPMI with 5% FCS) in the total IgG-coated wells to bring volume to 100 µL per well (*see* **Notes 8** and **10**).

19. Cover the plate with aluminum foil and place in 5% CO_2 incubator at 37 °C for 20 h. Do not disturb the cells during the incubation period (*see* **Note 11**).

3.8 Assay Development (see Note 12)

1. For assay development, please refer also to the manufacturer's protocol (Mabtech).

2. After the 20-h incubation, remove the media from the ELISPOT plate.

3. Using a 50–300 µL multichannel pipette, wash the plate five times with sterile PBS (250 µL/well, allow the wells to soak for 1–2 min at each wash step).

4. Remove wash buffer by "flicking" the plate. Pat the plate dry on paper towels between washes.

5. Dilute the detection biotinylated mAb MT78/145 to 1 µg/mL in PBS-0.5% FBS (20 µL in 10 mL). Add 100 µL/well and incubate the plate for 2 h at room temperature.

6. Remove the detection antibody by "flicking" the plate in the sink. Pat the plate dry on paper towels.

7. Wash wells five times with sterile PBS (250 µL/well), as described above.

8. Before use, dilute the Streptavidin-HRP enzyme conjugate (dilution 1:1000) by adding 10 µL of Streptavidin-HRP concentrate into 10 mL of Dilution Buffer (PBS-0.5% FBS). Add 100 µL of diluted Streptavidin-HRP into each well and incubate for 1 h at room temperature (*see* **Note 13**).

9. Wash wells 5× with sterile PBS (250 µL/well), as described above.

10. Add 100 µL of substrate solution (TMB Substrate) to each well. Incubate the plate in the dark for 5–20 min at room temperature (*see* **Note 14**).

11. Remove the chromogen by "flicking" the plate into sink. Invert the plate and blot dry on paper towels.

12. Rinse the ELISPOT plate 3× with deionized water. Remove the plastic drain and rinse the bottom of the plate. Invert the plate and blot dry on paper towels. Wipe the bottom of the plate dry with paper towels.

13. Invert the plate and allow to dry overnight in the dark. Once the plate is dry, cover it with the original lid.

3.9 Determination of Memory B Cell Frequencies (in SFUs per 2 × 10⁵ Cells)

Once the microplate is completely dry, the spots per well can be analyzed/counted using pre-optimized counting parameters on an automated ELISPOT reader, or manually using a stereomicroscope (*see* **Note 15**). The results are presented in spot forming units (SFUs) per 2×10^5 cells as subjects' medians (i.e., median of influenza virus-specific response, measured in quadruplicate) or means. Alternatively (or in addition), the results for antigen-specific IgG memory B cells can be presented as % of total IgG-secreting B cells (*see* **Note 16**).

4 Notes

1. Do not add more than 20 mL of whole blood into the Accuspin™ tube in order to achieve good cell separation.

2. Required volume (mL) freezing medium = 1×10^7/total number of cells.

3. Keep the cells on dry ice during handling to prevent thawing.

4. At this point, if you have multiple tubes for one subject/sample, then they should be pooled into one 50 mL conical centrifuge tube before cell counting.

5. If any cells remain (with a volume <2 mL) after the 2 mL/well addition, add remaining cells to a new well and bring the volume (per well) up to 2 mL with RPMI culture medium supplemented with 5% FCS.

6. The rhIL-2 provided in the Mabtech ELIspot^PLUS kit for human IgG should be reconstituted in advance with 1 mL PBS to obtain 1 μg/mL concentration. The stock solution should be used immediately or stored in aliquots at −20 °C.

7. Warm 0.25% Trypsin-EDTA in a 37 °C water bath for a minimum of 15 min prior to usage.

8. The desired cell concentration for this assay is 2×10^6 cells/mL for plating the influenza virus-coated wells of the ELISPOT plate, and 2×10^5 cells/mL for plating the total IgG-coated wells of the ELISPOT plate. Alternatively, higher or lower cell concentrations can be used for detection of the antigen-specific memory B cells, depending on the expected frequency of these cells.

9. Cells should be plated within 30 min after counting in order to maintain optimal viability.

10. Mix the cells well while pipetting; ensure the cells are in a homogenous suspension.

11. Wrapping microplate in aluminum foil during incubation reduces well-to-well variability.

12. The assay setup requires work in a biosafety hood; however, assay-development steps do not require aseptic conditions and can be performed outside of the hood.

13. During the incubation, warm the chromogen to room temperature.

14. Five to 20 min is usually sufficient for plate development, but longer incubation periods can be used if needed.

15. In larger studies, quality control (QC) needs to be performed by a single operator (visual checking for abnormalities/errors and QC of the plates on the ELISPOT reader) to ensure uniform QC and consistency of results. The scanning and counting of multiple plates (in larger studies) needs to be performed with set parameters/gating of the ELISPOT reader for all plates.

16. In larger studies, statistical analysis should be used to assess assay drift, inter-operator differences, and study design variables (e.g., shipment of samples, time of year assay was performed), which could cause bias, distribution of raw data, etc.

Acknowledgments

We would like to thank the Mayo Clinic Vaccine Research Group personnel for their technical assistance during the development and execution of these assays. We also thank Caroline L. Vitse for her editorial assistance. This work was supported by the National Institute of Allergy And Infectious Diseases of the National Institutes of Health under award number U01AI089859.

Dr. Poland is the chair of a Safety Evaluation Committee for novel investigational vaccine trials being conducted by Merck Research Laboratories. Dr. Poland offers consultative advice on vaccine development to Merck & Co. Inc., Avianax, Adjuvance, Alopexx, Sanofi Pasteur, GlaxoSmithKline, and Emergent Biosolutions. Drs. Poland and Ovsyannikova hold four patents related to vaccinia and measles peptide research. Dr. Kennedy has received funding from Merck Research Laboratories to study waning immunity to mumps vaccine. These activities have been reviewed by the Mayo Clinic Conflict of Interest Review Board and are conducted in compliance with Mayo Clinic Conflict of Interest policies. This research has been reviewed by the Mayo Clinic Conflict of Interest Review Board and was conducted in compliance with Mayo Clinic Conflict of Interest policies.

References

1. Thompson MG, Shay DK, Zhou H, Bridges CB, Cheng PY, Burns E, Bresee JS, Cox NJ (2010) Estimates of deaths associated with seasonal influenza-United States, 1976–2007. Morb Mortal Wkly Rep 59(33):1057–1062

2. Poland GA (2009) Valuing influenza vaccine: medical, economic, and social benefits. Clin Infect Dis 48(3):299–301

3. Wrammert J, Koutsonanos D, Li GM et al (2011) Broadly cross-reactive antibodies dominate the human B cell response against 2009 pandemic H1N1 influenza virus infection. J Exp Med 208(1):181–193

4. Li GM, Chiu C, Wrammert J et al (2012) Pandemic H1N1 influenza vaccine induces a recall response in humans that favors broadly cross-reactive memory B cells. Proc Natl Acad Sci U S A 109:9047

5. Ovsyannikova IG, White SJ, Albrecht RA et al (2014) Turkey versus guinea pig red blood cells: hemagglutination differences alter hemagglutination inhibition responses against influenza A/H1N1. Viral Immunol 27(4):174–178. https://doi.org/10.1089/vim.2013.0111

6. Lambert ND, Ovsyannikova IG, Pankratz VS et al (2012) Understanding the immune response to seasonal influenza vaccination in older adults: a systems biology approach. Expert Rev Vaccines 11(8):985–994

7. Painter SD, Haralambieva IH, Ovsyannikova IG et al (2014) Detection of influenza A/H1N1-specific human IgG-secreting B cells in older adults by ELISPOT assay. Viral Immunol 27(2):32–38. https://doi.org/10.1089/vim.2013.0099

8. Haralambieva IH, Painter SD, Kennedy RB et al (2015) The impact of immunosenescence on humoral immune response variation after influenza A/H1N1 vaccination in older subjects. PLoS One 10(3):e0122282. https://doi.org/10.1371/journal.pone.0122282

9. Haralambieva IH, Ovsyannikova IG, Kennedy RB et al (2016) Transcriptional signatures of influenza A/H1N1-specific IgG memory-like B cell response in older individuals. Vaccine 34(34):3993–4002. https://doi.org/10.1016/j.vaccine.2016.06.034

10. Poland GA, Ovsyannikova IG, Jacobson RM (2008) Immunogenetics of seasonal influenza vaccine response. Vaccine 26S:D35–D40

11. Ovsyannikova IG, Oberg AL, Kennedy RB et al (2016) Gene signatures related to HAI response following influenza A/H1N1 vaccine in older individuals. Heliyon 2(5):e00098. https://doi.org/10.1016/j.heliyon.2016.e00098

12. Umlauf BJ, Pinsky NA, Ovsyannikova IG et al (2012) Detection of vaccinia virus-specific IFN-g and IL-10 secretion from human PBMC and CD8+ T cells by ELISPOT. In: Kalyuzhny AE (ed) Handbook of ELISPOT. Springer, New York, NY, pp 199–218

13. Ryan JE, Ovsyannikova IG, Poland GA (2005) Detection of measles virus-specific interferon-gamma-secreting T-cells by ELISPOT. Methods Mol Biol 302:207–218

14. Salk HM, Haralambieva IH, Ovsyannikova IG et al (2013) Granzyme B ELISPOT assay to measure influenza-specific cellular immunity. J Immunol Methods 398-399:44–50. https://doi.org/10.1016/j.jim.2013.09.007

15. Jahnmatz M, Kesa G, Netterlid E et al (2013) Optimization of a human IgG B-cell ELISpot assay for the analysis of vaccine-induced B-cell responses. J Immunol Methods 391(1-2):50–59. https://doi.org/10.1016/j.jim.2013.02.009

Chapter 20

Towards a Full Automation of the ELISpot Assay for Safe and Parallelized Immunomonitoring

J. C. Neubauer, I. Sébastien, A. Germann, H. von Briesen, and H. Zimmermann

Abstract

The ELISpot assay, as a sensitive and specific method, enables the detection of cytokines for immunological purposes and in vaccine development. Here we describe the successful transfer of the manual procedure to a commercially available automated liquid handling platform, based on the work described in Neubauer et al. (Cytotechnology 69:57–73, 2017). Different kinds of technical issues (dead volume reduction, instrumental handling limitations, liquid class improvement) have been solved and biological effects (reagents concentration, selectivity tests, dispensing way, etc.) have been controlled during the implementation process. At the end a maximum of 6% mean delta difference and a lower mean dispersion than the manual assay were reached as well as a turnaround time of four to six times higher than the manual process.

Key words ELISpot, Peripheral blood mononuclear cells, PBMCs, Automation, Standardization

---

1 Introduction

The ELISpot assay is an important immunomonitoring method for the detection, measurement, and characterization of immune cell activities in clinical and cancer trials [1]. Such a worldwide used technique requires a high level of standardization and reproducibility to enable comparability of multi-site research studies. The highest limitation of the method is the inter-operator and inter-assay inconsistency besides assay-specific parameters like motion sensitivity, operator pipetting accuracy, or spot evaluation [2–6]. Over the last decades, reagents and protocols were simplified and standardized and automated cell counters and spot readers were developed [7, 8] in order to reduce the human factor on variability [9]. Due to its high potential, automation solutions became more and more important for process standardization [10]. An automated system guarantees (or at least improves) reproducibility, high-throughput, process control, and operator safety [11], and

Alexander E. Kalyuzhny (ed.), *Handbook of ELISPOT: Methods and Protocols*, Methods in Molecular Biology, vol. 1808, https://doi.org/10.1007/978-1-4939-8567-8_20, © Springer Science+Business Media, LLC, part of Springer Nature 2018

reduces in addition the inter-operator and inter-assay variability to their technical minimum.

We demonstrated that the ELISpot assay can be performed with high quality and comparable results on an automated platform, the Tecan Freedom EVO 200 [12]. We were able to negociate the technical issues and biological limitations and to transfer the procedure completely (besides cells/reagents preparation) to a commercially available, freely programmable automated system. In this process, the following issues have been addressed: (1) manual procedure was adapted, (2) liquid classes were optimized, (3) dead volume was minimized, and (4) reagent consumption and concentrations were determined and adapted [12]. Thus, we describe here now the final, optimized protocol for a full automation of the ELISpot assay using a commercially available liquid handling platform with safer and more reproducible results than the manual procedure.

2 Materials

2.1 Isolation of Human PBMCs

1. Ficoll solution LSM 1077.

2. Phosphate-buffered saline (PBS) without calcium and magnesium, pH 7.2.

3. R10 medium: RPMI 1640 containing 2 mM L-Glutamin supplemented with 10% heat-inactivated Fetal Bovine Serum (FBS), 1% Glutamax, 1% Penicillin/Streptomycin, and 2.5% 1 M HEPES.

4. Centrifuge allowing spinning 50 ml tubes at $850 \times g$.

5. Automated cell analyzer (e.g., Vi-Cell XR, Beckman Coulter, Krefeld, Germany) or hemacytometer to count lymphocytes.

6. Cell culture incubator (37 °C, 5% CO_2).

2.2 ELISpot Assays

1. Antibody-coated 96 well plate (anti-IFN-gamma mAb 1 D1k pre-coated, Mabtech, Nacka Strand, Sweden).

2. PBS.

3. R10 medium.

4. 50 µl/well peptides or unspecific stimulation reagent to stimulate the release of cytokines (e.g., IFN-gamma) from cultured PBMCs: 1 µg/ml CEF (cytomegalovirus, Epstein–Barr virus, influenza virus) peptide pool (CTL, Bonn, Germany), 2 µg/ml CMV (cytomegalovirus) (PepMix HCMVA pp65, JPT, Berlin, Germany), and 4 µg/ml lectin PHA.

5. Sterile and (0.45 µm) filtered PBS containing 0.5% FBS (*see* **Note 1**).

6. Anti-human IFN-gamma detector antibody 7B6-1 HRP conjugated (Mabtech, Nacka Strand, Sweden). Prepare manually a 1:200 dilution of the detector antibody in the PBS-FBS solution before use (*see* **Note 2**).

7. 50 µl/well substrate (Nova Red, Biozol, Eching, Germany). Substrate solution consists of a mixture of four different components in a specific order and amount according to the operating manual. Prepare manually 15 ml of the substrate in a foil-wrapped tube and incubate for 20 min in the dark at room temperature before use.

8. Automated ELISpot Analyzer including ImmunoScan and ImmunoSpot software (CTL, Bonn, Germany) as well as plate transfer kit.

9. Paper towels and container for liquid waste remaining from the flicking of the plate.

10. Distilled and tap water.

2.3 Pipette Robot Assembly

1. Tecan Freedom EVO 200 consisting of a 2 m worktable, a liquid handling arm (LiHa) with four steel fixed needles and four needles with single-use tips allowing liquid level detection through conductivity, a robotic manipulator arm (RoMa) with gripper, dark chamber (TIG, Tecan, Crailsheim, Germany), cell culture incubator (37 °C and 5% CO_2, StoreX500, Liconic, Mauren, Liechtenstein), a Carousel (CarouselNT, Liconic, Mauren, Liechtenstein), and a sterile laminar flow cabinet housing the whole system (Fig. 1).

2. Free dispense mode for dispensing liquids in the air without contact with the hardware or medium.

3. Tecan software EVOware Standard.

4. Vessel for up to 100 ml liquid transfer (Tecan, Crailsheim, Germany).

5. 2 ml cryovials as recipient for antibody and cell suspension solutions, held in a 48 well plate (Greiner, Kremsmünster, Österreich).

3   Methods

3.1 Configuration of Tecan Freedom EVO 200

1. Configurate the Tecan software in accordance with the specifications and geometric dimensions of all devices and labware used. All information are combined and visualized on the worktable editor (Fig. 2). For further information on this topic, please refer to the software manual [13].

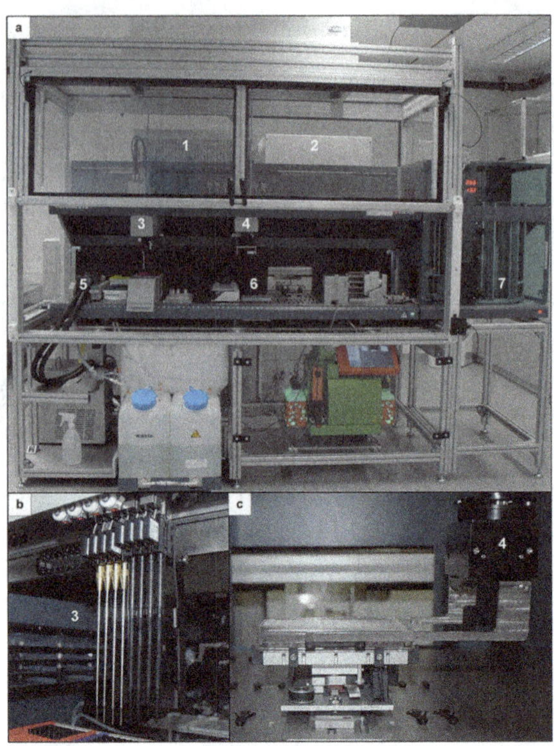

Fig. 1 Tecan Freedom EVO 200 assembly as commercially available liquid handling platform: (**a**) Whole system with incubator, carousel, cell counter, and laminar flow among other devices. (**b**) LiHa (Liquid Handling Arm) including the four fixed needles and the four needles with single-use tips. (**c**) RoMa (Robot Manipulator Arm). Cell culture devices are numbered: (1) Refrigerator, (2) Incubator, (3) LiHa, (4) RoMa, (5) Wash station, (6) Dark room incubator, (7) Carousel. Reprinted from Neubauer et al. [12] with permission from Springer (http://creativecommons.org/licenses/by/4.0/)

2. Example for pre-coated 96 well plate (Mabtech, Nacka Strand, Sweden): membrane area of 0.26 cm^2, plate dimensions of 127.8 mm × 85.5 mm × 14.4 mm (L × W × D).

3. Teach the approach (wide or narrow) and set displacement vectors of the gripper arm for the labware transfer between two devices (i.e., 96 well plate moved from dispensing platform to the incubator).

4. For the 96 well plate, set the lowest aspirate position so-called z-max without touching the membrane to ≤1 mm gap (*see* **Note 3**) and the dispense height to 1 cm above the membrane (*see* **Note 4**).

5. Perform gravimetrical analysis for fixed (1000 μl) and disposable tips (200 μl) to guarantee accurate and precise liquid distribution. The motion accuracy should reach 1 mm and the volume accuracy 1–10 μl, depending on the tip capacity.

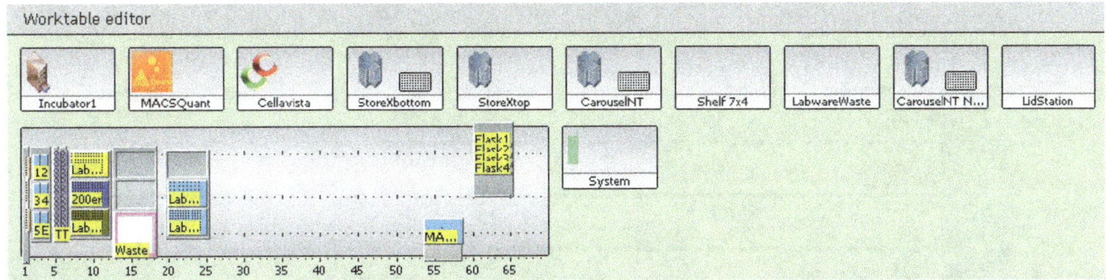

Fig. 2 Visualization of the used worktable editor: All available devices, configured labwares, and predefined recipients are integrated in the software EVOware Standard and summarized in the digital visualization of the platform, so-called worktable editor. It allows a technical overview about the system and the representation shows all necessary information for the script programming

6. Define the aspirate and dispense commands in "liquid classes." The flow speed (in μl/s) and air gap (in μl) parameters influence the correct and accurate treatment of the liquid, based on its conductivity and viscosity (*see* **Note 5**).

7. In the aspirate and dispense settings, turn off the liquid level detection option (*see* **Note 6**).

8. Write a script as a digital transfer of the standard protocol (*see* **Note 7**). A section of our script is represented in Fig. 3 as an example. To enable multi-plates handling and scheduling, include variables for the position of the plates on the dispensing platform and in the incubator. A detailed list and description of the available commands can be found in the software manual [13].

9. Determine the system-specific minimum volume (dead volume) in the different vials and vessels that is required for successfully performing the pipetting steps (*see* **Note 8**). For example with our system configuration, at least 50 μl or 10% extra volume on top of the necessary volume were calculated for the cryovial to allow safe liquid handling without wastage.

3.2 Isolation of Peripheral Blood Mononuclear Cells (PBMCs) from Citrated Buffy Coats

1. Transfer the citrated buffy coat in a cell culture flask and dilute the blood cells with PBS at a ratio of 1:1 (one part PBS per one part blood).

2. Mix gently the solution by inverting the flask 4–6 times.

3. Transfer 20 ml of Ficoll solution LSM per 50 ml tube and overlay slowly each tube with 30 ml of the blood-PBS solution.

4. Centrifuge the tubes for 30 min at $850 \times g$ without brake.

5. After centrifugation four different layers are formed. The thin white layer between the PBS and the LSM solution is characteristic for the PBMC interphase layer. Collect this layer carefully with 10 ml serological pipette to a fresh 50 ml tube.

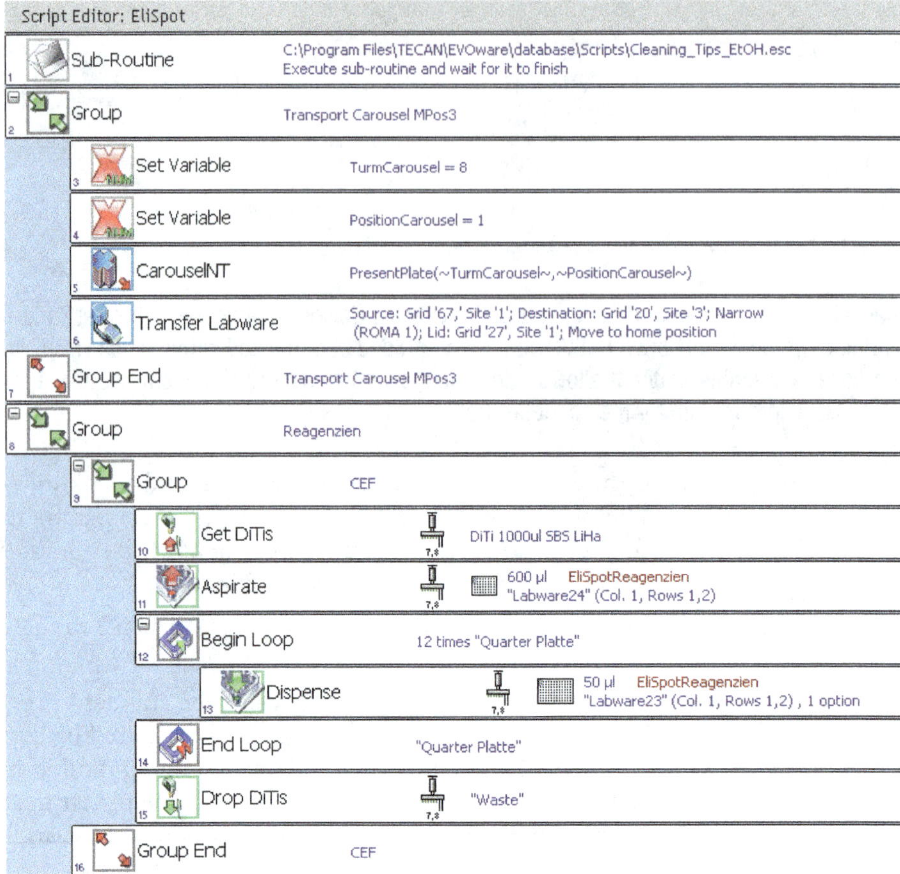

Fig. 3 Example of programming: The figure represents a short impression how the automated script of the ELISpot assay can be programmed. Modules like "sub-routine" or "group" are included, as well as variables, loops, and the standard basic commands "aspirate" and "dispense"

6. Wash the PBMCs with PBS for a total volume of 45 ml and mix gently by inverting the tube 4–6 times.

7. Centrifuge 10 min at $400 \times g$ with maximum brake.

8. Remove the supernatant and resuspend the pellet gently in an appropriate volume of PBS for cell counting and viability determination.

9. Resuspend the cells in 10 ml R10 medium with a concentration of 1×10^6 cells/ml and cultured overnight at 37 °C and 5% CO_2 for direct use. Alternatively, freeze PBMCs with cryomedium at a concentration of 1×10^7 cells/ml for later application.

10. On the next day, centrifuge the cells at $400 \times g$ for 10 min and resuspend the cell pellet in an appropriated volume (600–1000 μl) of R10 medium.

11. Determine the cell concentration and viability, adjust the PBMC suspension to an appropriate concentration,

e.g., 2×10^6 PBMC/ml, with R10 medium, and store the cells in the incubator for at least 30 min before use.

3.3 Performance of Automated ELISpot

1. Place the antibody-coated 96 well plate (*see* **Note 9**) into the carousel of the Tecan system (*see* **Note 10**).

2. Fill manually designated vessels with enough PBS, R10 medium, and ethanol.

3. Place two cryovials of each stimulation reagent (CEF, CMV, PHA) and two cryovials of R10 medium as negative control to the designated 48 well plates as well as one cryovial per PBMC donor suspension (*see* **Note 11**).

4. Start the script with the blocking part: Wash the plate four times with 200 µl PBS/well from the vessel, using fixed needles four rows at a time (*see* **Note 12**). All repeating washing steps were performed with aspirate flow rate of 100 µl/s and dispense flow rate of 200 µl/s to treat the membrane with care.

5. Replace PBS with R10 medium following the same settings than PBS (fixed tips, 100 µl/s aspirate rate and 200 µl/s dispense rate). Incubate 30 min at room temperature in order to block unspecific binding on the plate. Remove the solution afterwards (*see* **Note 13**).

6. Dispense 50 µl/well of the 4 µg/ml CEF peptide pool solution using the disposable needles (*see* **Note 14**) with an aspirate flow rate of 150 µl/s and a dispense rate of 600 µl/s. Use at least triplicates per donor, e.g., dispense the solution to the wells A1–D3 for four donors (*see* **Note 15**).

7. As described in Subheading 3.2, **step 6** dispense 50 µl/well of the 2 µg/ml CMV peptide pool for the wells A4–D6, 50 µl/well of the 8 µg/ml PHA peptide pool for the wells A7–D9, and 50 µl/well R10 medium for the wells A10–D12.

8. Mix 600 µl cell suspension three times with a dispense flow rate of 400 µl/s at the bottom of the cell container using fixed tips. In our case, the concentration is set to 2×10^6 cells/ml.

9. Aspirate donor PBMCs with a low flow rate of 100 µl/s using the disposable needles for the plate loading and dispense 50 µl suspension per well (with our plate design, one donor per row) with a flow rate of 400 µl/s.

10. Transfer the plate from the pipetting platform to the StoreX incubator and incubate for 24 h. During this period, avoid agitation of the plate (*see* **Note 16**).

11. On the next day, transfer the plate back to the pipetting platform and remove the cells with the fixed needles and 150 µl/s aspirate rate. Perform a plate wash with PBS (five times) with 200 µl/well each time using fixed tips as well as 100 and 200 µl/s as aspirate and dispense flow rate (*see* **Note 17**).

12. For the cytokine detection step, fill manually the designated vessel with the detector antibody-PBS-FBS solution and add 50 µl antibody solution per well with the disposable tips and aspirate and dispense flow rate of 150 and 600 µl/s, respectively.

13. Transfer the plate to the dark room and incubate at room temperature for 2 h.

14. Before the end of the incubation, transfer manually the Nova Red solution in a (preferably disposable) vessel of the system.

15. After antibody incubation, transfer the plate back, remove the antibody solution (*see* **Note 18**) with the fixed tips and an aspirate flow rate of 100 µl/s and wash the plate five times with PBS with the same settings as already described in Subheadings 3.2, **steps 4** and **11**.

16. Add 50 µl of Nova Red substrate solution to each well with the disposable tips and a flow speed of 150 µl/s during aspiration and 600 µl/s during dispension (*see* **Note 19**). Wait for 5 min in the dark (*see* **Note 20**).

17. Bring the plate back with the gripper arm to the user and stop the reaction immediately by manually holding the plate in a 45° angle under water-tap. Wash the plate subsequently with distilled water.

18. Remove the bottom of the plate and rinse its back.

19. Remove excess of liquid on a paper towel and dry the plate overnight in the dark at room temperature.

20. On the following day, wells were transferred and if necessary stuck to a glass plate.

3.4 ELISpot Analysis

1. Set parameters at the ELISpot Analyzer to: e.g., Spot separation: 0; Minimal manual gating: 0.0041 mm^2; Counted area: 95%. These parameters can have critical influences on the spot evaluation as described in Janetzki [2] and must be adapted for each assay and reader.

2. Scan the plate with the automated EliSpot Analyzer ImmunoScan.

3. Analyze the scan with the software ImmunoSpot.

4. Control each well for false-positive hits like dust or agglomerated spots.

5. Export the scan with the amount of spots (Spot Forming Cells or SFC).

6. Represent results in graphs with the donors and antigens as *x*-axis and the relative amount of spot (SFC/10^6 PBMCs) as *y*-axis.

4   Notes

1. Used FBS lot has been inactivated (at 56 °C for 30 min) and tested for EliSpot low background activity and appropriated reactivity against the stimulating reagent or used peptides.

2. The 1:200 dilution of the antibody is related to the manual procedure and must be adapted to the own system. In our case, we prepared a 1:155 dilution based on the remaining dead volume per well after a washing step. Each new configuration of the pipetting system would need a new labware and z-max teaching and requires a unique concentration factor.

3. Teaching of the z-max in the 96 well plates is absolutely crucial. It should be as close as possible to the membrane but has to enable pipetting commands without damaging the membrane or creating under-pressure. At least the tips should never touch the bottom of the plate. Many plates (they all show minimal differences in their dimensions) were tested to find the optimal z-max value, in our case 0.45 mm above the set membrane height. This height results in a remaining volume of about 14 µl that was used for the later antibody concentration recalculation.

4. Empirical value to avoid cross-contamination.

5. Depending on the multipipetting parameters defined in the liquid classes, the dispensed volume of the last well of a loop or row can show some variances. Different combinations of air gap, speed, exceed volume, and delay have to be tested for each liquid type.

6. The detection of the liquid level is time-consuming (in a time critical protocol). In our configuration, all liquid levels during the different processes are known and are controlled by the liquid classes and the well-defined z-max and z-dispense heights.

7. The utilization of loops, user comments, washing subscripts, and incubation times are essential for the correct and safe process as well as an easy understanding of the script.

8. The extra volume results from the dead volume of the reservoir plus the volume lost during the process. The dead volume, as the minimum remaining volume in the reservoir that cannot be aspirated, can be calculated using the formula $\pi R^2 H$, with R being the inner radius of the reservoir and H the safety gap between the vessel base and the lowest aspiration position z-max.

9. Always use a fresh and properly stored plate to guarantee the intact coating of the membrane.

10. The orientation of the plate in the carousel determines the pipetting order inside the plate.

11. Place cryovials containing the same peptide in the same column of a 48 well plate. Additionally, take care that in one column of the plate cryovials with cells from different donors are arranged. This assures simultaneous and fast aspirating steps (parallel to the pipette head) and is easier to handle in the programming script regarding loop commands.

12. The aspiration volume during the washing steps was increased from 200 µl (dispensed volume) to 230 µl in order to avoid surplus volume. The constant z-max as lowest aspiration position guaranteed comparable start volumes in the well.

13. Take care to remove liquid only short time before the next solution is added in order to avoid any dehydration of the coated membrane.

14. If using non-original disposable tips for pipetting reagents or antibodies, extensive pre-testing is crucial. Tips from other manufacturers often have slightly different diameters and lengths, resulting in incorrect pipetting processes. The difference can also lead to collisions of the pipet head or to damages of the plate membrane.

15. Plate design used is the following: CEF peptide pool is pipetted in wells of the columns 1–3, CMV in columns 4–6, PHA in columns 7–9, and R10 in columns 10–12. Each row is designated for one tested donor.

16. Agitation of the plate can lead to irregular or diffuse spots caused by rolling cells. Due to this motion-sensitive state during the incubation, the Liconic maintenance script had to be consequently adapted. An extra incubator program was written by the Liconic technical support and was installed on our system in order to remove the recurrent maintenance rotation of the StoreX carousel.

17. Loops of automated washing steps are time-consuming compared to the manual process but they are necessary due to the remaining volume in wells. The repeat of the washing steps avoids false-positive results.

18. As well as for the washing steps, the aspiration volume of the antibody solution was increased from 50 µl (dispensed volume) to 70 µl to ensure that as much as possible unbound antibodies is removed.

19. The addition of the Nova Red substrate is critical in terms of time and should be pipetted as fast as possible to minimize well-to-well development discrepancy.

20. During standard programming of the script, it is possible to control either actions of the LiHa (pipet head) or actions of

the RoMa (gripper arm) but not both simultaneously due to security and collision reasons. To minimize the total script time, subscripts were written to e.g., wash tips during the time RoMa was moving labware to incubation places. This programming is sensitive and should only be used in specific situation where both arms will not meet at any time for sure.

References

1. Cox JH, Ferrari G, Janetzki S (2006) Measurement of cytokine release at the single cell level using the ELISPOT assay. Methods 38(4):274–282. https://doi.org/10.1016/j.ymeth.2005.11.006

2. Janetzki S, Price L, Schroeder H et al (2015) Guidelines for the automated evaluation of Elispot assays. Nat Protoc 10(7):1098–1115. https://doi.org/10.1038/nprot.2015.068

3. Janetzki S, Schaed S, Blachere NEB et al (2004) Evaluation of Elispot assays. Influence of method and operator on variability of results. J Immunol Methods 291(1–2):175–183. https://doi.org/10.1016/j.jim.2004.06.008

4. Maecker HT, Moon J, Bhatia S et al (2005) Impact of cryopreservation on tetramer, cytokine flow cytometry, and ELISPOT. BMC Immunol 6:17. https://doi.org/10.1186/1471-2172-6-17

5. Moodie Z, Price L, Janetzki S et al (2012) Response determination criteria for ELISPOT. Toward a standard that can be applied across laboratories. Methods Mol Biol 792:185–196. https://doi.org/10.1007/978-1-61779-325-7_15

6. Maecker HT, Hassler J, Payne JK et al (2008) Precision and linearity targets for validation of an IFNgamma ELISPOT, cytokine flow cytometry, and tetramer assay using CMV peptides. BMC Immunol 9:9. https://doi.org/10.1186/1471-2172-9-9

7. Hawkins N, Self S, Wakefield J (2006) The automated counting of spots for the ELISpot assay. J Immunol Methods 316(1–2):52–58. https://doi.org/10.1016/j.jim.2006.08.005

8. Zadorozhny SS, Martynov NN (2012) Mathematical algorithms for automatic search, recognition, and detection of spots in ELISPOT assay. Methods Mol Biol 792:145–153. https://doi.org/10.1007/978-1-61779-325-7_12

9. Janetzki S, Panageas KS, Ben-Porat L et al (2008) Results and harmonization guidelines from two large-scale international Elispot proficiency panels conducted by the Cancer Vaccine Consortium (CVC/SVI). Cancer Immunol Immunother 57(3):303–315. https://doi.org/10.1007/s00262-007-0380-6

10. Almeida C-AM, Roberts SG, Laird R et al (2009) Automation of the ELISpot assay for high-throughput detection of antigen-specific T-cell responses. J Immunol Methods 344(1):1–5. https://doi.org/10.1016/j.jim.2009.02.007

11. Franscini N, Wuertz K, Patocchi-Tenzer I et al (2011) Development of a novel automated cell isolation, expansion, and characterization platform. J Lab Autom 16(3):204–213. https://doi.org/10.1016/j.jala.2011.01.002

12. Neubauer JC, Sébastien I, Germann A et al (2017) Towards standardized automated immunomonitoring. An automated ELISpot assay for safe and parallelized functionality analysis of immune cells. Cytotechnology 69(1):57–73. https://doi.org/10.1007/s10616-016-0037-4

13. Tecan Schweiz AG (2009) Freedom EVOware Software Manual. 393172, en, version 2.3

INDEX

Alexander E. Kalyuzhny (ed.), *Handbook of ELISPOT: Methods and Protocols*, Methods in Molecular Biology, vol. 1808,
https://doi.org/10.1007/978-1-4939-8567-8, © Springer Science+Business Media, LLC, part of Springer Nature 2018

CPSIA information can be obtained
at www.ICGtesting.com
Printed in the USA
BVHW01*1701290718
522919BV00015B/6/P